MEDICAL
NEUROANATOMY

A PROBLEM-ORIENTED MANUAL
WITH ANNOTATED ATLAS

MEDICAL
NEUROANATOMY

A PROBLEM-ORIENTED MANUAL
WITH ANNOTATED ATLAS

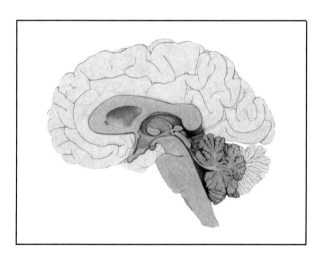

Frank H. Willard, PhD

Associate Professor, Department of Anatomy, University of New England, College of Osteopathic Medicine, Biddeford, Maine

Clinical Commentary by
Daniel P. Perl, MD

Professor of Pathology and Psychiatry, Mount Sinai School of Medicine; Director, Neuropathology Division, Mount Sinai Hospital, New York, New York

J. B. LIPPINCOTT COMPANY
Philadelphia

Acquisitions Editor: Richard Winters
Assistant Editor: Jody M. Schott
Project Editor: Dina K. Rubin
Indexer: David Amundson
Designer: Doug Smock
Cover Designer: Ilene Griff
Production Manager: Caren Erlichman
Production Coordinator: Sharon McCarthy
Compositor: Bi-Comp, Incorporated
Printer/Binder: Arcata Graphics/Kingsport

6 5 4 3 2 1

Library of Congress Cataloging in Publications Data

Willard, Frank H., 1948–
    Medical neuroanatomy: a problem-oriented manual with annotated
atlas/Frank H. Willard, Daniel P. Perl.
        p.   cm.
    Includes bibliographical references and index.
    ISBN 0-397-51171-X
    1. Neuroanatomy—Problems, exercises, etc.   2. Neuroanatomy—
Atlases.   I. Perl, Daniel P.   II. Title.
    [DNLM: 1. Neuroanatomy—Case studies.   2. Nervous System—anatomy
& histology—atlases.   3. Nervous System—anatomy & histology—
problems.   4. Nervous System Diseases—atlases.   5. Nervous System
Diseases—problems.   WL 18 W692m]
    QM451.W697   1992
    611′.8—dc20
    DNLM/DLC
    for Library of Congress   92-49837
                                                                        CIP

The authors and publisher have exerted every effort to ensure that drug selection and dosage set forth in this text are in accord with current recommendations and practice at the time of publication. However, in view of ongoing research, changes in government regulations, and the constant flow of information relating to drug therapy and drug reactions, the reader is urged to check the package insert for each drug for any change in indications and dosage and for added warnings and precautions. This is particularly important when the recommended agent is a new or infrequently employed drug.

PREFACE

Medical Neuroanatomy: A Problem-Oriented Manual With Annotated Atlas represents a regional approach to the central nervous system. It is aimed at first- and second-year medical students; however, it should also be useful to dental, veterinary, and graduate students as well as anyone seeking to correlate the neural sciences with clinical presentations in neurology.

The manual is designed as an annotated atlas arranged around a series of clinical case studies. A major effort has been made to relate the geographic features of the central nervous system to clinical presentations resulting from lesions such as vascular accidents, tumors, cysts, and degenerative processes. This approach to the subject has been made all the more important by the amazing advances in imaging and rehabilitation therapy that have occurred in the past few years.

The manual is arranged in a spiral. The first chapter makes a quick passage along the caudal-to-rostral axis of the central nervous system, introducing its major characters. The second chapter returns to the spinal cord level and begins a more detailed approach. Subsequent chapters ascend the neuraxis systematically, extending this detailed treatment to the brain stem, cerebellum, thalamus, cerebral cortex, and basal ganglia. Each chapter is composed of several clinical case studies followed by an analysis of the neuroanatomic features with reference to the appropriate atlas sections. A litany of general questions is included after each case to help guide the student toward a consistent, methodic approach to a clinical problem. Strong emphasis is placed on the distribution of cerebral vasculature and any associated vascular syndromes.

The teaching method used in this manual has evolved from a series of mock case presentations given by second-year students for critique by faculty at the University of New England. To assist in their understanding of a patient's presentation, students could be observed eagerly relearning material that they had just laboriously worked through in their standard neuroanatomy course. Watching this activity, it was evident that the learning process for a medical student became far more exciting when a practical endpoint or goal was the motivating force. In addition, it seemed more logical to approach students saying "Here is a problem, go find the answers," than "Here are a lot of answers. In a few years you will be seeing the problems."

Ideally, in this educational process students should be presented with case histories, or the patients themselves, from which they will develop and pursue their own questions and learning objectives; however, given the time constraints of many medical curricula, this extremely open-ended approach is not always practical. In an attempt to compromise, this manual is composed of a series of extensive case studies, each of which is accompanied by a structured litany of general questions that can be used to initiate and guide the learning process. Although the manual can complement a standard human neuroanatomy text, it can also stand alone, or function as a review of the subject for medical board exams.

This manual takes a contemporary approach to the classical spinal cord sensory systems. The view presented in most texts and reviews, that of the three clinically important sensory pathways: ([1] the dorsal columns system carrying vibratory and conscious position sense, and discriminative touch, [2] the spinocerebellar tracts carrying proprioceptive information from the muscle spindles and tendon organs, and [3] the anterolateral tract carrying nociception), can no longer be squared with the current literature (Davidoff RA. The dorsal columns. Neurology 1989, 39:1377–1385). Based on numerous clinical examinations, it appears that humans do not permanently lose vibratory and position sense after complete transection of the doral column system as long as the lateral and ventral funiculi are intact. The functions ascribed to these major spinal cord sensory pathways, as presented in Chapter 2, have been altered to reflect redundancy in the systems; consequently, shared functions are described in all three of these tracts.

Frank H. Willard, PhD

► How to Use This Manual: A Suggestion to Instructors

The teaching approach taken in this manual is conducive for small-group study sessions. As a suggestion, the method used at the University of New England will be briefly outlined. Most of the chapters in the manual are treated in two, 2-hour, small-group study sessions. In the first session, 8 or 9 students meet with a facilitator (upper-classmate or faculty member, often a family practitioner) to examine the case and the accompanying questions. As the case is opened for discussion, issues are raised by the students and identified for further study outside of the group. The atlas sections related to the chapter are examined, the structures listed in the text are identified, and the comments on their clinical deficits are studied. At the end of the session, the students assign themselves specific issues for outside study.

The second session of the group resolves the case studies and re-examines the learning issues. The session begins with a brief summary of the case and student reports on the learning issues raised from the first session. The atlas sections are re-examined to make sure the group has mastered the organization of the particular brain region under consideration. Students propose answers to specific questions accompanying each case, and group discussion follows. It should be appreciated that some of the questions do not have concrete answers; for this reason it is exciting to have several clinicians of varied training involved as resources in the course (the neurologist's view of the case may well differ from that of the pathologist or the general practitioner).

The questions accompanying each case are arranged in a specific litany designed to lead the student toward a reasonable conclusion regarding the pathophysiology occurring in the patient. (Seeds for the development of this approach can be found in Daube JR, Ragan TJ, Sandok BA, Westmoreland BF. *Medical Neurosciences*. Boston: Little, Brown, 1986.) The questions initially attempt to guide thinking toward the correct level on the neuraxis for localizing the pathologic process(es): supratentorial, posterior cranial fossa, vertebral canal, or peripheral nervous system. Subsequently, the student is asked to examine the distribution of the damage and clinicotemporal profile of the process. From this analysis, it is possible to hypothesize what type of events are, or have, occurred in the patient. Additional questions, specific to the case under consideration, usually are added to the end and the students are encouraged to raise their own learning issues.

The information necessary to answer the case-related questions is *not* always present in the text of this manual by any means. This is particularly so concerning the analysis of neurologic deficits. Students are encouraged to seek and discuss conflicting opinions from texts or resource persons. In some places I have attempted an explanation or description of a specific neurologic symptom; for others, only the name of the symptom and a reference citation is given. This was done because many neurologic symptoms require detailed explanations well beyond the scope of this text; furthermore, it makes no sense to simply rewrite what has already been defined and is accessible in other sources. At all times in the small group sessions, it is beneficial to have an internal medicine text, a neurology text, and a medical dictionary available for consultation. Finally, to develop an understanding of some of the learning issues, students should be encouraged to consult some of the references cited at the end of each chapter.

The general references at the end of each chapter contain a list of neuroanatomy/neuroscience and neurology texts and atlases. Usually two books in each category are listed and specific chapters, figures, or sections are cited. This is an attempt to account for diversity in learning styles and approaches. These books contain many excellent diagrams, plates, and descriptions that will be of much value in interpreting the case studies and the material presented in this manual. I encourage students to have access to at least one book in each category as they work in their study groups.

This method of teaching neuroanatomy has developed on the strength of student criticism and continues to evolve with each year of our curriculum. Undoubtedly, through the scrutiny of reviewers, faculty, and additional students, further improvements can be made. I would greatly appreciate comments aimed at improving case histories and the litany of questions as well as correcting mistakes in the text.

► How to Use This Manual: A Suggestion to Students

Modern techniques of rehabilitative medicine demand a careful analysis of neurologic patients; recent advances in neuroimaging have begun providing data necessary to support this type of analysis. This manual is designed to help you master the neuroanatomic details necessary for an understanding of brain function, while learning to associate specific groupings of neurologic signs and symptoms with dysfunction at distinct levels of the neuraxis.

Each chapter in the manual analyzes a level of the central neuraxis. The basic pattern of organization features the presentation of a clinical problem followed by the information necessary to begin an understanding of the problem. Each chapter opens with a case study and associated questions. Understanding the patient's presentation represents the major problem. The section after the case examines the Atlas Plates, describing the structures present, listing their functions, and any known clinical deficits that appear when the structure is damaged. By assembling this information, an understanding of the clinical presentation can be obtained. The questions associated with the case are arranged in an outline of the thought process frequently used by clinicians in approaching neurologic problems. They are designed to help organize your thinking as you approach an understanding of the case.

Neuroanatomy in the first or second year of medical school is often considered one of the more difficult subjects to master. The following steps will be helpful in organizing your approach to the material in this manual.

1. Read the case carefully and make an outline or list of the patients neurologic signs and symptoms. If you are working in a group with other students, place this list on the board or a large sheet of paper for all to see. Include in this list the sequence of events happening to the patient, and the time intervals between the events.
2. Read the questions and begin framing answers. Where difficulty arises in developing an answer, make this a learning issue to be resolved.
3. Once issues have been raised, begin examining the Atlas Plates associated with the chapter. Locate, on each plate, the structures listed in the text, paying specific attention to the dorsal-ventral and medial-lateral position in the central nervous system of each structure, as well as to its blood supply. Read the annotations associated with each structure concentrating on the ascribed function and on the deficit expressed in dysfunctions.
4. Compare the descriptions of deficits to the list of the patient's neurologic presentation, and decide which neuroanatomic structures have been affected in this individual's central nervous system.

Summary of Major Relationships Between Temporal and Spatial Features in Neurologic Presentation

	ACUTE	SUBACUTE	CHRONIC
FOCAL	Vascular (infarct or intraparenchymal hemorrhage)	Inflammatory (abscess, myelitis)	Neoplasm
MULTIFOCAL	Vascular (embolic shower)	Inflammatory (autoimmune)	Neoplasm (metastic spread from primary)
DIFFUSE	Vascular (subarachnoid hemorrhage or anoxia)	Inflammatory (meningitis, encephalitis)	Degenerative

(Modified from Daube JR, Sandok BA. Medical Neurosciences. Boston: Little, Brown, 1978)

5. Examine and answer questions 1 to 4, and, based on these answers, decide where on the neuraxis the patient's damage lies (question 5).

6. Question 1 asks you to evaluate functions typically related to the supratentorial portion of the nervous system. Question 2 asks you to evaluate cranial nerve functions typical of the posterior cranial fossa; in each case you need to ask, "Are these signs due to suprasegmental or segmental damage, and if the latter is true, is it occurring in the central or peripheral nervous systems?" Question 3 concerns the motor functions of the patient (exclusive of the cranial nerves); again, it is important to determine whether the lesion involves suprasegmental or segmental damage (or both) and if the signs are from segmental levels, whether the damage is central or peripheral in location. Finally, question 4 considers the sensory integrity of the patient; the pattern of sensory losses can assist in determining whether the damage is central or peripheral in the nervous system.

7. Compile a list of the neurologic structures damaged in this patient, then decide whether they resulted from focal or multifocal damage, or a diffuse process (question 6).

8. Examine the time line or chronology of events for the patient and decide if this is an acute or rapidly occurring event (seconds to minutes), a subacute or slowly occurring event (hours to days), or a chronic or very slowly occurring event (weeks to months).

9. By combining the information required in questions 6 and 7 and the chart in Table 1, decide what type of process is occurring in this patient: a vascular event, a tumor or cyst, or a degenerative or inflammatory process.

10. Discuss the case and the answers to the questions with your peers and with faculty until you have gained confidence in your explanation of the problem faced by the patient. (A useful exercise at this point is to formulate an explanation that you would be willing to give to the patient or family.)

By approaching the subject in this manner, you are building a knowledge of neuroanatomy in the context of its clinical applications. However, you are also developing an underlying thought process for topological diagnosis of neurologic cases. The mechanics of this process also have useful applications in any differential diagnosis course.

ACKNOWLEDGMENTS

Medical Neuroanatomy: A Problem-Oriented Manual With Annotated Atlas is based on the concept that student learning is best facilitated when they seek answers to problems, especially those problems that will confront them throughout the rest of their professional lives. Design and construction of the manual has received immeasurable help from the many students who have been subjected to medical neuroanatomy at the University of New England since 1983. I especially thank four students: Ingrid Schmedtje DO, Patricia Lampugnale, DO, Teresa Such, DO, and Trish Campbell, DO, who spent their summertime editing, researching, and outlining various problems in this text. Also, I extend my appreciation to Liz Havu for her secretarial assistance. I thank Steve Freedman, PhD, for supplying the brain stem section used for Atlas Plate 25, and for letting me teach in his course at the University of Vermont as a graduate student. Two people have made invaluable contributions to the construction of this manual: Tom McCoy, DO, provided much assistance in the design of the questions following each case; and Bruce P. Bates, DO, Associate Clinical Dean, Family Practitioner, and good friend, has provided many details in the construction of the case histories.

Frank H. Willard, PhD

CONTENTS

MEDICAL
NEUROANATOMY

A PROBLEM-ORIENTED MANUAL
WITH ANNOTATED ATLAS

INTRODUCTION TO NEUROANATOMY

► Introduction

Of all the organs in the body, the central nervous system has by far the most varied surface topography and internal structure. Encased in a bony vault that limits its expansion during development, the tissue of the central nervous system has formed numerous convoluted folds. From the intricate structure of the brain and spinal cord arise the complexities of human reflexive, emotional, and motivational behavior. The primary goal of this manual is to approach an understanding of these functions by studying the deficits in human performance resulting from neurologic damage.

From embryologic studies, it is known that the adult central nervous system can be partitioned into a hierarchy of levels.[1] Specific neurologic functions can be associated with each level in the hierarchy. Furthermore, each level is located within one of three meningeal compartments: supratentorial, infratentorial, or vertebral (Table 1-1). At any level on the neuraxis, alterations in structure due to vascular accidents, mass occupying events (*e.g.,* tumors or abscesses), or degenerative processes can occur. These events, which generally are destructive to neural tissue, have been referred to as **lesions.** When a lesion occurs in the nervous system, the patient presents neurologic signs and symptoms that represent clues to the location of the damage. Associating these clinical signs with lesions of specific levels of the neuraxis requires knowledge of the neuroanatomy of a given area and of what happens when the brain attempts to work with damaged structures.[2] Knowledge of the meningeal compartments and their contents can assist in localizing the general region of neurologic damage in a patient.

This chapter examines both the major neural components in each meningeal compartment and a gen-

Table 1-1.
The Six Major Levels of the Central Nervous System, Their Embryonic Origin, and the Meningeal Compartment in Which They Are Located

EMBRYO	ADULT	MENINGEAL LOCATION
Spinal cord ——	Spinal Cord ————————————	Vertebral
Myelencephalon ——	Medulla ⎤	
Metencephalon ——	Pons/cerebellum ⎦ ——	Infratentorial
Mesencephalon ——	Midbrain———————————	Tentorium
Diencephalon ——	Thalamus ⎤	
Telencephalon ——	Cerebral hemispheres ⎦ ——	Supratentorial

eral scheme of cerebral vascularization. *Although at this point you may not understand the function of the structures presented, gaining familiarity with their location will greatly help you in the remaining chapters.* In keeping with the goal of the text (described in the preface), our exploration will be done in the context of a case study involving damage somewhere along the human neuraxis.

GENERAL OBJECTIVES

The major objective of Chapter 1 is simply an overview of central nervous system anatomy. **It is not intended for memorization at this time.** A general knowledge of this material will be helpful in organizing material presented in later sections. The specific objectives of this chapter are as follows:

1. To describe the nervous system in terms of its six major levels of organization and function (Table 1-1)
2. To learn general types of clinical defects resulting from damage in each of the six major levels in the neuraxis
3. To understand where extravasated blood accumulates in the cerebral vault

INSTRUCTIONS

In this chapter you will be presented with one or more clinical case studies. *Each one will be followed by a list of questions that can best be answered by using a knowledge of regional and functional neuroanatomy and by referring to outside reading material.* Following the questions will be a section devoted to structures from a specific region of the central nervous system. Before attempting to answer the questions, compile a list of the patient's neurologic signs and symptoms; then examine the structures and their functions and study their known clinical deficits. After you are familiar with the material, reexamine the list of neurologic signs and symptoms and formulate answers to the questions. Be aware that some of the questions can have multiple responses or require information beyond the scope of this manual. It may be necessary to obtain material or advice from additional resources, such as specialty texts, a medical dictionary, or clinical personnel.

MATERIALS

1. One complete human brain and spinal cord
2. One brain sectioned in the midsagittal plane
3. A medical dictionary

UNIT A

Case Study 1-1

A 74-year-old man with a history of hypertension, onset neurologic signs, and progressive demise

A 74-year-old retired lawyer was brought into a small community clinic in northern Maine complaining of a pain on the right side of his head and weakness on the left side of his body.

He had had mild hypertension for several years but was otherwise in excellent health. He had been in Maine on a hunting trip for the previous 3 days. On the day of admission he had been walking back to camp in a heavy snowfall when he suddenly developed pain behind the right ear, along with weakness of the left side of his body and dysarthria. He was brought immediately to the clinic, where he was examined by a physician's assistant. He was observed to be afebrile, to have a pulse rate of 88 beats per minute, regular breathing at a rate of 16 respirations per minute, and blood pressure of 200/112 mmHg. He was awake, oriented, and followed commands. He was dysarthric and complained of a steady, moderately severe pain above and behind the right ear. His head and eyes deviated moderately to the right, and there was a left homonymous hemianopsia.

The patient denied any recent history of trauma, headaches, or dizzy periods. He admitted to consuming one to two bottles of beer each evening on the hunting trip but denied consistent use of alcohol in his daily life. He also denied the use of any illicit drugs and was not taking any prescription medications.

He was able to deviate his eyes just past the midline to the left, volitionally; however, with the doll's head maneuver, his eyes could be directed into the left visual hemisphere. The pupils were unequal, the right being 2 mm and the left, 3 mm; both reacted to light. Sensation was reduced in the left side of the face and cornea. There was a moderately severe, flaccid left hemiparesis interrupted intermittently by clonic movements of the leg and tonic flexor movements of the left arm. Stretch reflexes on the left side were reduced, but the plantar response was extensor.

Within an hour of admission, the patient was having periodic decorticate posturing on the left side. The right plantar response had become extensor. He gradually lost consciousness; within 4 hours of admission he was unresponsive except to noxious stimuli. At first, painful stimuli produced extensor responses on the left but decorticate responses on the right; however, this pattern finally matured into bilateral extensor posturings, slightly more pronounced on the left than on the right. By this time, the right pupil had dilated and fixed in an oval shape, being 7 mm vertically and 3 mm horizontally. Minimal oculomotor responses could be elicited to cold caloric stimulation, and the patient was hyperventilating. Blood pressure had risen to 235/150 mmHg.

One hour after entering the clinic, preparations were begun for emergency transfer to Bangor, Maine, the closest major medical center; however, because of the snowstorm, air travel was impossible and ground transportation was slow. Treatment with mannitol was started, and during the next hour the patient's condition stabilized, except that the right pupil became round and regained a minimal reaction to light. En route to Bangor, the patient's blood pressure dropped to 160/60 mmHg, he began to vomit, and his temperature rose to 39.6°C. He began to sweat profusely, and within 6 hours of initial presentation at the clinic, the decerebrate responses had become less intense; the pupils were fixed, slightly irregular at 3 to 4 mm in diameter, and unequal; oculocephalic responses were absent; and respiration was quiet and shallow. Within 8 hours of admission to the clinic (2 hours into the trip to Bangor), respiration was ataxic; the pupils remained slightly unequal, with no oculovestibular responses; and the patient was diffusely flaccid but had bilateral extensor plantar responses and mild flexor response in the legs to noxious stimulation of the soles of the feet. He died 30 minutes later while still en route.

QUESTIONS

1. Does the patient exhibit a language or memory deficit or an alteration in consciousness or cognition?

2. Are signs of cranial nerve dysfunction present?

3. Are there any changes in motor functions, such as reflexes, muscle tone, movement, or coordination?

4. Are any changes in sensory functions detectable?

5. At what level in the central neuraxis is this lesion probably located?

6. Is the pathology focal, multifocal, or diffuse in its distribution within the nervous system?

7. What is the clinical–temporal profile of this pathology: acute or chronic; progressive or stable?

8. Based on your answers to the previous two questions, decide whether the patient's symptoms are most likely caused by a vascular accident, a tumor, or a degenerative or inflammatory process.

9. If you feel this is the result of a vascular accident, what vessels are probably involved?

10. Is this patient's initial damage occurring in epidural space, between dura and cerebrum, or intracerebrally?

11. Are the patient's neurologic sequelae due to the initial damage or to other processes?

12. What does the progress of events in this patient's demise reveal concerning the hierarchy of the central nervous system?

► DISCUSSION
Coverings of the Brain and Spinal Cord

The tissue of the central nervous system is contained within a bony vault called the cranium and vertebral canal. Between nervous tissue and bone can be found three general layers of protective coverings or meninges (Fig. 1-1). A rich vasculature supply perfuses the tissue within the cranial vault. Abnormal accumulation of fluids, such as extravasated blood, either between meningeal layers (epidural, subdural, or subarachnoid) or within the nervous tissue itself (intracerebral) will increase the pressure within the cranial vault or vertebral canal (see p. 16). This increased pressure can compromise function in surrounding neural tissue.

MENINGEAL STRUCTURES

Dura

The dura mater is a tough outer covering of dense irregular connective tissue surrounding the brain and spinal cord. The cerebral dura is divided into two layers. The **outer dura** forms the periosteum of the cranial vault (see Fig. 1-1). The **inner or meningeal dura** for the most part is fused with the outer; however, in specific regions it separates to create venous sinuses such as the superior sagittal sinus (see Fig. 1-1). The **falx cerebri** and **tentorium cerebelli** are formed by the fusion of meningeal dural sheets derived from the inner border of the venous sinuses.

In the vertebral canal the organization of the dural sheath changes. The outer dural layer of the cranial vault fuses with the periosteum of the vertebral canal. A thickened lip of outer dura wraps around the edge of the foramen magnum to fuse with the periosteum of the outer cranium. Only the meningeal dural layer of the cranial vault is continuous with the spinal dura through the foramen magnum. An **epidural space** containing a venous plexus (Batson's plexus of veins) and adipose tissue separates the periosteum from the spinal dura. As cranial and spinal nerves exit the dural sac they acquire sheaths of meningeal dura, called **epineurium** (Fig. 1-2).

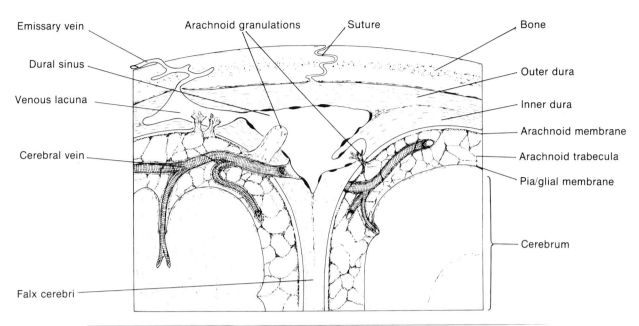

Emissary vein

Dural sinus

Venous lacuna

Cerebral vein

Falx cerebri

Arachnoid granulations

Suture

Bone

Outer dura

Inner dura

Arachnoid membrane

Arachnoid trabecula

Pia/glial membrane

Cerebrum

Figure 1-1. A diagram of a midline, coronal section through the cerebrum illustrates the three layers of meninges with respect to the bony cranium. Note the split in the dura as the outer dura adheres to the cranium and the two inner layers of dura pass around the sagittal sinus to form the falx cerebri. Arachnoid granulations are seen connecting the subarachnoid space with the lumen of the sinus. The position of the bridging veins as they pass from the cerebrum through the meninges to the sinus is also illustrated. (Modified from Carpenter MB, Sutin, J. Human neuroanatomy. 8th ed. Baltimore: Williams & Wilkins, 1983; and Nieuwenhuys R, Voogd J, van Huijzen C. The human central nervous system. Berlin: Springer-Verlag, 1988)

Arachnoid

The arachnoid can be divided into two layers, the outer of which is a delicate membrane located internal to, but not adherent to, the inner dura. A potential space exists between these two layers of tissue. This space is crossed by many bridging veins. During a traumatic event, the dura moves with the cranium and the arachnoid moves with the brain. The shearing forces developed between these two meningeal layers can rupture some of the bridging veins, initiating a subdural hematoma (see p. 17).

The inner layer of arachnoid consists of many delicate trabeculae that extend through the subarachnoid space to reach the pial surface. Blood vessels traverse the inner portion of the arachnoid supported by the labyrinthine trabecular network. It is around the arachnoid trabeculae that cerebrospinal fluid circulates.

Pia

The pia is a thin layer of connective tissue closely adherent to the surface of the brain and spinal cord. Its inner surface is fused to the end-feet of astrocytes and thus becomes closely adherent to the central nervous system. Thin sheets of pia, called **denticulate ligaments**, extend outward from the lateral margin of the spinal cord and attach to the dura (see Fig. 1-2). As such, denticulate ligaments serve to anchor the cord within the dural sac and are a surgical landmark separating the dorsal and ventral roots of the spinal cord. The most superior denticulate ligament extends upward through the foramen magnum to attach to the inner wall of the occipital bone.

MENINGEAL COMPARTMENTS

Major folds in the dura help delineate several meningeal compartments in the cranial vault. The **falx cerebri** divides the cranial cavity into left and right **supratentorial compartments,** and the **tentorium cerebelli** separates the supratentorial from the **infratentorial compartments.** The foramen magnum marks the transition from the compartments of the cranial vault to the **vertebral compartment.**

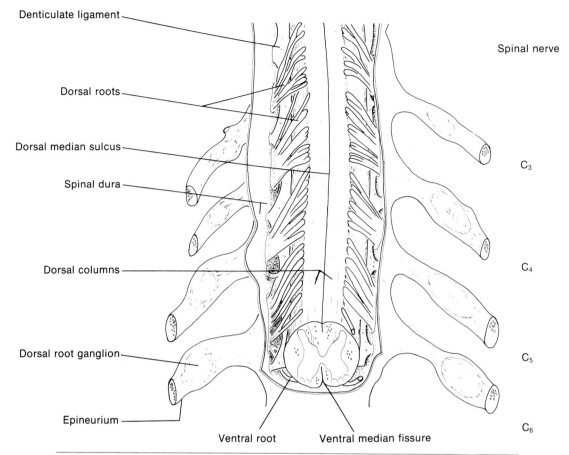

Denticulate ligament

Dorsal roots

Dorsal median sulcus

Spinal dura

Dorsal columns

Dorsal root ganglion

Epineurium

Ventral root

Ventral median fissure

Spinal nerve

C_3

C_4

C_5

C_6

Figure 1-2. Dorsal view of the cervical enlargement of the spinal cord with the meningeal layers opened. The dorsal root ganglia and the corresponding roots of the spinal nerve are also present. Some of the major surface landmarks of the spinal cord are indicated.

Supratentorial Compartment

The floor of the supratentorial compartment includes the orbital plate of the frontal bone, the wings of the sphenoid, the squamae and anterior petrous wall of the temporal bone, and tentorium cerebelli. It is bounded laterally and superiorly by the calvarium (made up of the squamae of the frontal, parietal, temporal, and occipital bones). Medially, the falx cerebri divides this compartment into two partitions. The supratentorial compartment contains the cerebral hemispheres, subcortical nuclei, and thalamus.

Infratentorial Compartment

The infratentorial compartment represents the posterior cranial fossa. The tentorium cerebelli and the foramen magnum form the superior and inferior boundaries, respectively. The posterior aspect of the petrous temporal bone and portions of the occipital bone inferior to the transverse sinus complete the an-

terior, lateral, and posterior compartmental boundaries. The cerebellum and most of the brain stem are contained in this compartment. The midbrain passes through the opening at the apex of the tentorium (the incisor cerebelli) to enter the supratentorial compartment.

Vertebral Compartment

The foramen magnum is the rostral boundary of the vertebral compartment. Caudally, this meningeal compartment extends to the second sacral vertebra, where the dural sac fuses with the periosteum of the sacral canal. The lateral border of the vertebral compartment extends to the entrance of the **intervertebral foramina**, where the dura fuses with the spinal roots, forming the epineurium.

Between the foramen magnum and vertebral level S_2 the anterior surface of the spinal dura is intermittently adherent to the posterior longitudinal ligament of the vertebral canal. Occasional straps of dura ex-

6

tend from the posterior surface of the dural sac to pass through the epidural space and attach to the periosteum of the vertebral canal. These dural adhesions and straps have been implicated as a source of discogenic pain[3] and sciatica[4] in the lumbar region.

The spinal cord and the dorsal and ventral spinal roots are contained within the vertebral compartment. The dorsal root ganglia are located within the intervertebral foramina at each vertebral level. The intermingling of fibers from dorsal and ventral roots to form the spinal nerve also occurs in the intervertebral foramen, at a point distal to the dorsal root ganglion.

► The Organization of the Central Nervous System

The brain and spinal cord contain an enormous three-dimensional network of connections between neurons. (The general features of this network are succinctly reviewed by Nauta and Feirtag.[5]) At first glance, attempting to understand this organization appears overwhelming. However, guiding principles, established through phylogeny, can help sort out nervous system structure and function. One of these principles states that the major components of the brain develop in a hierarchic array; each level of the hierarchy supplements and influences, but does not replace, those below it.[6] A list of the general levels and their location by meningeal compartment is presented in Table 1-1. We will examine each level in the central nervous system and formulate a general statement concerning the neurologic deficits that occur when that level is damaged. *It is important to familiarize yourself with these general deficits, since later chapters will give a more detailed treatment of the lesion-induced deficits.*

SPINAL CORD

The spinal cord is contained within the vertebral meningeal compartment and transmits somatic sensory information to the brain that is collected from peripheral nerves. It also transmits descending instructions from the cerebral cortex and brain stem to individual cord segments.

Each spinal segment represents that region of the cord serviced by a **spinal nerve.** The spinal nerve enters the vertebral canal through an intervertebral foramina; as it approaches the cord, it separates into **dorsal and ventral roots** that subsequently fan out into rootlets. The latter enter the cord over the space of approximately 1 inch (Fig. 1-2), a value that de-

creases in the lower sacral and coccygeal regions of the spinal cord. The entry zone for an individual root constitutes a **spinal segment.** Sensory (or afferent) axons enter the spinal cord over the dorsal root, and motor (or efferent) axons leave the cord over the ventral root. Cell bodies for the sensory axons are found in the **dorsal root ganglion** located in the dorsal root at its junction with the ventral root in the intervertebral foramen.

At each segmental level, a cross section of the spinal cord will reveal an H-shaped core of gray matter surrounded by vertical columns of white matter. The ventral gray, or **ventral horn**, contains motoneurons that innervate skeletal muscle fibers; the dorsal gray matter, or **dorsal horn**, contains tract cells for communication with the brain and interneurons for communication with other portions of the spinal cord. The surrounding white matter contains ascending sensory and descending motor tracts.

The spinal cord has two **enlargements, cervical** and **lumbar,** to house the neural circuitry necessary to service the upper and lower extremities, respectively. The narrowing of the cord in its thoracic portion reflects the reduced skin sensitivity and reduced muscle mass of this body region. Distal to the lumbar enlargement, the cord is tapered (the **conus medullaris**) and ends in a thin thread (the **filum terminale).** Since the spinal cord is shorter than its bony canal and ends at approximately vertebral level L$_2$, the lumbar and sacral nerve roots must course considerable distances along the vertebral canal before reaching their appropriate intervertebral foramina. This arrangement gives these nerve roots the appearance of a horse's tail, called the **cauda equina.**

CLINICAL DEFICIT

Injury of the spinal roots, either in the vertebral compartment or as they pass out of the intervertebral foramen into the periphery, can lead to a radicular (root) distribution of altered sensory experience and weakness. The altered sensory experience can be in the form of decreased sensibility (hypoesthesia), increased sensibility (hyperesthesia), abnormal quality of sensation (paresthesias), or pain.[7] The areas affected reflect the afferent distribution of the root or peripheral nerve injured.

Transection of sensory tracts in the spinal cord can result in the loss of pain and temperature sensation, discriminative touch, and proprioception. In general, the loss of sensation consequent to cord damage is more broadly distributed, usually occurring below the segmental level of the lesion, than that resulting from a specific root or peripheral nerve lesion. The horizontal line across the body, below which sensory functions are diminished in a cord lesion, is called a

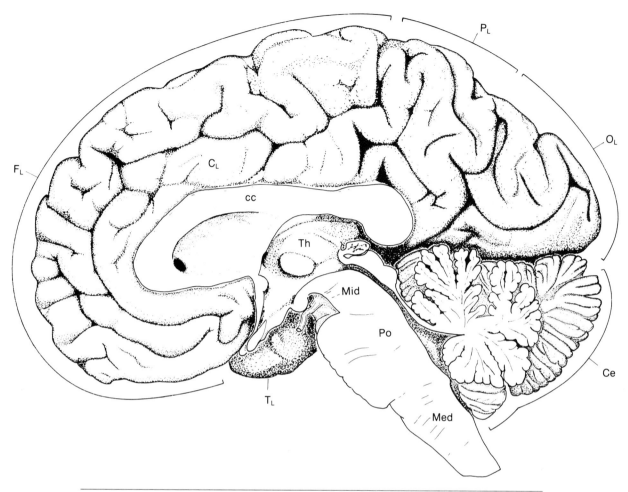

Figure 1-3. A sagittal view of the brain illustrates brain stem, cerebellum, thalamus, and cerebral cortex. (cc, corpus callosum; Ce, cerebellum; C_L, cingulate gyrus; F_L, frontal lobe; Med, medulla; Mid, midbrain; O_L, occipital lobe; P_L, parietal lobe; Po, pons; Th, thalamus; T_L, temporal lobe.)

sensory level. Irritation, as opposed to transection, of sensory tracts in the spinal cord can present with pain and paresthesias instead of sensory loss.[8]

Damage to the motoneurons of individual spinal segments can present as weakness and flaccidity of the muscles innervated from that segment. Damage to the descending fiber tracts from suprasegmental structures can result in weakness and spasticity for muscles innervated by motoneurons located below the level of the lesion (see Chap. 2 for further discussion of this concept).

MEDULLA

The medulla is located in the infratentorial compartment and represents the most caudal portion of the brain stem (Fig. 1-3). It contains major ascending sensory tracts to the cerebrum and cerebellum, de-

scending motor tracts to the spinal cord, and the central nuclei related to the fifth, eighth, ninth, tenth, eleventh, and twelfth cranial nerves.

The ventral surface of the medulla is characterized by two longitudinal ridges along the midline; these are the **pyramids** containing corticospinal fibers (Fig. 1-4). Lateral to each pyramid is a tubercle called the **olive,** which marks the location of the massive inferior olivary nucleus. The **hypoglossal nerve** exits the brain stem between the olivary tubercle and the pyramid. The **glossopharyngeal, vagus,** and **cranial root of the accessory nerve** leave the brain stem dorsal to the olivary tubercle and the **vestibulocochlear nerve** exits the brain stem at the pontomedullary junction.

The salient features of the dorsal surface of the medulla (Fig. 1-5) are the **gracile** and **cuneate tubercles** along the inferior portion of the **fourth ven-**

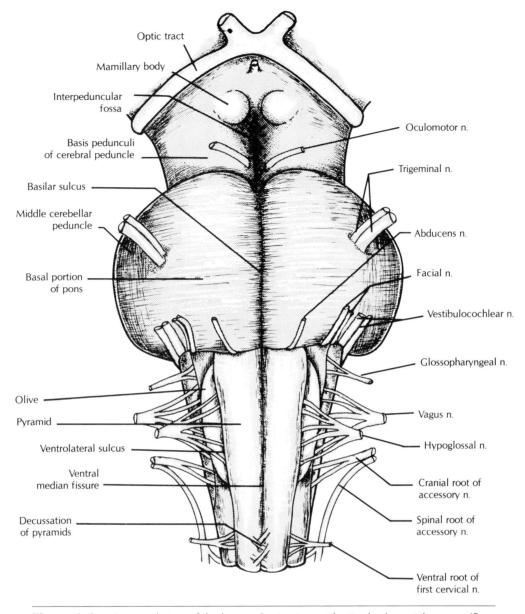

Optic tract

Mamillary body

Interpeduncular fossa

Basis pedunculi of cerebral peduncle

Basilar sulcus

Middle cerebellar peduncle

Basal portion of pons

Olive

Pyramid

Ventrolateral sulcus

Ventral median fissure

Decussation of pyramids

Oculomotor n.

Trigeminal n.

Abducens n.

Facial n.

Vestibulocochlear n.

Glossopharyngeal n.

Vagus n.

Hypoglossal n.

Cranial root of accessory n.

Spinal root of accessory n.

Ventral root of first cervical n.

Figure 1-4. A ventral view of the human brain stem with attached cranial nerves. (Barr ML, Kiernan JA. The human nervous system: an anatomical viewpoint. 5th ed. Philadelphia: JB Lippincott, 1988:85)

tricle. These tubercles are located at the superior end of the gracile and cuneate fiber tracts, respectively, and mark the site of two large, sensory nuclei in the brain stem, the **nucleus gracilis** and **cuneatus.** The walls of the fourth ventricle approximate themselves inferiorly to form the **obex,** a surgical landmark. At the lateral extremes of the fourth ventricle and lying on the surface of the eighth cranial nerve is the dorsal cochlear nucleus, a component of the auditory system.

The core of the medulla (as well as the pons and midbrain) is composed of the reticular formation. Its

neuronal circuits are involved in the control of cardiovascular tone and respiratory rate, pharyngeal and laryngeal musculature, gastrointestinal secretions and mobility, and emesis (see Chap. 3).

CLINICAL DEFICIT

Large lesions of the medulla will most likely result in coma and death due to compression of surrounding brain stem structures. Smaller, more confined lesions in the medulla generally do not result in coma[9] but can present as primary sensory loss (proprioception and vibratory sense) from the body and face; loss of

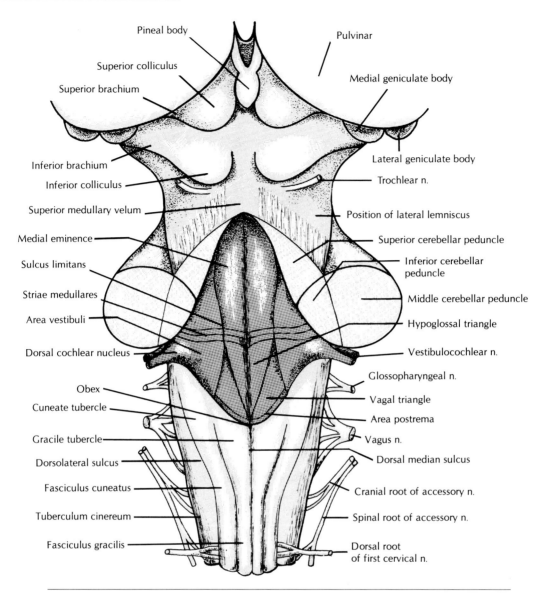

Figure 1-5. A dorsal view of the human brain stem with attached cranial nerves. (Barr ML, Kiernan JA. The human nervous system: an anatomical viewpoint. 5th ed. Philadelphia: JB Lippincott, 1988:88)

motor control (spastic paralysis) in the limbs; loss of pain and temperature sensations from the body and face; loss of hearing or balance; speech (dysarthria) and swallowing (dysphagia) disorders; and paralysis of tongue movement.

Since the medulla also contains respiratory and cardiovascular control circuits, their damage can result in cardiac arrhythmias and dyspnea, eventually leading to death. The unfortunate patient can remain conscious throughout much of this process.[9] Descending fiber tracts from the hypothalamus involved with the autonomic nervous system pass through the medulla; hence, medullary lesions can also result in dysautonomic symptoms.

PONS

The pons is located ventral to the cerebellum in the infratentorial compartment (see Fig. 1-3). Its external features are dominated by the cerebellar peduncles (see Figs. 1-4 and 1-5). The pons contains major ascending sensory and descending motor fiber tracts interconnecting spinal cord, cerebral cortex, and cerebellum. In addition, it contains the central nuclei related to the fifth, sixth, seventh, and portions of the eighth cranial nerves. The reticular formation of the pons contains the caudal portion of a major cerebral activating system. This system functions to arouse and maintain the level of activity in the supratentorial structures, such as the thalamus and cerebral cortex.

The dorsal surface of the pons forms the floor of the **fourth ventricle.** It is marked by the median eminence, sulcus limitans, and several transverse bands called the stria medullares (see Fig. 1-5). On the ventral surface of the brain stem, the large **middle cerebellar peduncle** is seen wrapping around the pons. The **vestibulocochlear** and **facial cranial nerves** leave the pons laterally along the pontomedullary border; the **abducens nerve** exits medially. The **trigeminal nerve** exits the pons by penetrating the middle cerebellar peduncle laterally. The neuronal circuitry surrounding the cranial nerve structures of the pons is involved in controlling postural musculature and in directing horizontal (lateral) eye movements (see Chap. 4).

CLINICAL DEFICIT

Large, bilateral lesions of the pons that damage the reticular activating system most likely will result in coma and death.[9] Smaller, more confined lesions, especially if they are unilateral, can present as loss of primary sensory modalities (vibratory sense, discriminative touch, and proprioception) as well as pain and temperature sensations from the body and face, aberrant motor control (ataxia or paralysis) of the limbs, facial paralysis, paralysis of the jaw, lateral gaze palsies, and internal strabismus (esotropia) of the eye.

CEREBELLUM

The cerebellum is located in the infratentorial compartment in the angle between the brain stem and tentorium cerebelli (Fig. 1-3). It is divided into two large **hemispheres** and a midline **vermis.** The cerebellum is connected to the brain stem through three major structures, the **superior, middle,** and **inferior cerebellar peduncles** (see Figs. 1-4 and 1-5).

Through its peduncles, the cerebellum receives proprioceptive information from muscles and joints via the spinal cord as well as instructions from the cerebral cortex. It functions in motor control, computing the timing of muscle contractions for coordinated movements (see Chap. 5).

CLINICAL DEFICIT

Lesions involving the cerebellum result in defects in the timing of muscle contractions. They can present as a breakdown of rapid hand or finger movement, ataxia, dysmetria, loss of balance, swaying, staggering, and intention tremor (see Chap. 5).

MIDBRAIN

The midbrain is located at the rostral end of the brain stem (see Fig. 1-3). It passes through the **incisura cerebelli** (the large opening in the tentorium), thus straddling the border between the supratentorial and infratentorial compartments. The midbrain contains major ascending sensory and descending motor tracts similar to other portions of the brain stem. In addition, it contains structures related to the third and fourth cranial nerves. Its reticular formation has neural circuits involved in controlling vertical eye movements. The midbrain reticular activating system regulates the level of neural activity in the thalamus and cerebral cortex, it is involved in controlling sleep and arousal.

The ventral surface of the midbrain is characterized by two large cerebral peduncles (see Fig. 1-4). Between the peduncles is the interpeduncular fossa; the **oculomotor nerve** emerges from the midbrain along the walls of this fossa. Dorsally, the midbrain is identified by the two pairs of **colliculi** (inferior and superior; see Fig. 1-5). The **trochlear nerve** emerges from the dorsal surface at the base of the inferior colliculus (see Chap. 6).

CLINICAL DEFICIT

Both large and small paramedian lesions in the midbrain reticular formation or its ascending projections can result in coma and sleep dysfunctions.[9] Smaller lesions, especially those occurring more laterally, can present as loss of primary sensory modalities (vibratory sense, discriminative touch, and proprioception), as well as pain and temperature sensations from the body and face, abnormal motor control (ataxia and paralysis), and eye movement dysfunction (third and fourth nerve palsies and vertical gaze palsies). Lesions at the midbrain level can separate the cerebral and midbrain controls of the motor system from the motor regions of the lower brain stem and spinal cord. In such cases the patient can experience decerebrate posturing, with the upper and lower limbs going into an extreme, extensor-dominated positions.

THALAMUS

The thalamus is located in the supratentorial compartment, positioned rostral to the midbrain and nestled under the cerebral cortex (see Fig. 1-3). Laterally, it is bordered by the white matter of the **internal capsule.** The ventral surface of the thalamus is exposed externally and presents the **optic chiasm** and **optic tracts** rostrally, the **mamillary bodies** caudally, and in between, the **infundibulum** (stalk) of the pituitary.

Dorsally, the thalamus is covered by the massive **corpus callosum.** The dorsal surface of the thalamus can be seen by sectioning this fiber bundle at the base of the longitudinal fissure. It presents the two **thalamic hemispheres** laterally, separated by the narrow opening to the **third ventricle.** The roof of the third ventricle is formed by the **fornix,** a fiber bundle connecting the hippocampus in the temporal lobe to the hypothalamus.

The rostral boundary of the thalamus extends to the anterior commissure; its caudal boundary lies at the **pineal gland** and midbrain. The thalamus is divided into two symmetric hemispheres by the third ventricle; its medial or ventricular surface contains the **massa intermedia** or thalamic adhesion (see Fig. 1-3 and Chap. 7).

The thalamus is reciprocally connected by axons to most areas of cerebral cortex. Through these connections it relays ascending sensory information to the primary sensory areas of the cortex. It also contains pathways involved in cortical motor control systems. Thus, through the thalamocortical and corticothalamic connections, the thalamus is intimately involved in the functioning of the overlying cortical mantle. In addition, several pathways from the brain stem to the thalamus influence memory processing, consciousness, and arousal.

The ventral portion of thalamus, called the **hypothalamus,** is separated from the (proper or dorsal) thalamus by the hypothalamic sulcus. The hypothalamus controls the autonomic nervous system and, through the infundibulum and pituitary gland, modulates the endocrine system. Through these connections with the autonomic nervous system and the endocrine glands the hypothalamus can also influence the operation of the immune system.[10,11]

CLINICAL DEFICIT

Damage to the thalamus can present as loss of primary sensory modalities as well as pain and temperature sensation, abnormal motor control (ataxia, hyperkinesia, hypokinesia, or paralysis), intractable intense pain, memory loss, confusion and altered behavioral patterns, sleep disorders, coma, endocrine imbalances, and autonomic dysfunction (see Chap. 7).

CEREBRUM

The cerebral hemispheres are contained in the supratentorial compartment. They are separated by the falx cerebri lying in the **longitudinal fissure.** At the base of this fissure, the hemispheres are interconnected by the **corpus callosum** (see Fig. 1-3). The rostral-most portion of each hemisphere is the **frontal lobe,** it extends caudally to the **central sulcus** and is separated from the **temporal lobe** laterally by the **lateral fissure** (Fig. 1-6). Nestled deep within the lateral fissure is the **insula lobe.** The **parietal lobe** extends from the central sulcus to the **parieto-occipital sulcus.** The caudal-most portion of the hemisphere is the **occipital lobe** (see Chap. 8).

The ventral surface of the cerebrum presents a long, curved, medially placed gyrus, the **parahippocampal gyrus,** which wraps around the brain stem. Rostrally, this gyrus ends in an enlarged mass, the **uncus.** The medial surface of the hemisphere displays the profile of the corpus callosum arched over the thalamus (see Fig. 1-3). Dorsally, the corpus callosum is bordered by the **cingulate gyrus.** The parahippocampal gyrus and cingulate gyrus are continuous around the caudal end of the corpus callosum and form the limbic lobe.

Subcortical structures are buried within the cerebral hemispheres; two of these structures are located in close approximation to the ventral surface landmarks. The **hippocampus** is found internal to the parahippocampal gyrus, and the **amygdala** is positioned internal to the uncus (see Chap. 9). The **corpus striatum** is located rostral and lateral to the thalamus, embedded deep in the white matter of the cerebral hemisphere (see Chap. 10). It cannot be seen from the external surface of the brain.

The cerebral cortex has specific areas for receiving sensory information and for developing motor activity. However, its largest portion is called the **association cortex** and is devoted to such cognitive functions as understanding written and spoken language, mechanicospatial relationships, attention, perceptions, and memory, as well as the guidance of socially appropriate behavior. However, as a caveat, the cerebral cortex should not be thought of as containing specific centers for our individual cognitive functions; rather, these activities arise out of the combined interactions of multiple cortical association areas as well as those of the sensory and motor cortex.[2] This arrangement is called *parallel distributed processing* and represents a network analysis of cerebral cortical function.[12,13] It will be discussed further in Chapter 8.

Subcortical structures such as the basal ganglia receive a significant portion of their input from the cerebral cortex and, through their connections with the thalamus, modulated cerebral cortical activity. They are therefore involved in controlling or scaling the

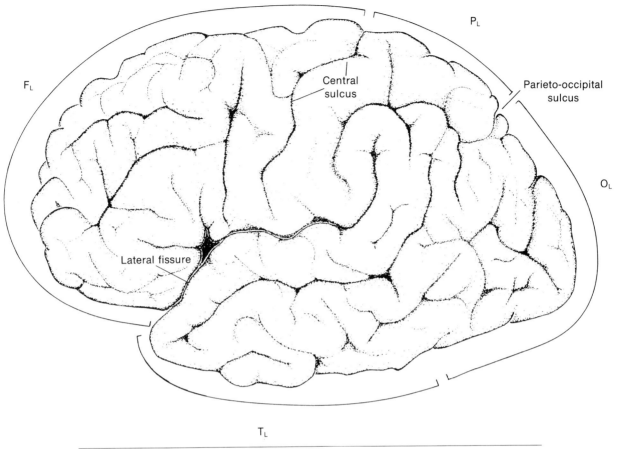

Figure 1-6. A lateral view of the brain illustrates the lobes and several major landmarks of the cerebral hemisphere. (Ce, cerebellum; F_L, frontal lobe; LF, lateral fissure; Med, medulla; O_L, occipital lobe; P_L, parietal lobe; T_L, temporal lobe.)

intensity of emotional behavior and of motor activity and cognitive functions.[14] The basal ganglia will be discussed further in Chapter 10.

CLINICAL DEFICIT

When the cerebral cortex is damaged, clinical deficits range from specific sensory and motor losses to alterations of cognitive functions—language, speech, writing, and reading—as well as changes in awareness, social mores, memory, or consciousness. Damage to the subcortical structures can result in memory loss, aberrant emotional behavior, and personality changes. Movement disorders can also occur, such as hyperkinesia or hypokinesia (see Chaps. 8-10).

When the cerebral cortex comes under increased pressure, for example, from a space-occupying lesion or a bleeding intracranial vascular accident, its function can diminish. The patient becomes obtunded or unconscious. Cerebral control of the brain stem motor regions is diminished and the patient displays varying degrees of decorticate posturing, with the upper extremity dominated by the flexor muscles and the lower extremity dominated by the extensor muscles.

► Cerebral Vasculature

Cerebral arteries supply blood to the central nervous system. Occlusion or rupture of a cerebral vessel (artery or vein) can compromise the blood flow to a specific region of the central neuraxis, resulting in infarction or hemorrhage and, ultimately, damage to neural tissue. Based on the signs and symptoms displayed by the patient, it may be possible to localize the vascular accident on the neuraxis. This information is important when considering where to look with sophisticated and expensive imaging techniques and when designing rehabilitative therapy. An understanding of cerebral vascular distribution is critical for the localization process.

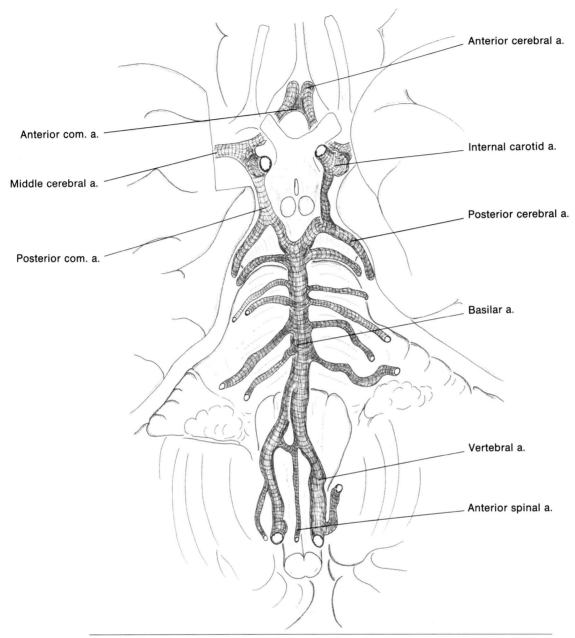

Anterior cerebral a.

Anterior com. a.

Internal carotid a.

Middle cerebral a.

Posterior cerebral a.

Posterior com. a.

Basilar a.

Vertebral a.

Anterior spinal a.

Figure 1-7. A ventral view of the blood supply to the brain demonstrates the union of four large arteries. The two vertebral arteries unite to form the basilar which splits to form the posterior aspect of the circle of Willis. The anterior aspect of this circle is derived from the two internal carotid arteries. The circle of Willis surrounds the optic chiasm and hypothalamus.

Cerebral circulation can be divided into anterior and posterior sources. The anterior circulation derives from the **internal carotid arteries**; the posterior circulation comes from the **vertebral arteries.** These two sources anastomose at the base of the brain in the **circle of Willis** (Fig. 1-7).

ANTERIOR CIRCULATION

The anterior circulation is generally confined to the supratentorial compartment. It arises from the bifurcation of the **internal carotid arteries** to form the **anterior cerebral artery** and the **middle cerebral**

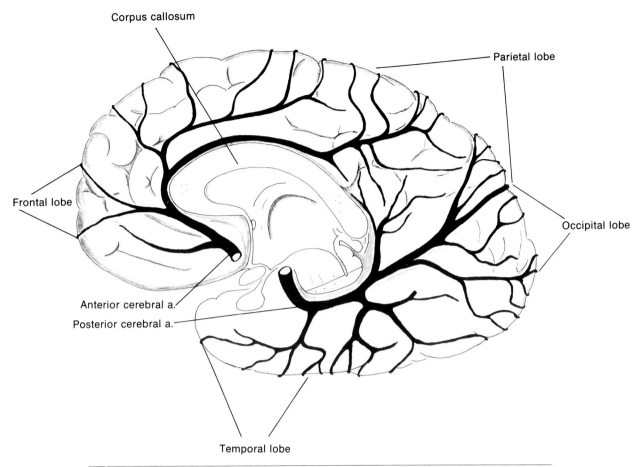

Corpus callosum

Parietal lobe

Frontal lobe

Occipital lobe

Anterior cerebral a.

Posterior cerebral a.

Temporal lobe

Figure 1-8. Distribution of anterior and posterior cerebral arteries as seen on the medial surface of the brain. The distal tips of the middle cerebral artery can be seen as they pass around the edge of the cerebrum to anastomose with the tips of the anterior and posterior cerebral arteries.

artery (see Fig. 1-7). The two anterior cerebral arteries are connected by the **anterior communicating artery.** The anterior cerebral artery perfuses the cingulate gyrus, portions of the medial frontal lobe, and the corpus callosum (Fig. 1-8); the middle cerebral artery perfuses the lateral aspect of the frontal lobe and portions of the temporal lobe (see Figs. 1-8 and 1-9). Penetrating branches of both anterior and middle cerebral arteries reach the corpus striatum and anterior thalamus.

POSTERIOR CIRCULATION

The **anterior** and **posterior spinal arteries** join with the **vertebral artery** to form the source of the posterior circulation (see Fig. 1-7). Subsequently, both vertebral arteries unite on the midline to form the **basilar artery**, which, after giving off vessels to the

cerebellum, divides to form the **posterior cerebral arteries.** The posterior circulation supplies the spinal cord in the vertebral compartment, most of the brain stem and cerebellum in the infratentorial compartment, and the medial and caudal aspect of the temporal and occipital lobes in the supratentorial compartment (see Figs. 1-8 and 1-9). Penetrating branches of the posterior cerebral artery reach the hippocampus and posterior thalamus.

► Intracranial Hemorrhages

EPIDURAL HEMORRHAGE

The dura is closely adherent to the inner table of the cranium; wedged snugly in a groove in the inner cranium and bordered by the dura is the middle me-

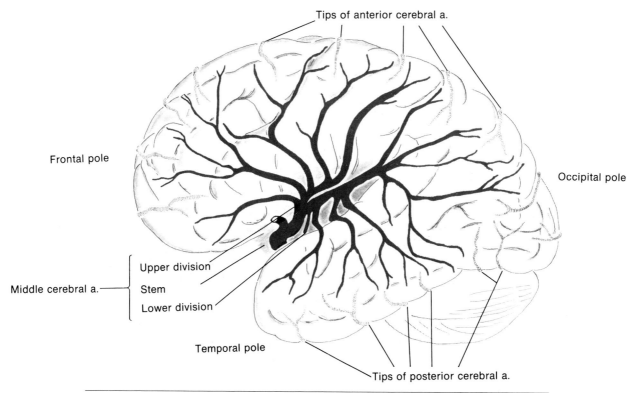

Tips of anterior cerebral a.

Frontal pole

Occipital pole

Middle cerebral a.
Upper division
Stem
Lower division

Temporal pole

Tips of posterior cerebral a.

Figure 1-9. Distribution of the branches of the middle cerebral artery on the lateral surface of the brain. The distal tips of the anterior and posterior cerebral arteries can be seen as they pass around the edge of the cerebrum to anastomose with the tips of the middle cerebral artery.

ningeal artery. A traumatic blow to the lateral convexity of the head, resulting in a fracture of the temporal or parietal bone, can rupture the middle meningeal artery or its branches. The result is an epidural hematoma (Fig. 1-10). During this process extravasated blood accumulates between the dura and inner table of the cranium.[15,16] In addition to laterally located hematomas resulting from the middle meningeal artery, frontal and posterior epidural hematomas have been reported.

A "lucid interval" without neurologic symptoms can occur following traumatic injury as the nascent hematoma grows in size. Generally, after reaching 50 mL in volume, drowsiness, confusion, and headache appear; these can progress into obtundation and coma in patients with supratentorial hematomas.[17]

The increased intracranial pressure accompanying the epidural hematoma can cause transtentorial herniation of the uncus. Medial displacement of the uncus compromises the third cranial nerve. Pupillary responses can be sensitive indicators of the progress of the herniation in an unconscious patient. The side of the dilated pupil is an indicator of the hematoma's laterality. Continued progression of the hematoma can lead to tonsillar herniation (downward displacement of the cerebellum through the foramen magnum), compression of the medulla, and respiratory arrest resulting in death.[16]

SUBDURAL HEMORRHAGE

The dura mater is adherent to the calvarium and the arachnoid is adherent to the cerebral hemispheres. The dura and arachnoid are adjacent but not adherent to one another; numerous cerebral (bridging) veins pass between these two layers. Trauma to either the frontal or posterior aspect of the skull can result in rebound shearing of the cerebral veins, with extravasated blood accumulating in the potential space between dura and arachnoid and forming a subdural hematoma.

When the head strikes a stationary object with force, a subdural hematoma frequently results. If the force is applied across the long axis of the cranium (*e.g.,* the forehead striking a windshield), the resulting hematoma can be bilateral, as bridging veins tear along both sides of the brain. If the arachnoid layer

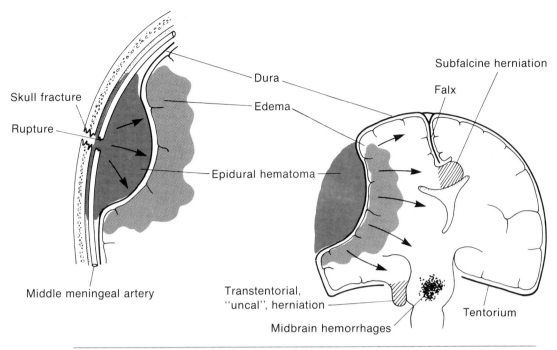

Figure 1-10. Epidural hematoma. A fracture of the parietal bone can result in rupture of the middle meningeal artery. The bleeding slowly dissects the dura from the calvarium. The resulting hematoma can compress the underlying tissue of the central nervous system. (Vogel FS, Bouldin TW. The nervous system. In: Rubin E, Farber JL, eds. Pathology. Philadelphia: JB Lippincott, 1988:1419)

preserves its integrity, the blood initially compartmentalizes without contact with the cerebrospinal fluid (CSF) (Fig. 1-11). Since the hemorrhage is from low-pressure venous blood, it can discontinue after 25 to 30 mL have accumulated.[18]

Acute subdural hematomas have a latency period between the traumatic event and the onset of neurologic sequelae of up to 3 days. Chronic subdural hematoma, which has an age-related and alcohol-associated predisposition, can have a longer latency period to the onset of neurologic sequelae.[19]

SUBARACHNOID HEMORRHAGE

Subarachnoid hemorrhages are usually due to trauma, rupture of an intracranial aneurysm, or leakage from an arteriovenous malformation.[16,19] Extreme hemorrhage may cause shock, coma, and death in a few hours; limited bleeding, on the other hand, may present as only a slight headache. The patient may appear confused, irritable, and semicomatose. Neck rigidity and signs of meningeal irritation can be present. Blood will discolor the CSF.

The discolorization of the CSF by the breakdown products of blood is called xanthochromia. This process is characterized by a colored pigment, a product of the breakdown of oxyhemoglobin and bilirubin, appearing in the CSF. Within 2 hours of entry into the CSF, red blood cells release hemoglobin. The hemoglobin breaks down to oxyhemoglobin, thus initiating xanthochromia in the CSF. Oxyhemoglobin is broken down into bilirubin within 10 hours.[20]

Following a subarachnoid bleed, red blood cells can be seen in the CSF. Conversely, subdural bleeding generally will not show red blood cells in the CSF, although the degradation products may traverse the arachnoid membrane and result in xanthochromia. This process may be detected up to 3 weeks after the initiating incidence.

INTRACEREBRAL HEMORRHAGE

Rupture of blood vessels within the central nervous system can result in intracerebral hemorrhage. The concomitant loss of circulation in the surrounding area can initiate a period of hypoxia and ischemia.

17

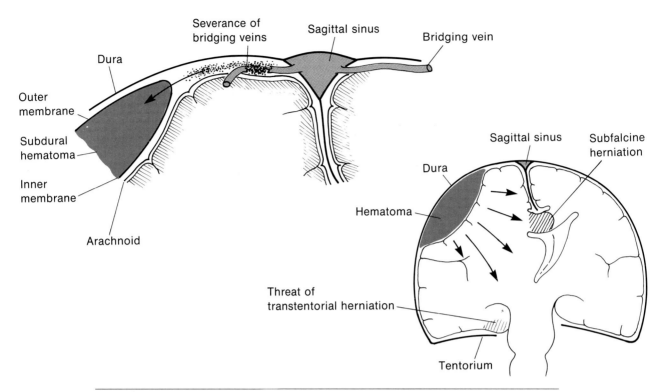

Figure 1-11. Subdural hematoma. Rupture of the bridging veins between the arachnoid and dura can result in extravasation of blood into the potential space between these two meningeal layers. The slow venous bleeding creates an expanding hematoma. The resulting herniation of the central nervous system is life threatening. (Vogel FS, Bouldin TW. The nervous system. In: Rubin E, Farber JL, eds. Pathology. Philadelphia: JB Lippincott, 1988:1423).

Tissue damage is also compounded by the irritating effects of extravasated blood.

The ischemic event and the extravasated blood in an intracranial hemorrhage can produce immediate neurologic sequelae, usually of rapid onset. Subsequent to the initial presentation, the hemorrhaging vessel may continue to release blood, resulting in gradually increasing intracranial pressure. A progression of neurologic signs and symptoms can compound the initial presentation as the central nervous system tissue attempts to herniate out of the cranial compartment affected by the bleeding vessel.

Increased intracranial pressure is said to occur when the CSF pressure exceeds 200 mm water (15 mmHg) with the patient lying in the lateral decubitus position.[16] The pressure inside the cranium increases for several reasons, such as the presence of an expanding tumor, an active hemorrhage, a ventricular occlusion, or an inflammatory and edematous process. The consequence of prolonged increase in intracranial pressure can be devastating. CNS tissue, being soft and pliable, usually herniates out of the more rigid cranial spaces as the surrounding pressure increases. Various types of herniations have been described.[21] Performing a lumbar puncture on a patient with increased intracranial pressure can have extremely serious consequences. The medulla and cerebellum attempt to herniate through the foramen magnum in response to the rapidly diminished pressure in the vertebral compartment.

The effects of a hernia on cerebral function depend on its location. Supratentorial expanding lesions can produce a shift of the falx cerebri toward the contralateral side, a process that can be monitored with computerized imaging. An index of this shift is seen in the lateral displacement of the pineal (which is in close juxtaposition with the falx; its calcium deposits are usually detectable in CT scans). No displacement or one of up to 3 mm of the pineal and midline can be present in an alert patient. Displacement of 3 to 4 mm is associated with drowsiness; one of 6 to 8.5 mm, with stupor; and one of 8 to 13 mm, with coma.[22]

Unlike intracranial bleeding, where hypoxia and ischemia occur, the expression of neurologic signs and symptoms in epidural and subdural hematomas is due primarily to the effect of an expanding mass as well as compression. Consequently, there is usually a time delay between the injury and the onset of neurologic sequelae as the volume of blood accumulates in the hematoma.[20] This lag time in the onset of neurologic signs can help to distinguish patients with epidural and subdural hematomas from those with intracranial hemorrhage.

► Bibliography

Barr ML, Kiernan JA. The human nervous system: an anatomical viewpoint. Philadelphia: JB Lippincott, 1988: Chap. 1.

Daube JR, Ragan TJ, Sandok BA, Westmoreland BF. Medical neurosciences. Boston: Little, Brown, 1986: Chaps. 2–5.

Haines DE. Neuroanatomy: an atlas of structures, sections, and systems, Baltimore: Urban & Schwarzenberg, 1987 *(see especially Figs. 2-1 to 4-3).*

Nieuwenhuys R, Voogd J, van Huijzen C. The human central nervous system. Berlin: Springer-Verlag 1988: Parts I and II.

► References

1. Moore KL. The developing human. Philadelphia: WB Saunders, 1988.

2. Damasio H, Damasio AR. Lesion analysis in neuropsychology. New York: Oxford University Press, 1989.

3. Parke WW, Watanabe, R. Adhesions of the ventral lumbar dura: an adjunct source of discogenic pain? Spine 1990;15:300.

4. Spencer DL, Irwin GS, Miller JAA. Anatomy and significance of fixation of the lumbosacral nerve roots in sciatica. Spine 1983;8:672.

5. Nauta WJH, Feirtag M. The organization of the brain. Sci Am 1979;241(3):88.

6. Sarnat HB, Netsky MG. Evolution of the nervous system. New York: Oxford University Press, 1981.

7. Spence AM. Pain and sensory disturbances in the extremities: radiculopathies, plexopathies, and mononeuropathies. In: Swanson PD, ed. Signs and symptoms in neurology. Philadelphia: JB Lippincott, 1984:245–281.

8. DeMyer W. Anatomy and clinical neurology of the spinal cord. In: Joynt RJ, ed. Clinical neurology, Vol III. Philadelphia: JB Lippincott, 1979:1–32.

9. Plum F, Posner JB. The diagnosis of stupor and coma. Philadelphia: FA Davis, 1982:377.

10. Freier S. The neuroendocrine-immune network. Boca Raton, FL: CRC Press, 1990.

11. Goetzl EJ, Spector NH. Neuroimmune networks: physiology and diseases. New York: Alan R Liss, 1989.

12. Goldman-Rakic P. Topography of cognition: parallel distributed networks in primate association cortex. Ann Rev Neurosci 1988;11:137.

13. Mesulam M-Marsel. Large scale neurocognitive networks and distributed processing for attention, language, and memory. Ann Neurol 1990;28:597.

14. Alexander GE, DeLong MR, Strick PL. Parallel organization of functionally segregated circuits linking basal ganglia and cortex. Ann Rev Neurosci 1986;9:357.

15. Dacey RG, Jane JJ. Craniocerebral trauma. In: Joynt RJ, ed. Clinical neurology. Philadelphia: JB Lippincott, 1984:1–61.

16. Morris JH. The nervous system. In: Cotran RS, Kumar V, Robbins SL, eds. Robbin's pathologic basis of disease. Philadelphia: WB Saunders, 1989:1385–1449.

17. Ritchie AC. Boyd's textbook of pathology. Philadelphia: Lea & Febiger, 1990.

18. Vogel FS, Bouldin TW. The nervous system. In: Rubin E, Faber JL, eds. Pathology. Philadelphia: JB Lippincott, 1988:1416–1499.

19. Hardman JM. Cerebrospinal trauma. In: Davis RL, Robertson DM, eds. Textbook of neuropathology. Baltimore: Williams & Wilkins, 1985:842–882.

20. Adams RD, Victor M. Principles of neurology. New York: McGraw-Hill, 1989.

21. McComb JG, Davis RL. Choroid plexus, cerebrospinal fluid, hydrocephalus, cerebral edema, and herniation phenomena. In: Davis RL, Robertson DM, eds. Textbook of neuropathology. Baltimore: Williams & Wilkins, 1985:147–175.

22. Ropper AH. Lateral displacement of the brain and level of consciousness in patients with acute hemispheral mass. New Engl J Med 1986;314:953.

2 *SPINAL CORD*

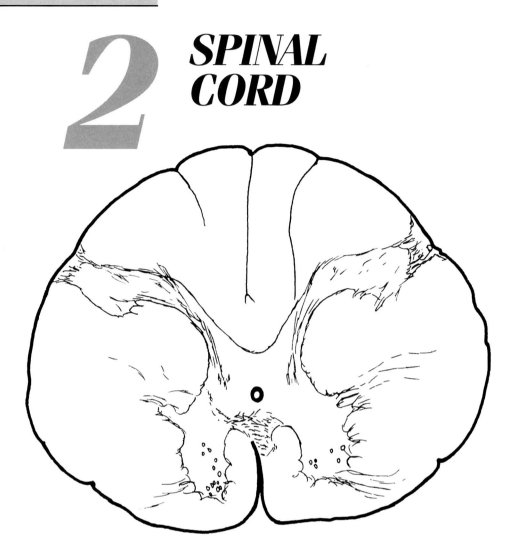

► Introduction

The spinal cord, a caudal extension of the brain stem, lies within the vertebral canal reaching from the foramen magnum at the base of the skull to the L_{1-2} vertebral level. This elongated portion of the central nervous system represents the major conduction pathway for motor and sensory information and links the brain to the body.

Two different but interconnected levels of activity occur in the spinal cord. At each nerve entry/exit zone, or **segmental level,** neuronal circuitry exists that can mediate spinal reflexes. These reflexes can withdraw a limb from pain or alter muscle tone in response to shifting forces. Yet daily living requires more than simple reflexes; the **suprasegmental system** controls these more complex activities.

21

The suprasegmental system involves ascending connections from each of the spinal segments to the brain stem and thalamus and is relayed ultimately to the cerebral cortex, carrying information about activity in the body and its environment. Descending connections from each of these areas return to the spinal cord segments, influencing their output and controlling their intake of sensory information. These reciprocal connections mediate suprasegmental control of the spinal cord and strongly influence the complex activity patterns that characterize our lives.

The division between segmental and suprasegmental levels in spinal cord organization is both a functional and a clinical distinction. Damage to the spinal cord can present as sensory loss and weakness; the weakness can be accompanied by either hypotonia (segmental damage) or hypertonia (suprasegmental damage). Making the distinction between these two clinical presentations can provide important information that can help to identify the locus of damage in a patient.

GENERAL OBJECTIVES

1. To identify cross-section profiles of spinal cord taken through the four major vertebral levels
2. To locate, within a given spinal segment, the circuitry of the gray matter
3. To examine and understand the neuronal circuitry underlying spinal reflexes (segmental level activity)
4. To learn the major spinal tracts and describe their origin, laterality, termination, and function

(suprasegmental activity) and to describe any deficit associated with their lesion (suprasegmental activity)
5. To use the clinical manifestations of a lesion to locate accurately the position, level, and extent of any spinal cord pathology

INSTRUCTIONS

In this chapter you will be presented with one or more clinical case studies. *Each study is followed by a list of questions that can be answered best by using a knowledge of regional and functional neuroanatomy and by referring to outside reading material.* Following the questions is a section devoted to structures from a specific region of the central nervous system. Before you attempt to answer the questions, compile a list of the patient's neurologic signs and symptoms, then examine the structures and their functions and study their known clinical deficits. After becoming comfortable with the material, reexamine the list of neurologic signs and symptoms and answer the questions. Be aware that some of the questions can have multiple responses or require information beyond the scope of this manual. It may be necessary to obtain material or advice from additional resources such as specialty texts, a medical dictionary, or clinical personnel.

MATERIALS

1. A human spinal cord and its dural covering
2. Spinal cord histology sections
3. Spinal cord atlas plates

UNIT A

Case Study 2-1

A 68-year-old man with progressive weakness and atrophy

This 68-year-old, left-handed, married businessman was referred by the family physician to a neurologist for evaluation of progressive weakness and atrophy of both lower extremities.

Past Medical History

He is married and has two children no longer living in his house. He has enjoyed good health up until 9 months prior to admission. At this time the patient had noticed an abnormal weakness in his legs; over the 9-month period since onset the weakness has become progressively worse, spreading to his arms. Three months prior to admission, his wife noted a change in his speech; in addition, he began to have difficulty swallowing. Recently, he has had difficulty dressing and eating. At present, he no longer feels capable of driving the family car.

General Physical Examination

He is an awake, oriented, well-hydrated man who appears slightly older than his stated age. Significant loss of muscle mass was noticeable in the shoulders, arms, and legs. His heart rate and blood pressure were within normal ranges. Peripheral pulses were intact at the wrists and ankles. Abdomen was soft with no masses; normal bowel sounds were present.

Neurologic Examination

Mental Status. He was awake and oriented for time and place. His fund of knowledge and memory functions were appropriate. He could recite a list of the last five presidents and accurately follow four-step commands. His speech was slow and pronunciation of words was slurred; however, speech patterns and content were meaningful. He gave an accurate history.

Cranial Nerves. His visual fields were full and he had a complete range of eye movements. Facial expression was appropriate; the corneal, jaw-jerk, and gag reflexes were present but sluggish. His tongue protruded on the midline but was weak; fasciculations were present on the surface of the tongue. Response to pinprick was intact throughout his face.

Motor Systems. Strength was diminished in all extremities and in the trunk musculature. Deep tendon reflexes were elevated (4/5) at the knees and ankles and depressed at the elbows and wrists (1/5). Significant atrophy was present bilaterally in the shoulder muscles and the muscles of the upper and lower extremities. Widespread fasciculations were noted at rest in all four extremities. The patient was able to rise from a chair and walk a short distance unassisted. A fine tremor was present in the upper extremities when they were held in the extended and pronated position. The tremor diminished when his arms were lowered into a resting position. Finger-to-nose and heel-to-shin testing was normal in all extremities. No pronator drift was observed. His bowel and bladder functions were intact.

Sensation. Discriminative touch, vibratory sense, proprioception, and pain and temperature sensation were intact throughout his body.

QUESTIONS

1. Does the patient exhibit a language or memory deficit or an alteration in consciousness or cognition?

2. Are signs of cranial nerve dysfunction present?

3. Are there any changes in motor functions, such as reflexes, muscle tone, movement, or coordination?

4. Are any changes in sensory functions detectable?

5. At what level in the central neuraxis is this lesion most likely located?

6. Is the pathology focal, multifocal, or diffuse in its distribution within the nervous system?

7. What is the clinical–temporal profile of this pathology: acute or chronic; progressive or stable?

8. Based on your answers to the previous two questions, decide whether this patient's symptoms are most likely caused by a vascular accident, a tumor, or a degenerative or inflammatory process?

9. If you feel this is the result of a vascular accident, what vessels are most likely involved?

10. What is the significance of the muscular fasciculations in this patient?

11. How can obvious motor deficits be present at a given segmental level while sensory function seemingly remains unimpaired?

12. What is the significance of the tremor observed in this patient?

13. What spinal cord neurons are degenerating in this patient?

► DISCUSSION
Spinal Cord Segmental Organization

The spinal cord receives approximately 32 pairs of spinal nerves. The entry of each nerve root into the cord defines the spinal segment. The area of skin (cutaneous distribution) of each spinal nerve is referred to as a **dermatome,** the muscles innervated by that nerve constitute a **myotome,** and the connective tissue structures so innervated belong to the corresponding **scleratome.** Dermatomes, myotomes, and scleratomes do not necessarily lie in register in the body; often, because of embryonic migration, these three components of a given spinal nerve can be separated from one another, sometimes by considerable distances.

Each spinal cord segment is composed of an inner column of gray matter containing nerve cell bodies, surrounded by an outer sheath of white matter composed of neuronal processes. A cross section (taken transverse to its long axis) of a fresh spinal cord preparation reveals a gray, H-shaped area at the center (Plates 1 to 4), which extends the entire rostral-to-caudal length of the cord. The dorsal portion of the "H," or **dorsal horn,** is involved with processing the sensations of pain, temperature, and light touch, as well as visceral sensory information. The ventral portion of the "H," or **ventral horn,** is involved in the motor system, containing the neurons that innervate skeletal muscle. Between the dorsal and ventral horns is an intermediate zone composed of interneurons linking the sensory, suprasegmental, and motor systems together. Between cord segments T_1 and L_{2-3} a lateral horn of the gray matter can be seen; it is involved with the sympathetic outflow from the autonomic nervous system.

In the older literature, the spinal gray matter was described as containing discrete clusters of neurons, called nuclei; however more recently, it has been divided into several distinct layers or laminae.[1] Each lamina represents a slab of neurons and fibers that, in most cases, extends the full length of the spinal cord (Figs. 2-1 to 2-3). In general, the individual laminae of spinal gray matter have a unique cellular and chemical composition, establish differential connections, and serve differing functions.[2–4]

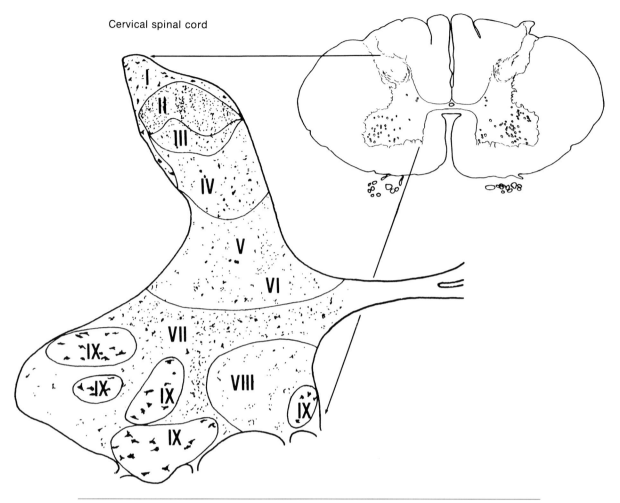

Cervical spinal cord

Figure 2-1. Gray matter of the cervical spinal cord segments. Dots indicate the relative size and distribution of neurons within the laminae.

LAMINA I

The first lamina forms a thin cap perched on the apex of the dorsal horn. It was referred to previously as the posterior marginal nucleus. Lamina I cells receive synapses from small, unmyelinated cutaneous primary afferent fibers carrying the sensations of prickling pain, tickling, and coolness. Axons from some lamina I neurons cross to the contralateral side of the spinal cord and ascend to the brain stem and thalamus. These fibers contribute to the perception of painful stimuli.

LAMINAE II AND III

Small, unmyelinated, primary afferent fibers carrying sensations of burning pain, itch, and warming from cutaneous receptors terminate in laminae II and

III. (Lamina II corresponds to the **substantia gelatinosa** of older terminology.) This type of sensory input is called **nociception.** Axons from neurons in these two laminae innervate surrounding neurons or exit the dorsal horn and travel up or down the spinal cord several segments in a thin band of fibers, the **propriospinal tract,** which surrounds the spinal gray matter (Plates 1 to 4). In general, the neurons of laminae II and III do not project axons out of the spinal cord, contributing instead to the integration of multiple segments.

LAMINA IV

The afferent fibers to lamina IV are mostly of the large-caliber type, carrying low-threshold stimuli referred to as light touch. Axons from some of these cells cross to the contralateral side of the spinal cord

25

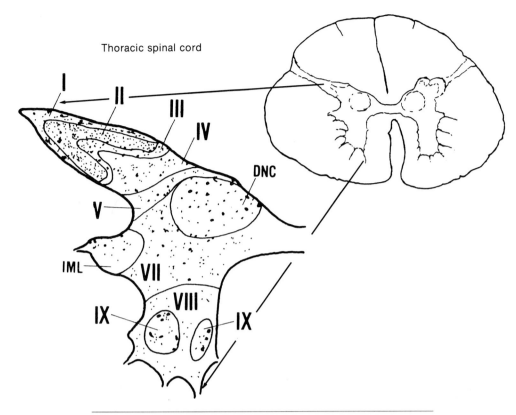

Thoracic spinal cord

Figure 2-2. Gray matter of the thoracic spinal cord segments.

and ascend to the brain stem and thalamus. Laminae III and IV correspond to the **nucleus proprius** of older terminology.

LAMINAE V AND VI

Laminae V and VI are positioned at the ventral portion of the dorsal horn. Afferent fibers to these laminae arise from peripheral cutaneous and visceral sources as well as from descending fiber systems, such as the corticospinal and rubrospinal tracts. Some of the large-caliber primary afferent fibers from muscles, entering the cord in the dorsal roots, end by projecting into lamina VI; thus, this region receives a mixture of sensory information. Also, convergence of somatic and visceral input onto individual lamina V cells has been documented.[5] Cells in this lamina contribute to the phenomenon of referred pain. Axons from cells in laminae V and VI cross to the contralateral side of the spinal cord and ascend in the anterolateral system to reach the brain stem and thalamus. Lamina VI is present only in the enlargements of the spinal cord and is absent from segments T_4 to L_2.

LAMINA VII

The seventh lamina receives large-caliber, myelinated primary afferent fibers that originate in the encapsulated receptors of skeletal muscle and tendon. Its neurons have axons that innervate motoneuron cell columns of lamina IX. In addition, several regions of lamina VII are differentiated into specific cell clusters: the **dorsal nucleus of Clarke** and the **intermediolateral nucleus.**

The *dorsal nucleus of Clarke* is located in the medial aspect of lamina VII at the ventromedial base of the dorsal horn of spinal segments C_8–L_3 (Plate 3). It receives large caliber, myelinated, primary afferent fibers from muscle spindle receptors. Large neurons in Clarke's nucleus give rise to axons that ascend in the dorsal spinocerebellar tract (Plates 3 and 4) to reach the ipsilateral cerebellum. These fibers carry information concerning the positioning of limb muscles (proprioception).

The *nucleus intermediolateralis* is found in a lateral protuberance off of lamina VII, called the lateral horn. This region is present in spinal segments T_1 to L_2 and S_2 to S_4. These areas receive information both

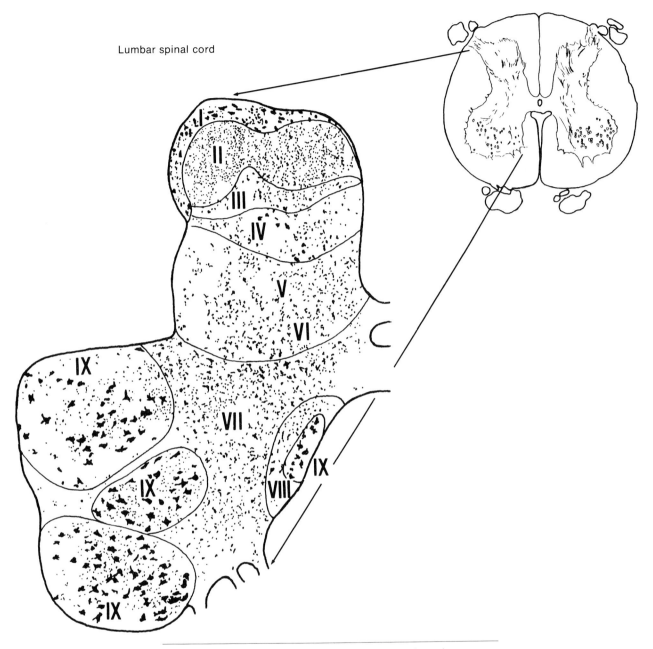

Lumbar spinal cord

Figure 2-3. Gray matter of the lumbar spinal cord segments.

from visceral and somatic primary afferent fibers and from descending fibers from the hypothalamus and brain stem. Preganglionic neurons of the sympathetic nervous system (T_1–L_2) and parasympathetic nervous system (S_2–S_4) are contained within the lateral horn.

LAMINA VIII

Lamina VIII surrounds the ventromedial motoneuron column of lamina IX. Its afferent fibers are derived from descending systems originating in the cerebral cortex, vestibular nuclei, and reticular formation of the brain stem. Lamina VIII interneurons function to integrate activity in the medial columns of motoneurons, controlling the axial musculature.

LAMINA IX

The columns of motoneurons in the ventral horn constitute lamina IX. Several prominent cell columns are identified by their position in the ventral horn.

Dorsolateral Motor Columns

The dorsolateral motor columns occupy the dorsal and lateral portions of the ventral horn and contain alpha and gamma motoneurons. These cells have axons that travel in peripheral nerves to innervate appendicular muscles. Large, myelinated, primary afferent fibers from muscle spindles form synaptic endings on the motoneurons. The monosynaptic connections established between the primary afferent fibers and the ventral horn motoneurons mediate the myotatic reflex. Other inputs to the dorsomedial column of motoneurons include the corticospinal tract and the medullary reticulospinal tract.

The motoneuron columns are arranged in a topographic fashion with those innervating proximal limb musculature located medially and those innervating distal limb musculature situated laterally. Columns innervating flexor muscles are found dorsally; those innervating extensor muscles are located more ventrally in the ventral horn.

Ventromedial Motor Columns

The ventromedial motor column occupies the ventral and medial portion of the ventral horn. It contains alpha and gamma motoneurons whose axons innervate axial (truncal) musculature. Inputs to this column of motoneurons are complex. It receives descending projections from the corticospinal, vestibulospinal, and pontine reticulospinal tracts. Coordination with other regions of the spinal cord is accomplished through its connections with the propriospinal tract. Feedback from the muscles (proprioception) is obtained through large-caliber primary afferent fibers (Table 2-1). Much of this input does not reach lamina IX directly, but is filtered instead through the interneurons of lamina VIII.

Table 2-1.
Classification of Primary Afferent Fibers

FIBER TYPE	SOURCE	INFOR-MATION
Group I	Muscle spindles and tendon organs	Position sense
Group II	Mechanoreceptors	Discriminative touch
Group III	Naked nerve endings	Fast pain
Group IV	Naked nerve endings	Slow pain

CLINICAL DEFICIT

Damage to the dorsal horn or its efferent projections, which can occur with occlusion of the central branch of the anterior spinal artery (see Fig. 2-10), will result in the loss of pinprick and temperature sensation over the affected body dermatomes (see pp. 46–47).

Damage to the ventral horn, which occurs in occlusion of the anterior spinal artery (see Fig. 2-10) or in motoneuron disease, can result in the loss of the ventral horn motoneurons. Death of the motoneurons denervates the skeletal muscle related to that spinal segment. Since the nerve terminal normally provides a trophic substance(s) to the muscle, denervated skeletal muscle becomes flaccid and atrophies. Clinically, this presents as weakness, muscle wasting, and fasciculations. Affected muscles do not resist passive stretch and have diminished deep tendon reflexes or hyporeflexia (see pp. 41–43).

DORSAL ROOT ENTRY ZONE

Between the end of the dorsal root and the apex of the dorsal horn is a complex area called the dorsal root entry zone. It can be partitioned into *lateral* and *medial* divisions based on a segregation of fiber sizes in the dorsal roots (see Fig. 2-8). The medial division contains large, myelinated fibers (groups I and II; see Table 2-1) carrying precise sensory information concerning body (muscle and joint) position and discriminatory touch from the dermis. The lateral division contains small myelinated (group III) and unmyelinated (group IV) fibers that carry information concerning light touch, thermal sense, pain (nociception), and visceral sensations. Because of this segregation of primary afferent fibers in the dorsal root entry zone, nociception, light touch, and thermal senses are conducted into the dorsal horn, whereas proprioception and the discriminative senses are diverted medially around the apex of the dorsal horn. These large fibers can (1) enter the dorsal columns to ascend the length of the spinal cord, (2) enter the base of the dorsal horn where they can innervate tract cells, or (3) continue into the ventral horn where they participate in segmental reflex arcs.

CLINICAL DEFICIT

The presentation of pain is common when pathology affects the spinal cord or its roots and spinal nerves. Often the quality of the pain and its distribution can reveal its origin. Several different pain presentations have been defined.[6] *Radicular pain* is described as usually unilateral and dermatomal in its distribution; its quality is a lancinating, or shooting, sharp pain.

This type of pain, typical of extradural (outside the spinal cord) lesions, can be caused by pressure on the nerve root or spinal nerve in and around the intervertebral foramen. *Funicular (central) pain* is described as a deep, poorly defined painful experience, not related directly to the distribution of any spinal nerves. It is more characteristic of intramedullary (inside the spinal cord) lesions.

Surgical lesions of the dorsal root entry zone have been used to treat intractable pain.[7] As such, the lesion interrupts the small-caliber primary afferent fibers as they enter the dorsal horn, thus preventing the transmission of nociceptive information to the spinal cord from that specific spinal nerve.

UNIT B

Case Study 2-2

A 27-year-old man suffering from a traumatic injury to the spinal cord

A 27-year-old, right-handed machinist was brought by ambulance into the emergency room after suffering a knife wound in the back during an argument in a local bar. He was conscious but somewhat intoxicated. A penetrating wound was present on his back, slightly off the midline and opposite the superior border of the right scapula.

Physical Examination

The patient is an awake, intoxicated male. He is muscular, well nourished, well hydrated, and appears his stated age. Blood pressure, heart rate, and respirations were slightly elevated; peripheral pulses were intact at the wrists and ankles.

Neurologic Examination

Mental Status. He was awake but somewhat intoxicated. Speech was slurred and rambling; however, no word substitution or word confusion was present. Memory and knowledge could not be tested adequately because of his level of intoxication.

Cranial Nerves. A full range of eye movements was present. Hearing was normal bilaterally. Pupillary, gag, and corneal reflexes were intact; facial movements were full; uvula and tongue were midline.

Motor Systems. Strength was completely absent and flaccid paralysis was present in the right lower extremity. Deep tendon reflexes were absent on the right lower extremity and the patient could make no voluntary movements in this limb. Strength was normal in the right shoulder and arm but diminished in the forearm; it was absent in the hand. Deep tendon reflexes were normal in the scapulohumeral, biceps, and brachioradialis muscles on the right but diminished in the triceps, wrist, and fingers. Strength, movement, and reflexes were appropriate in both left extremities.

Sensation. Complete loss of the sensation for pinprick and temperature was found over the left trunk below C_8 and in the left lower extremity. Loss of discriminatory touch and vibratory sense was found over the right half of the body below and including C_8.

Follow-up

Two weeks later a neurologic examination revealed no change in the distribution of sensory loss, and strength remained diminished in the forearm, hand, and complete lower extremity on the right. However, the following changes were seen: Deep tendon reflexes were elevated at the wrist, finger, knee, and ankle on the right side. A positive Babinski sign could be elicited from the right foot.

QUESTIONS

1. Does the patient exhibit a language or memory deficit or an alteration in consciousness or cognition?

2. Are signs of cranial nerve dysfunction present?

3. Are there any changes in motor functions, such as reflexes, muscle tone, movement, or coordination?

4. Are any changes in sensory functions detectable?

5. At what level in the central neuraxis is this lesion most likely located?

6. Is the pathology focal, multifocal, or diffuse in its distribution within the nervous system?

7. What is the clinical–temporal profile of this pathology: acute or chronic; progressive or stable?

8. Based on your answers to the previous two questions, decide whether the symptoms in this patient are most likely caused by a vascular accident, a tumor, or a degenerative or inflammatory process.

9. If you feel this is the result of a vascular accident, what vessels are most likely involved?

10. On follow-up, why is the patient's strength diminished on the right side when his deep tendon reflexes in these limbs are hyperactive?

11. Why were pain and temperature sensation lost on the left, whereas discriminatory touch and vibratory sense were lost on the right side of the body?

12. What is the significance of the presence of a Babinski sign?

Case Study 2-3

A 36-year-old man with sensory and motor loss

A 36-year-old man presented to his family physician with weakness and sensory loss in upper and lower extremities. He describes his arms as feeling limp and his legs as feeling stiff.

Past Medical History

He is a faculty member at a small liberal arts college, has never married, and currently lives alone. He does not smoke or consume alcohol and denies any sexual activity. He first noticed the weakness and loss of sensation to temperature in the upper extremity 3 years previously; the weakness in the lower extremity occurred recently. He has no history of blood transfusions, denies IV drug abuse, and has not been out of the country except for an occasional trip to Canada. He denies any recent history of noticeable viral or bacterial infections.

General Physical Examination

This is an awake, oriented male, appearing older than his stated age and with noticeable muscle wasting in the upper extremity. His heart rate, blood pressure, temperature, and respirations were normal; skin was moist and supple. His chest was clear to auscultation and abdomen was soft to palpation with no tenderness. No lymphadenopathy was detected in the axilla or groin area.

Neurologic Examination

Mental Status.   He was awake, oriented for time and place, and had an appropriate memory and knowledge base. Speech was clear and meaningful.

Cranial Nerves.   A full range of eye movements was present; visual acuity was 30/20 in the right eye and 40/20 in the left eye without glasses. Pupillary reflexes were present to direct and consensual light. Gag and corneal reflexes were intact and facial movements were full. The uvula was symmetric and the tongue protruded on the midline.

Motor Systems.   Strength in the upper extremities was +2/5 on the right and +1/5 on the left. Both upper extremities were areflexic at the elbow, and wrist, muscular fasciculations, and atrophy were present bilaterally. Strength in the lower extremities was reduced and both lower extremities had elevated deep tendon reflexes.

Sensation.   He lacked sensation to temperature and pinprick in a cape-like distribution over the chest and shoulders extending throughout the upper extremity to the fingertips. Vibratory sense, discriminative touch, and proprioception were intact throughout his chest and upper extremities. Normal sensation was found elsewhere over the body.

QUESTIONS

1. Does the patient exhibit a language or memory deficit or an alteration in consciousness or cognition?

2. Are signs of cranial nerve dysfunction present?

3. Are there any changes in motor functions, such as reflexes, muscle tone, movement, or coordination?

4. Are any changes in sensory functions detectable?

5. At what level in the central neuraxis is this lesion most likely located?

6. Is the pathology focal, multifocal, or diffuse in its distribution within the nervous system?

7. What is the clinical–temporal profile of this pathology: acute or chronic; progressive or stable?

8. Based on your answers to the previous two questions, decide whether the symptoms in this patient are most likely caused by a vascular accident, a tumor, or a degenerative or inflammatory process.

9. If you feel this is the result of a vascular accident, what vessels are most likely involved?

10. What are the distinctive features between flaccid and spastic paralysis?

11. Which extremity illustrates signs of suprasegmental level damage?

12. Which extremity illustrates signs of segmental level damage?

13. How can the discriminative sense be intact while the nociceptive and thermal senses are diminished?

▶ DISCUSSION
Spinal Cord Suprasegmental Organization

The white matter of the spinal cord is partitioned into three large divisions called **dorsal, lateral,** and **ventral funiculi.** Each funiculus is further divided into several smaller bundles, called **fasciculi.** Individual fasciculi are composed of fiber tracts containing ascending or descending axons. Ascending fiber tracts have their cell bodies of origin in the spinal gray or dorsal root ganglia and project their axons up the spinal cord toward the brain stem and thalamus. Conversely, descending fiber tracts have cell bodies in the cerebral cortex or brain stem and project their axons down the spinal cord.

The ascending somatic and visceral sensory information passes from the segmental level of the spinal cord to the brain through the ascending fiber systems. Descending fiber systems carry motor and sensory control information caudalward from the cerebral cortex and brain stem. Within a given fiber tract, its axons tend to share a common function, such as conducting sensory information of a similar modality or specific aspect of the motor control signals.

Axons within a tract are often arranged in an orderly fashion, such that those carrying information from the distal end of the extremity are found on one border of the tract, and those involved with the proximal end of the extremity course along the opposite border.

This general organization is called *topography* or, when referring specifically to the somatic sensory system, *somatotopy.* Arranging axons in an orderly fashion helps the nervous system maintain fidelity in its sensory and motor pathways. Interruption of portions of either sensory or motor tracts within the spinal cord results in neurologic signs and symptoms localized to a specific region of the body; understanding the somatotopic maps can help predict the extent to which the central nervous system has been damaged by a lesion.

DORSAL FUNICULUS

Fasciculus Gracilis and Cuneatus
(Ascending)

The axons in the fasciculus gracilis are said to carry proprioception, two-point discrimination, and vibratory sensation from the lower extremity to the brain stem and thalamus for relay into the somatic sensory portion of the cerebral cortex. The cell bodies for fibers in the fasciculus gracilis are located in the dorsal root ganglia of vertebral levels T_6 and below (Fig. 2-4). The tract begins in the sacral cord (see Plate 1) and ascends to the caudal medulla (Plates 2 to 7), where it terminates in the ipsilateral nucleus gracilis.

In a similar organization, axons of the fasciculus cuneatus are said to carry information concerning two-point discrimination, vibratory sense, and proprioception from the upper extremity. The cell bodies

Figure 2-4.
Diagram of the dorsal column pathway. (**Source:** Large primary afferent fibers, group II fibers; **function:** discriminatory touch, vibratory sense, stereognosis; **laterality:** crosses the midline at the level of the internal arcuate fibers in caudal medulla.)

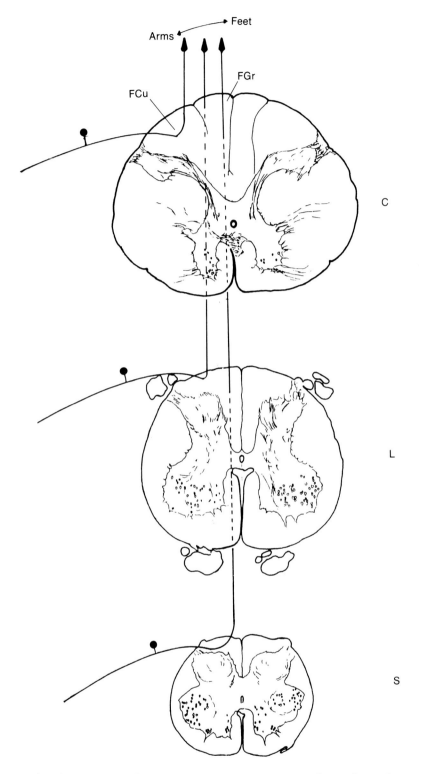

of these fibers are found in dorsal root ganglia above T_6 (see Fig. 2-4). The tract first appears as a thin band in the spinal cord at, or slightly above, T_6, expanding in thickness as it extends rostrally to reach the nucleus cuneatus in the caudal medulla (Plates 3 to 8).

The two tracts are referred to collectively as the **dorsal column system.** The cell bodies of neurons giving rise to the axons in the dorsal column tracts are located in the dorsal root ganglia. Their peripheral processes are group I and group II fibers that arise in encapsulated nerve endings in skin, fascia, bone, and muscle.

The axons in fasciculus gracilis and cuneatus are organized in a topographic fashion. The sacral dermatomes, starting with S_5, are represented most medially in the fasciculus gracilis. Successive ascending dermatomes are added laterally, such that at the cervicomedullary junction, the C_1 dermatome is located at the lateral extreme of the fasciculus cuneatus. The division between gracilis and cuneatus is found at T_6. In summary, the somatotopic map of the human dorsal column system is arranged so that the person's feet are represented toward the midline and the arms lie laterally.[8]

CLINICAL DEFICIT

Pure lesions of either of the dorsal column tracts *do not* completely eliminate vibratory or position sense in the human. It appears that these modalities are also carried by axons in the adjacent dorsolateral fasciculus and in the anterolateral system[9,10] as well as in the dorsal spinocerebellar tracts.[11] (See the discussions of the anterolateral system [p. 38] and the dorsal spinocerebellar system [p. 34], and the summary [p. 41].)

The clinically demonstrable deficit resulting from isolated lesions of the dorsal columns appears to be astereognosis. Thus, tests for stereognosis and graphesthesia have been proposed as appropriate clinical tests of dorsal column system integrity.[9,12]

Dorsolateral Fasciculus

A thin band of fibers, forming a cap over lamina I, represents the zone of Lissauer, or dorsolateral fasciculus (labeled DLatF in Plates 1 to 4). It contains small- and large-caliber ascending axons as well as the axons of dorsal horn neurons traveling between segments. These latter fibers are part of the propriospinal system for integrating segmental-level activities. The fasciculus contains a mixture of sensory modalities. The smallest-caliber fibers are involved in nociception, whereas some of the larger-caliber fibers carry modalities similar to those in the dorsal columns. It has been proposed, on the bases of lesion studies, that the dorsolateral fasciculus can at least blunt, if not mask, the effects of lesions restricted to the dorsal column system.[9,10] At the level of the medulla, the dorsolateral fasciculus becomes the tract of the spinal trigeminal nucleus (labeled SpTT in Plate 5).

CLINICAL DEFICIT

The results of damage to the dorsolateral fasciculus are discussed with those involving the fasciculus gracilis and cuneatus (see pp. 32–34).

LATERAL FUNICULUS—SUPERFICIAL

Dorsal and Cuneate Spinocerebellar Tract (Ascending)

The cerebellum utilizes proprioceptive information from muscles and joints to coordinate sequences of muscle contractions during limb movement. It receives this information from a complex series of tracts called the spinocerebellar system. The sensory information carried in the dorsal spinocerebellar tract informs the cerebellum of the position in space of individual muscles in the lower extremity. This information is gathered from large-caliber, primary afferent fibers arising in muscle spindle organs located in the lower-extremity muscles. The cell bodies of origin for this tract are located in the dorsal nucleus of Clarke, which extends from spinal segments L_3 to C_8 (Fig. 2-5 and see Plate 3). Primary afferent fibers entering the spinal cord below L_3 ascend to this level in the fasciculus gracilis to reach the caudal border of Clarke's nucleus. Axons from Clarke's neurons gather into the dorsal spinocerebellar tract located in the lateral fasciculus (DSCT in Plates 3 to 7). In the medulla, these axons join the inferior cerebellar peduncle and ascend into the ipsilateral cerebellum (see Plates 8 to 14).

Since the nucleus of Clarke does not extend rostral to C_8, it cannot receive primary afferent fibers from the upper extremity. Instead, the large-caliber axons from these upper spinal levels join the fasciculus cuneatus, where they form the cuneospinocerebellar tract, and course upward to terminate in the lateral cuneate nucleus of the medulla (Plates 8 and 9). Axons from the lateral cuneate nucleus enter the inferior cerebellar peduncle, delivering proprioceptive information from the upper extremity to the ipsilateral cerebellum.

Many of the axons in the dorsal spinocerebellar tract send collateral branches to the **nucleus Z** located in the lower medulla close to the cuneate nucleus. This nucleus projects its axons to the contralateral thalamus through the medial lemniscus along with those from the cuneate and gracile nuclei. Thus, the spinocerebellar projections to the cerebellum provide this structure with proprioceptive information, while their collateral branches to nucleus Z and its subsequent projections to thalamus provide the cerebral cortex with proprioceptive information.

CLINICAL DEFICIT

Lesions of the spinocerebellar tracts have received little attention in the clinical literature; however, the few that have been reported demonstrate ataxia[13] and loss of vibratory and position sense[11] as presenting

34

Figure 2-5.
Diagram of dorsal spinocerebellar pathway. (**Source:** Large primary afferent fibers, group Ia; **function:** muscle and joint position (proprioception); vibratory sense; **laterality:** uncrossed.)

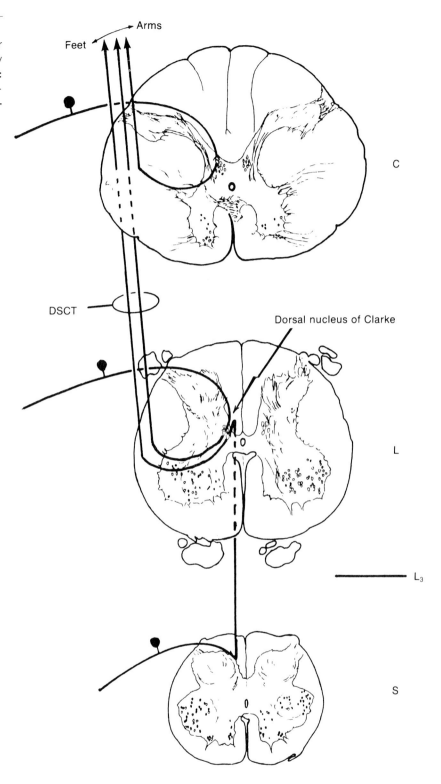

symptoms. Lesions of the spinocerebellar fibers in the brain stem also contribute to dysmetria, ataxia, and a loss of position sense of the extremities. Based on these and other studies,[9] it has been speculated that vibratory and position senses are also carried in the spinocerebellar system rather than completely by the dorsal column system.[11] The conduction of vibratory and position sense in both the dorsal column system and the spinocerebellar tracts represents a form of redundancy.

Profound ataxia and intense loss of position and vibratory senses are the salient symptoms of combined spinocerebellar and dorsal column degeneration such as that which occurs in syphilis and other degenerative diseases that affect the large-caliber-fibers of peripheral nerve and spinal cord. The patient is effectively stripped of somatic proprioceptive information. Although visual cues can combine with vestibular information to mask the deficit created by the loss of these fibers during the day, affected individuals will become unstable and ataxic at night or when asked to close their eyes.[14] This phenomenon forms the basis for the **Romberg test** and, when present, is called **sensory ataxia.**

Ventral (Anterior and Rostral) Spinocerebellar Tract
(Ascending)

A second component of the spinocerebellar system carries information concerning the activity of local circuit neurons in the intermediate portion of the spinal cord to the cerebellum. This information reflects the spinal pattern of motor activity and is referred to as the *efference copy* of the spinal motor instructions. The ventral spinocerebellar tract carries this information from the lower extremity, and the rostral spinocerebellar tract carries it from the upper extremity. Thus, the cerebellum receives data on where the limb muscles are in space (dorsal and cuneospinocerebellar tract) as well as on what these muscles are being told to do (ventral and rostral spinocerebellar tracts). All these data are used to coordinate muscle activity during limb movement (see Chap. 5).

The cell bodies of origin for the ventral spinocerebellar tract are located in the deeper laminae of the dorsal horn in the lumbar and sacral spinal cord. Their axons cross the midline to form a fasciculus in the ventral and lateral aspect of the spinal cord, medulla, and pons (VSCT in Plates 3 to 14). In the cervical region this tract is joined by axons from cervical interneurons forming the rostral spinocerebellar tract. In the rostral pons, both spinocerebellar tracts join the superior cerebellar peduncle to enter the cerebellum (Plate 15). Upon entering the cerebellum, some of these spinocerebellar fibers cross back to the opposite side; others do not. Thus, the termination of these tracts is bilateral.

LATERAL FUNICULUS—DEEP

Raphe-Spinal Tract
(Descending)

The raphe-spinal system plays a role in the modulation of nociception transmission through the dorsal horn as well as in controlling motor activity in the ventral horn. It also influences the activity of preganglionic neurons in the lateral horn. The cell bodies of origin for the raphe-spinal tract are located along the midline in the caudal portion of the medulla (Plates 11 to 14). Some of their axons descend into the spinal cord, coursing in the dorsolateral fasciculus. In the spinal cord, axons from the raphe nuclei innervate cells in the dorsal, ventral, and lateral horns.

CLINICAL DEFICIT

Information on isolated lesions of the raphe-spinal system in humans is unavailable; however, chemically blocking this system with naloxone in human subjects can decrease their threshold of pain.[15]

Lateral Corticospinal Tract
(Descending)

The lateral corticospinal tract controls mastery of fine motor movements in the distal extremities.[16] This descending system contains the axons of pyramidal neurons located in the precentral gyrus of the cerebral cortex and to a lesser extent, the postcentral gyrus. Upon reaching the medulla in the pyramidal tract, these axons cross the midline in the pyramidal decussation and shift laterally to form the lateral corticospinal tract (Fig. 2-6 and see Plates 4 to 6). Since it has crossed the midline at the cervicomedullary junction, fibers of this tract terminate in the ventral horn, contralateral to their cell bodies of origin in the cerebral cortex.

The corticospinal neurons are part of a complex array of descending projections controlling the ventral horn motoneurons of the spinal cord. Collectively, the cells in these descending systems are referred to as *upper motoneurons,* thus distinguishing them from the *lower motoneurons* of the ventral horn. Upper motoneurons represent the *suprasegmental level* of control and, by definition, innervate lower motoneurons (or their surrounding interneurons). Lower motoneurons represent the *segmental-level* control. They directly innervate skeletal muscle through the neuromuscular junction. The distinction between upper and lower motoneuron is of clinical significance in localizing damage on the neuraxis and requires careful study (see pp. 41–43 for further discussion).

CLINICAL DEFICIT

The clinical results of damaged corticospinal fibers in the human spinal cord have been the subject of controversy. Lesions, restricted to the primary motor cortex of nonhuman primates resulted in a flaccid paresis of the affected limbs with no accompanying spasticity,[17] and the corticospinal tracts role, if any, in the genesis of spasticity has been questioned.[18] However, recent reports of seemingly isolated lesions of

Figure 2-6.
Diagram of lateral corticospinal tract. (**Source:** cerebral cortex; **function:** fine movements of the distal extremities; **laterality:** crosses the midline at the pyramidal decussation in the medulla.)

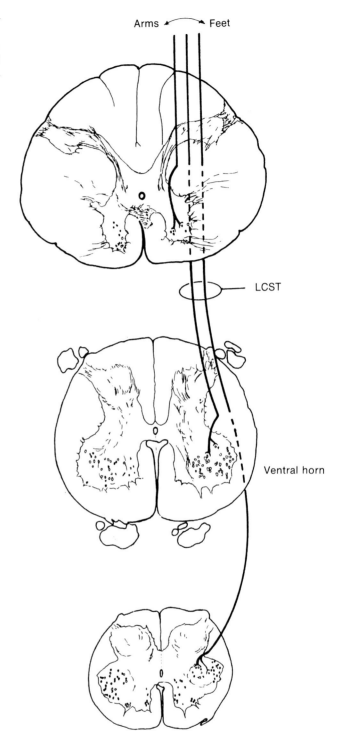

the human pyramidal tract in the medulla, involving destruction of axons in the lateral corticospinal tract, have demonstrated ipsilateral spastic paresis;[19,20] thus, the situation remains to be clarified.

Clinically, spasticity is defined as decreased dexterity, loss of strength, increased deep tendon reflexes, increased resistance to slow passive muscle stretch, and hyperactive flexor spasms.[21] The intense spastic

paralysis that follows severe brain stem or high spinal cord transections involves destruction of not only the corticospinal fibers but the other descending motor systems as well.

A complex pattern of suprasegmental- and segmental-level motoneuron degeneration can occur in diseases such as amyotrophic lateral sclerosis. Typically, the loss of ventral horn cells initially strikes in the cervical enlargement. Meanwhile, a broader spectrum of corticospinal fiber loss occurs that involves those to both upper and lower extremities. Consequently, the lower extremities present with elevated tendon reflexes and spasticity; however, these signs of suprasegmental-level involvement are masked in the upper extremity, where ventral horn cell loss results in decreased tendon reflexes and flaccid paralysis.

Rubrospinal Tract
(Descending)

The rubrospinal tract regulates ventral horn motoneuron activity, especially that of neurons innervating proximal flexor musculature of the upper extremity. In the spinal cord it courses in close association with the lateral corticospinal tract (Plates 3 to 5). It has been proposed that the rubrospinal tract is involved primarily in automated movements, whereas the lateral corticospinal tract is involved in the learning and mastering of new movements.[16]

The rubrospinal tract arises from neurons in the red nucleus of the midbrain (Plate 20). These axons cross the midline while still in the midbrain and descend toward the spinal cord. Most of its axons in the rubrospinal tract terminate in the caudal portions of the brain stem; however, a few of them descend into the cervical spinal cord, where they end in the contralateral gray matter between the dorsal and ventral horn.[22] Thus, the human rubrospinal tract can directly influence control of musculature in the upper extremity; however, any influence it has in the lower extremity has to be indirect (multisynaptic) at best.

CLINICAL DEFICIT

In terms of clinical signs and symptoms, the loss of the rubrospinal tract in humans is masked in large part by the function of the corticospinal tract. In nonhuman primates, isolated destruction of the rubrospinal tract results in some proximal limb weakness that eventually resolves.[17] Combined lesions of both tracts in nonhuman primates result in a more severe weakness and spastic paralysis.

Medullary Reticulospinal Tract
(Descending)

The medullary reticulospinal tract is involved in regulating somatic motor activity in the spinal cord. Its cell bodies of origin are located in the reticular formation of the medulla (Plates 8 to 11), and their axons form a tract that descends along the ventrolateral aspect of the ipsilateral ventral horn (Plates 1 to 4). At each segment, axons from the medullary reticulo-spinal tract enter the gray matter and terminate in the lateral aspect of the ventral horn. These axons can have either excitatory or inhibitory influences on motoneurons controlling limb muscles, depending on the particular phase of the locomotion cycle.[23]

CLINICAL DEFICIT

Isolated lesions of the medullary reticulospinal tract have not been reported for humans; however, lesions of the spinal cord involving this tract present with increased spasticity (see pp. 41–43). Most likely, the loss of this tract enhances the expression of spasticity by lessening the brain stem control over motoneurons involved in the myotatic reflex.

Anterolateral Tract or System
(Ascending)

The anterolateral system (a portion of which is called the spinothalamic tract) carries the modalities of crude touch in the anterior portion of the tract. (The distinction between light and crude touch is poorly made in the neurologic literature and often texts use the two synonymously. These modalities of touch sensation are carried in both anterolateral and dorsal column systems.) Pain and temperature are carried in the lateral portion. (In addition, it most likely carries some fibers with discriminative touch, vibratory sense, and proprioception.[9,10]) The cell bodies of origin for the anterolateral system are found in laminae I, IV, and V of the dorsal horn (Fig. 2-7). These tract cells receive information from small-caliber, unmyelinated or lightly myelinated, primary afferent fibers carrying the sensory modalities of pain, crude touch, and temperature. Their axons cross the midline in the **anterior white commissure** at or near the segmental level of origin and join the contralateral anterolateral system to ascend the spinal cord (see Plates 1 to 4). Termination of these axons occurs in the medullary and mesencephalic reticular formation as well as in the thalamus (see Plates 5 to 20).

CLINICAL DEFICIT

Lesions of the anterolateral system result in diminished sensation to pinprick, touch, and temperature below the segmental level of damage. The dermatome where the patient reports sensory diminution is referred to as a **sensory level.** Because of the overlap in dermatome distribution of primary afferent fibers for this system, the lesion can be one or two segmental levels below the presentation of the sensory levels.

Surgical lesions of the anterolateral system have been used to relieve intractable pain. Although initially successful, the pain often returns to these unfortunate

Figure 2-7.
Diagram of anterolateral tract. (**Source:** small primary afferent fibers, group III or A-delta, and group IV or C fibers; **function:** pain, temperature, and crude touch; **laterality:** crosses the midline at the segmental level.)

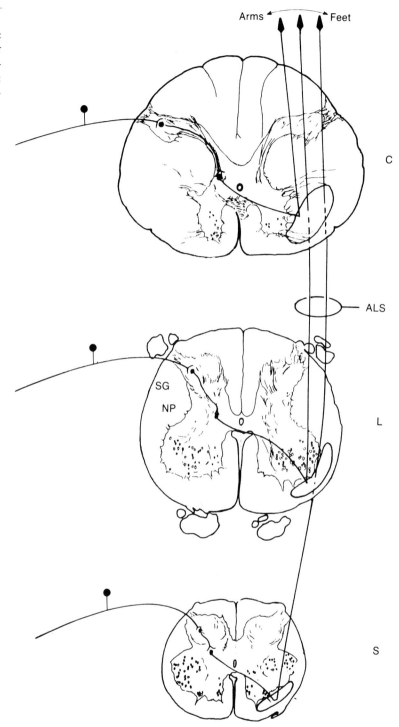

patients in a matter of weeks or months. The return of pain may be related to the presence of small-caliber, primary afferent fibers coursing in other ascending-fiber tracts,[24] such as the dorsal columns and proprio-spinal system (also see pp. 32–34).

An expanding lesion of the central canal of the spinal cord, called a syrinx, can compromise the ante-rior white commissure. When this happens in the cervical spinal cord it is called **cervical syringomyelia.** Initially, the patient experiences the loss of pain and temperature sensations over the shoulders and upper extremities in a cape-like distribution. This is a progressive disease, and with time, further expansion of the syrinx infringes upon the ventral horns, thus adding flaccid paralysis to the presenting signs of the patient. Finally, in extreme cases, the expanding syrinx, which often grows laterally more than anteriorly or posteriorly, reaches the anterolateral tract. At this point a sensory level develops; below this level the patient loses pain and thermal sensation but retains discriminative and proprioceptive senses, since the dorsal column system and dorsolateral fasciculus have not been affected. Because the syrinx first impinges on the medial aspect of the anterolateral system and then pushes laterally, the sensory level presents cervically and marches sacrally. This effect is due to the medial (cervical) to lateral (sacral) topography of the anterolateral system.[25]

VENTRAL FUNICULUS—SUPERFICIAL

Lateral Vestibulospinal Tract
(Descending)

The lateral vestibulospinal system functions to maintain posture against gravity; stimulation of the tract results in facilitation of motoneurons to extensor muscles and inhibition of motoneurons to flexor muscles. The cell bodies of origin for the lateral vestibulospinal tract are located in the ipsilateral lateral vestibular nucleus of the medulla (see Plates 11 to 14). These cells receive input from primary afferent fibers that arise in the utricle of the vestibular apparatus and carry information on head position with respect to gravity. Axons of the lateral vestibulospinal tract extend into the spinal cord to terminate in the medial portion of the ipsilateral ventral horn (see Plates 1 to 10).

CLINICAL DEFICIT
Isolated lesions of this tract in humans have not been reported. However, lesions of the spinal cord involving the lateral vestibulospinal tract present with the signs of damage to the suprasegmental control systems: weakness and spasticity.

Tectospinal Tract
(Descending)

The tectospinal tract mediates neck reflexes, especially those related to visual and acoustic stimuli. The cell bodies of origin for the tectospinal tract are located in the midbrain (tectum or superior colliculus; see Plates 18 and 19). The superior colliculus receives afferent fibers carrying visual, auditory, and somatic sensory information. These sensory modalities are combined into a neuronal map of external space used to guide the tectospinal neurons in mediating appropriate reflex responses. Tectospinal axons cross to the contralateral side in the brain stem and descend into

the cervical and thoracic spinal cord, where they terminate in the ventral horn (see Plates 4 to 16).

VENTRAL FUNICULUS—DEEP

Pontine Reticulospinal Tract
(Descending)

The pontine reticulospinal tract mediates facilitation of the gamma motoneurons controlling muscle spindles involved in the myotatic reflex; it is particularly excitatory to the neurons influencing spindles organs in extensor muscles. The cell bodies of origin for the pontine reticulospinal tract are in the pontine reticular formation (see Plates 12 to 16). Their axons form a tract descending along the ventromedial aspect of the medulla and spinal cord (see Plates 1 to 10). Most of these axons terminate medially in the ipsilateral ventral horn.

CLINICAL DEFICIT
Isolated lesions of this tract in humans have not been reported. However, lesions of the spinal cord involving the pontine reticulospinal tract result in increased spasticity. This tract—as with the other descending tracts from the brain stem reticular formation, red nucleus, and cerebral cortex—contributes to control of segmental (lower) motoneurons. Damage to these tracts deregulates the segment, resulting in muscles with tone but diminished strength.

Anterior (or Ventral) Corticospinal Tract
(Descending)

The anterior corticospinal tract influences the medial motor columns of the ventral horn, thereby controlling the axial musculature. Its cell bodies of origin are located in the motor area of the cerebral cortex; their axons travel with the corticospinal tract to the pyramidal decussation (see Plate 6). The majority of corticospinal axons cross the midline and shift laterally; however, a small number (approximately 8%) remain ventrally positioned to enter the cervical spinal cord in the ventral funiculus near the midline. These axons form the anterior corticospinal tract; they terminate bilaterally in the medial portion of the ventral horn of the cervical to lumbar cord (see Plates 2 to 5).

Medial Vestibulospinal Tract
(Descending)

The medial vestibulospinal tract is involved in coordinating neck and head movement with eye position. The cell bodies of origin for this tract are in the medial vestibular nucleus of the brain stem (see Plates

9 to 13). These nuclei receive input from primary afferent fibers that arise in the semicircular canals and carry information concerning the angular velocity of head movement. Axons from the medial vestibular nucleus join other fibers to form a tract along the midline of the brain stem called the **medial longitudinal fasciculus.** As this tract enters the spinal cord it is referred to as the medial vestibulospinal tract, and its fibers terminate bilaterally in the ventral horn of the cervical cord. The caudal extent of this tract in a human is not known.

► Summary

This section has presented the details of a number of fiber tracts in the spinal cord from a regional prospective. Each tract has been presented within the context of the three large funiculi of the spinal cord: dorsal, lateral, and ventral. Table 2-2 represents a summary of those tracts significant in clinical diagnosis. It is important that each tract, its origin, termination, topography, function, and deficit be thoroughly understood. It is also instructive to consider certain aspects of the spinal cord suprasegmental organization from a systematic perspective. This summary section reviews the general organization of sensory and motor systems.

SENSORY MODALITIES IN THE SPINAL CORD

Three major ascending systems for somatic sensory information have been presented: dorsal columns (FG&C), spinocerebellar tracts (DSCT), and anterolateral system (ALS, Fig. 2-8). Although each of these systems has been assigned distinct functions in the tertiary literature (Table 2-2), there is little in the primary literature to support this concept. Rather, it appears that vibratory and position (both conscious and unconscious) sense is carried in all three systems but primarily in the spinocerebellar tracts,[11] that nociception is carried at least in the anterolateral and dorsal column system,[9] and that the unique functions of the dorsal column system may be stereoagnosis and its action as a high-speed feedback pathway for the somatic motor system.[10]

MOTOR SYSTEMS

Two fundamentally different types of movements are possible in humans. The discrete and delicate movements of the distal extremities give us the ability to write, play musical instruments, or operate complex machinery. Conversely, postural and balance movements involve the axial and proximal limb musculature and serve to maintain our station, building a platform for the discrete movements of the distal limb musculature. To manage these two categories of movements, two motor systems, called lateral and medial, are contained in the brain and spinal cord.[26]

The **lateral motor system** consists of the lateral corticospinal tract and the rubrospinal tract. Their axons terminate in the lateral portion of the ventral horn, influencing the motoneurons that innervate the distal musculature of the limbs. It is through this system that fine movements of the fingers and hands are executed.

The **medial motor system** involves the anterior corticospinal tract, the reticulospinal tracts, and the vestibulospinal tracts. The axons of these tracts terminate on the medial portion of the ventral horn, influencing primarily the motoneurons that innervate the axial and proximal limb musculature. These tracts function in balance and postural movements.

FLACCID AND SPASTIC PARALYSIS

The descending somatic motor system can be divided into two operational and anatomic levels: **segmental** and **suprasegmental** (Fig. 2-9). The segmental level contains the neuronal circuits between muscle spindle apparatus, ventral horn motoneurons, and extrafusal muscle fibers, whereas the suprasegmental level includes the cortico-, rubro-, vestibulo-, and reti-

Table 2-2.
Summary of Fiber Tracts in the Spinal Cord and Their Ascribed Functions

TRACT	FUNCTION
ASCENDING	
Dorsal column system	Vibratory sense
	Discriminative touch
	Two-point discrimination
	Stereognosis
	Position sense
Anterolateral system	Crude touch
	Pain and thermal sense
Spinocerebellar tract	Position sense
	Vibratory sense
DESCENDING	
Lateral corticospinal tract	Volitional control

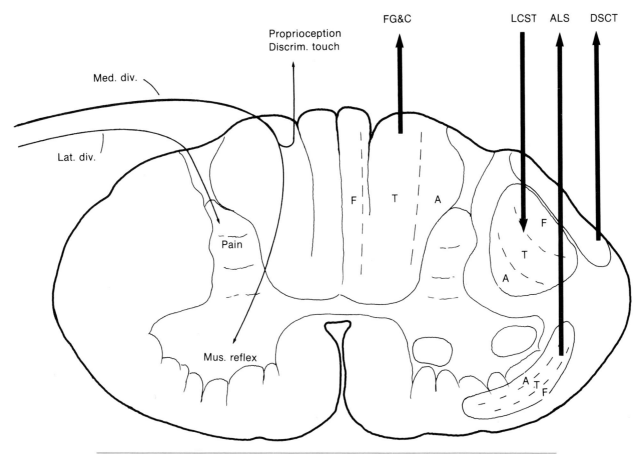

Figure 2-8. Diagram of clinically important spinal cord pathways and nuclei. The left side of the diagram illustrates the segmental divisions of primary afferent fibers to the spinal cord and their modalities; the right side illustrates the major suprasegmental tracts. The direction of the arrows indicates whether it is an ascending or descending tract. (F, feet; T, trunk; A, arm; FG & C, fasciculus gracilis and cuneatus; LCST, lateral corticospinal tract; ALS, anterolateral tract.)

culospinal tracts that control the segmental-level circuits. These levels reflect not only operation distinctions, but also differences in their clinical presentation subsequent to damage.

Damage to portions of the somatic motor system will present clinically as diminished strength and altered reflex tone in the affected muscles. The altered tone in affected muscles can be either hypotonic (flaccidity) or hypertonic (spasticity); the specific type is contingent on the location of damage in the motor system.

Interruption of a spinal segment interferes with the circuits containing ventral horn motoneurons (segmental level or lower motor neurons), thus denervating the musculature. Denervated muscles lack tone and control and are said to be in flaccid paralysis (lesion "B" in Fig. 2-9). In addition, the nerve terminal

(neuromuscular synapse) normally supplies a trophic substance to the muscle, in the absence of which the muscle atrophies.

Interruption of suprasegmental control pathways (upper motor neurons) will diminish the patient's control over the segmental circuit, *but without damaging the lower motor neurons*. The muscle is still connected to its ventral horn motoneurons, and these cells are still receiving information from the muscle spindle apparatus. Although the patient cannot control the muscle, it still has an intrinsic tone and is said to be in spastic paralysis (lesion "A" in Fig. 2-9). Since the circuit connecting spindle apparatus, motoneurons, and extrafusal muscle fiber is intact, tendon reflexes can still be elicited; however, the lack of control from suprasegmental sources renders the reflex hyperactive. The uncontrolled neural circuit is resistive to

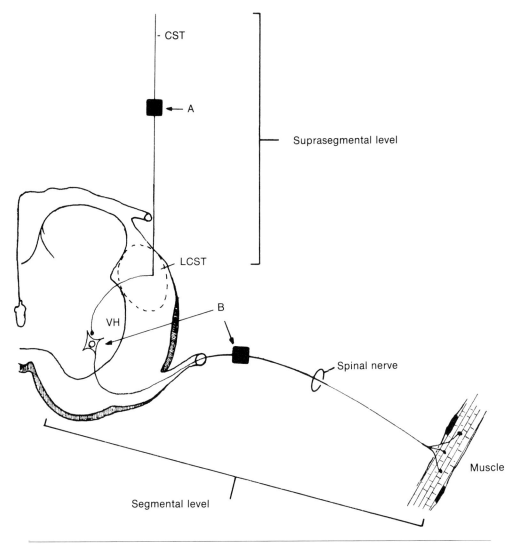

Figure 2-9. Diagram of a spinal cord segment illustrates difference between spastic and flaccid paralysis. A suprasegmental lesion at A interrupts descending control of segmental circuits and results in spastic paralysis. A segmental lesion at B (either within the cord or in the spinal nerve) denervates the muscle and results in flaccid paralysis. (CST, corticospinal tract; LCST, lateral corticospinal tract; VH, ventral horn.)

change; hence, the patient's limbs resist passive stretch.

Suprasegmental-level lesions can also unmask primitive reflexes that have been suppressed by the descending control. An example of this is the **extensor reflex** or **Babinski response** of the great toe following strong stimulus to the sole of the foot. This reflex is normally expressed in neonatal children and suppressed as the corticospinal tract develops its myelin sheaths. Damage to the corticospinal system can unmask the reflex.

Although the signs of suprasegmental, or upper motoneuron, lesions are pathognomonic for damage to the central nervous system, those of the segmental, or lower motoneuron, lesions can result from either central or peripheral nervous system damage. Although the presence of segmental- and suprasegmental-level signs in a patient strongly suggests a central nervous system lesion, it cannot rule out the possibility of an extradural process (*e.g.*, a herniated disk) that has progressed into a central lesion.[6]

Flaccid and spastic paralysis are important concepts in clinical medicine. The anatomic principles behind each of these clinical presentations need to be fully understood. Reread Case Study 2-3 and determine which portions of the patient's body are showing signs of suprasegmental-level injury and which are showing signs of segmental-level injury.

43

UNIT C

Case Study 2-4

An 82-year-old man with back pain and paralysis of the lower extremity

An 82-year-old, right-handed man was brought to the emergency room by his family; he was in acute distress with back pain and unable to walk.

History of Complaint

Patient experienced severe back pain radiating into both legs that remitted promptly when lying down. The next day he experienced similar transient pain in the back and the legs. Later that day, while experiencing an episode of severe back pain, his legs became paralyzed and he was rushed to the hospital.

Past Medical History

The patient had a previous history of transurethral prostatectomy and bilateral orchiectomy for carcinoma of the prostate, left hemicolectomy for adenocarcinoma of the rectum, and arteriosclerotic heart disease and congestive heart failure.

General Physical Examination

He was awake, cooperative, and afebrile and appeared older than his stated age. Funduscopic examination reveal bilateral ocular opacities obscuring visualization of the fundi. External auditory canal was patent. No cervical lymphadenopathy was detected. Blood pressure was 160/90 mmHg, pulse rate was 48 beats per minute with occasional premature beats. There was a grade 2 blowing apical systolic murmur. Bilateral basilar crackles were present in the lungs on inspiration and bilateral jugular venous distention was demonstrable in the neck. Peripheral pulses were intact and equal at the wrists and ankles. Pitting pretibial edema was present. A colostomy stoma was present in the lower left quadrant of the abdomen. Otherwise the abdomen was soft to palpation with normal bowel sounds and no aortic bruits.

Neurologic Examination

Mental Status. He was alert and oriented to time and place; memory and affect were appropriate for his age. Speech was clear and meaningful. He was a good historian.

Cranial Nerves. His visual fields were intact and eye movements were full; hearing, to finger rub, was diminished bilaterally. His pupillary, corneal, and gag reflexes were intact; facial expressions were appropriate; uvula elevated symmetrically; and tongue protruded on the midline. When asked, he could elevate his shoulders symmetrically with appropriate strength.

Motor Systems. His strength and muscle tone were absent in both lower extremities and deep tendon reflexes were absent at the knee and ankle. His strength and reflexes in the upper extremities were appropriate for his age. His urinary bladder was neurogenic; however, this had been present since his last surgery.

Sensation. There was a well-defined sensory level at T_{10}, below which he had lost sensation to pinprick and temperature. Touch, vibratory, and position sense were intact throughout his body and face.

Follow-up

He was treated with steroids and supportive measures without improvement. Five weeks after the onset of paraplegia he died from a sudden cardiorespiratory arrest.

QUESTIONS

1. Does the patient exhibit a language or memory deficit or an alteration in consciousness or cognition?

2. Are signs of cranial nerve dysfunction present?

3. Are there any changes in motor functions, such as reflexes, muscle tone, movement, or coordination?

4. Are any changes in sensory functions detectable?

5. At what level in the central neuraxis is this lesion most likely located?

6. Is the pathology focal, multifocal, or diffuse in its distribution within the nervous system?

7. What is the clinical–temporal profile of this pathology: acute or chronic; progressive or stable?

8. Based on your answers to the previous two questions, decide whether the symptoms in this patient are most likely caused by a vascular accident, a tumor, or a degenerative or inflammatory process.

9. If you feel this is the result of a vascular accident, what vessels are most likely involved?

10. Provide an explanation for the sensory dissociation present below T_{10}.

11. What type of paralysis is being expressed in the lower extremity and what is its source?

► DISCUSSION
Blood Supply to Spinal Cord

The spinal cord receives its blood supply from an array of spinal arteries. As each artery passes through the intervertebral foramen it gives off several branches to perfuse the spinal cord, spinal roots, and surrounding meninges (Fig. 2-10).

Spinal arteries represent a series of branches derived from the vertebral artery, thyrocervical trunk, intercostal arteries, lumbar arteries, and iliolumbar artery. They supply the spinal cord, spinal roots, meninges, and vertebral column. As the spinal artery negotiates the intervertebral foramen, it divides into radicular and medullary branches (based on descriptions presented by Gillilan[27]).

Radicular branches follow the nerve roots to the spinal cord supplying the roots, dorsal root ganglia, and dura. Eventually, the radicular branches end as small contributions to the arterial vasocorona surrounding the cord. These branches are not major contributors to the blood supply of the spinal cord proper.

Medullary branches tend to be larger than the radicular branches and travel along with the spinal nerve and roots to reach the anterior spinal artery or posterior spinal arteries. There are from seven to 10 of these arteries; the largest is the great medullary artery

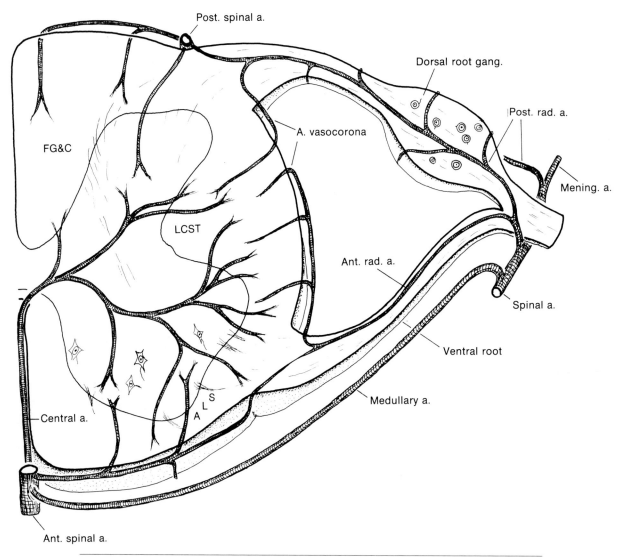

Figure 2-10. Arterial supply of the spinal cord. The cord has been sectioned through a spinal root and dorsal root ganglion. The blood plotted on to the section as if it was a whole spinal root.

of Adamkiewicz, which can occur at vertebral levels T_8 to L_4 and supplies the anterior spinal artery.

CLINICAL DEFICIT

Occlusion of a medullary branch can deprive the anterior spinal artery of blood over several segments of the spinal cord. Most notable is that of the medullary artery of Adamkiewicz, where occlusion can deny blood supply to the anterior spinal artery over a large portion of the lumbar spinal cord.[28]

Three arteries (the anterior and two posterior spinal arteries) are in close juxtaposition with the spinal cord and form the spinal plexus. They distribute small branches internally to perfuse the spinal parenchyma.

The **posterior spinal artery** is really a plexus of small, anastomotic vessels providing penetrating branches into the dorsal columns and a variable amount of the dorsal horn.

CLINICAL DEFICIT

Since this vascular system is a narrow, anastomotic plexus, one rarely sees a defined posterior spinal artery syndrome. However, when detectable infarctions occur, they can present with diminished vibratory sense and proprioception.[29]

The **anterior spinal artery** is well formed, and its occlusion or rupture can result in a distinct syndrome.[29] The major penetrating branch of the anterior spinal artery is the *central (or sulcal) artery,* which perfuses the central portion of the spinal cord supplying the ventral horn and anterior white commissure. The distal extreme of the central artery territory can include the lateral corticospinal tract.

The posterior plexus and anterior spinal artery are connected by an outer vascular ring called the *arterial vasocorona.* These vessels form an anastomotic channel surrounding the spinal cord. Venous drainage of the spinal cord occurs through the epidural (Batson's) plexus of veins.

CLINICAL DEFICIT

Damage to the anterior spinal artery or its central branch can present as paralysis and paresthesia below the level of the lesion.[29] Initially, the paralysis is flaccid because of spinal shock but resolves into a spastic form over a few weeks.

Infarction of the anterior spinal vessels usually occurs in a *watershed* area (*e.g.,* the anastomotic region between two medullary arteries). The paresthesia can present as an abrupt onset of a girdle of pain around the torso. A flaccid paralysis follows within minutes to hours and is bilateral, accompanied by loss of bowel and bladder function. A sensory level to pinprick develops below the level of the lesion.[6]

► Bibliography

Adams RD, Victor M. Principles of neurology. New York: McGraw-Hill, 1989: Chap. 36.

Barr ML, Kiernan JA. The human nervous system: an anatomical viewpoint. Philadelphia: JB Lippincott, 1988: Chaps. 5, 19.

Biller J, Brazis PW. The localization of lesions affecting the spinal cord. In: Brazis PW, Masdeu JC, Biller J, eds. Localization in clinical neurology. Boston: Little, Brown, 1990:69–92.

Brazis PW, Masdeu JC, Biller J. Localization in clinical neurology. Boston: Little, Brown, 1990: Chap. 4.

Daube JR, Ragan TJ, Sandok BA, Westmoreland BF. Medical neurosciences. Boston: Little, Brown, 1986: Chaps 7, 9, 13.

Haines DE. Neuroanatomy: an atlas of structures, sections, and systems. Baltimore: Urban & Schwarzenberg, 1987 *(see especially Figs. 5-1 to 5-8).*

Nieuwenhuys R, Voogd J, van Huijzen C. The human central nervous system. Berlin: Springer-Verlag, 1988 *(see especially Figs. 115 to 125).*

► References

1. Rexed B. The cytoarchitectonic organization of the spinal cord in the cat. J Comp Neurol 1952;96:415.
2. Schoenen J, Faull RLM. Spinal cord: cytoarchitectural, dendroarchitectural and myeloarchitectural organization. In: Paxinos G, ed. The human nervous system. San Diego: Academic Press, 1990:19–53.
3. Schoenen J, Faull RLM. Spinal cord: chemoarchitectural organization. In: Paxinos G, ed. The human nervous system. San Diego: Academic Press, 1990:55–75.
4. Schoenen J, Grant G. Spinal cord: connections. In: Paxinos G, ed. The human nervous system. San Diego: Academic Press, 1990:77–92.
5. Selzer M, Spencer WA. Convergence of visceral cutaneous afferent pathways in the lumbar spinal cord. Brain Res 1969;14:331.
6. Biller J, Brazis PW. The localization of lesions affecting the spinal cord. In: Brazis PW, Masdeu JC, Biller J, eds. Localization in clinical neurology. Boston: Little, Brown, 1990:69–92.
7. Friedman AH, Nashold BS. DREZ lesions for the relief of pain related to spinal cord injury. J Neurosurg 1986;65:465.
8. Smith MC, Deacon P. Topographical anatomy of the posterior columns of the spinal cord in man. Brain 1984;107:671.
9. Wall PD, Noordenbos W. Sensory functions which remain in man after complete transection of dorsal columns. Brain 1977;100:641.
10. Davidoff RA. The dorsal columns. Neurology 1989;39:1377.
11. Ross ED, Kirkpatrick JB, Lastimosa ACB. Position and vibration sensations: functions of the dorsal spinocerebellar tracts? Ann Neurol 1978;5:171.
12. Bender MB, Stacy C, Cohen J. Agraphesthesia. J Neurol Sci 1982;53:531.
13. Gudesblatt M, Cohn J, Gerber O, Sacher M. Truncal ataxia presumably due to malignant spinal cord compression. Ann Neurol 1987;21:511.
14. Schoene WC. Degenerative diseases of the central nervous system. In: Davis RL, Robertson DM, eds. Textbook of neuropathology. Baltimore: Williams & Wilkins, 1985:788–823.
15. Basbaum AI, Fields HL. Endogenous pain control mechanisms: review and hypothesis. Ann Neurol 1978;4:451.
16. Kennedy PR. Corticospinal, rubrospinal, and rubro-olivary projections: a unifying hypothesis. Trends Neurosci 1990;13:474.
17. Lawrence DG, Kuypers HGJM. The functional organization of the motor system in the monkey. I. The effects of bilateral pyramidal lesions. Brain 1968;91:1.
18. Davidoff RA. The pyramidal tract. Neurology 1990;40:332.
19. Paulson GW, Yates AJ, Paltan-Oritz JD. Does infarction of the medullary pyramid lead to spasticity? Arch Neurol 1986;43(1):93.
20. Jagiella WM, Sung JH. Bilateral infarction of the medullary pyramids in humans. Neurology 1989;39:21.
21. Landau WM. Spasticity: What is it? What is it not? In: Feldman RG, Young RR, Koella WP, eds. Spasticity: disordered motor control. Chicago: Yearbook Medical Publishers, 1980:17–24.
22. Nathan PW, Smith MC. The rubrospinal and central tegmental tracts in man. Brain 1982;105:223.
23. Martin GF, Holstege G, Mehler W. Reticular formation of the pons and medulla. In: Paxinos G, ed. The human nervous system. San Diego: Academic Press, 1990:203–220.
24. Briner RP, Carlton SM, Coggeshall RE, Chung K. Evidence for unmyelinated sensory fibres in the posterior columns in man. Brain 1988;111:999.
25. Brazis PW, Masdeu JC, Biller J. Localization in clinical Neurology. Boston: Little, Brown, 1990.
26. Kuypers HGJM. Anatomy of the descending pathways. In: Brookhart JM, Mountcastle VB, Brooks VB, eds. Handbook of physiology. The nervous system, Vol II: Motor control. Bethesda, MD: American Physiology Society, 1981:597–666.
27. Gillilan LA. The arterial blood supply of the human spinal cord. J Comp Neurol 1958;110:75.
28. Laguna J, Cravioto H. Spinal cord infarction secondary to occlusion of the anterior spinal artery. Arch Neurol 1973;28(2):134.
29. Moossy J. Vascular diseases of the spinal cord. In: Joynt RJ, ed. Clinical neurology. Philadelphia: JB Lippincott, 1988:1–19.

47

3 *MEDULLA*

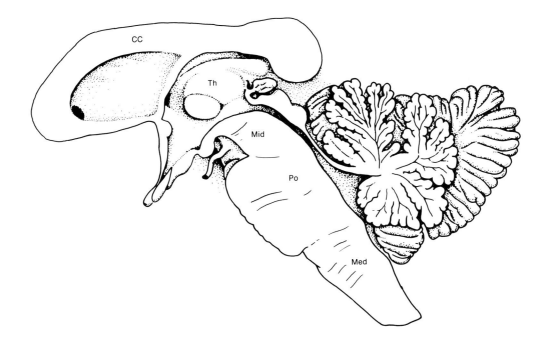

► Introduction

The medulla oblongata, the caudal extreme of the brain stem, is located in the posterior cranial fossa. This portion of the brain stem contains neural circuits regulating respiration, blood pressure, and cardiac rhythm, as well as nuclei for five cranial nerves: hypoglossal, accessory, vagus, glossopharyngeal, and acousticovestibular. The medulla receives its blood supply from branches of the vertebral and spinal arteries.

This chapter examines the organization of nuclei and tracts in the medulla. The blood supply to the medulla will be studied and several clinicopathologic cases concerning medullary lesions will be considered.

GENERAL OBJECTIVES

1. To learn the location and function of major nuclei and ascending and descending fiber tracts in the medulla

2. To learn the presenting signs and symptoms consequent to lesions involving major nuclei and tracts in the medulla
3. To apply the preceding knowledge to an understanding of the clinical manifestations of medullary vascular lesions
4. To distinguish between two vascular syndromes: the medial and lateral medullary syndromes

INSTRUCTIONS

In this chapter you will be presented with one or more clinical case studies. *Each study is followed by a list of questions that can be answered best by using a knowledge of regional and functional neuroanatomy as well as referring to outside reading material.* Following the questions is a section devoted to structures from a specific region of the central nervous system. Before you attempt to answer the questions, compile a list of the patient's neurologic signs and symptoms; then examine the structures and their functions and study their known clinical deficits. After becoming familiar with the material, reexamine the list of neurologic signs and symptoms and answer the questions. Be aware that some of the questions can have multiple responses or require information beyond the scope of this manual. It may be necessary to obtain material or advice from additional resources such as specialty texts, a medical dictionary, or clinical personnel.

MATERIALS

1. A human brain stem model
2. An atlas of the human brain stem
3. A medical dictionary

UNIT A

Case Study 3-1

A 59-year-old man with headaches, double vision, dizziness, and ataxia

A 59-year-old, right-handed male was admitted to the hospital with a chief complaint of occipital headaches of 3 weeks' duration. Two weeks prior to admission, the patient noted a sudden onset of diplopia on forward gaze and a sensation of dizziness. One day prior to admission he noted a relatively sudden onset of ptosis of the right eyelid.

Past Medical History

The patient had been under treatment for hypertension for 2 years with blood pressure in the range of 180/110.

General Physical Examination

The patient was alert, oriented, and cooperative. He was a well-nourished man of medium height who appeared his stated age. Funduscopic examination revealed clear optic disc with sharp borders. The external auditory canal was patent and uninflamed. Pharynx and larynx were nonreddened. A grade II/IV bruit was present over the right carotid artery. His blood pressure was elevated (192/96). Peripheral pulses were intact at the ankle and wrist. Respirations were normal. His chest was clear to auscultation; skin was warm and of normal texture; abdomen was soft with no tenderness, lumps, or masses. No edema was present in the extremities; no lymphadenopathy was present in the cervical or inguinal areas.

Neurologic Examination

Mental Status. The patient was awake and oriented with respect to person, place, and time. Memory was appropriate for his age. Speech was articulate and meaningful.

Cranial Nerves. Extraocular movements were full, but the patient complained of diplopia. Nystagmus was present on left lateral gaze. The right pupil measured 3 mm, the left was 5 mm, but both responded to light and accommodation. Ptosis of the right eyelid and decreased sweating on the right side of the face (anhidrosis) were also present. Hearing was diminished in both ears to high frequencies. Pain, but not touch sensation, was decreased on the right side of the face. The right corneal reflex was diminished. Facial expressions were full and symmetric. The uvula deviated to the left, and there was deficient elevation of the right side of the palate. There was also a suggestion of hoarseness.

Motor System. Strength was intact throughout the body; deep tendon reflexes were intact and symmetric. An ataxia was evident in the right upper extremity on finger-tapping, hand-patting, and finger-to-nose tests. A side-to-side intention tremor was present. Ataxia was also present in the right lower extremity on heel-to-shin and tibia-tapping tests.

Sensorium. There was decreased sensation to pinprick on the left side of the body, the left arm, and the left leg. The patient was unable to distinguish between hot and cold on the left side. Position, vibration, and touch modalities were intact throughout the entire body.

QUESTIONS

1. Does the patient exhibit a language or memory deficit or an alteration in consciousness or cognition?

2. Are signs of cranial nerve dysfunction present?

3. Are there any changes in motor functions, such as reflexes, muscle tone, movement, or coordination?

4. Are any changes in sensory functions detectable?

5. At what level in the central neuraxis is this lesion most likely located?

6. Is the pathology focal, multifocal, or diffuse in its distribution within the nervous system?

7. What is the clinical–temporal profile of this pathology: acute or chronic; progressive or stable?

8. Based on your answers to the previous two questions, decide whether the symptoms in this patient are most likely caused by a vascular accident, a tumor, or a degenerative or inflammatory process?

9. If you feel this is the result of a vascular accident, what vessels are most likely involved?

10. Explain the loss of pain and temperature sensation from the left side of the body but the right side of the face.

11. Explain the loss of pain sensation but not touch from the right side of the face.

12. Offer an explanation for the presence of ataxia in the right extremities.

13. Damage to what medullary structures can account for the patient's (1) dizziness, (2) deviation of the uvula, or (3) hoarseness?

► DISCUSSION
Medullary Structures

The medulla contains several long tracts interconnecting spinal cord, brain stem, and thalamus as well as numerous intrinsic nuclei related to the cranial nerves and reticular formation. The pertinent medullary structures, illustrated on each atlas plate, are described in this chapter. The abbreviation following the name of the structure corresponds to that used on the atlas plate. In reading through the material, you will find that the first time a given structure is encountered, a description will be provided along with comments on its function and, where possible, any clinical deficit consequent to its destruction. For subsequent sections, the structure will be listed by name and abbreviation only, unless significant changes have occurred in its location or composition to merit further comment.

▷ Atlas Plate 6

Atlas Plate 6 is taken from the cervicomedullary junction. Its salient features are the presence of the pyramidal decussation and three major sensory nuclei: spinal trigeminal, gracilis, and cuneatus.

GRACILE FASCICULUS AND NUCLEUS (FGr AND NuGr) AND CUNEATE FASCICULUS AND NUCLEUS (FCu AND NuCu)

The fasciculus gracilis and fasciculus cuneatus (dorsal columns) comprise the large, dorsal funiculus of the spinal cord. They contain the central axons of the group I and II primary afferent fibers from the dorsal roots as well as smaller-caliber axons from cells in the ipsilateral dorsal horn. The possible functions of these two fasciculi in carrying discriminative touch and detecting motion, as well as in providing feedback to the corticospinal system, have been discussed in Chapter 2.

The segregation of axons by size into the dorsal columns is not as homogeneous as previously thought. In addition to the large group I and II axons, numerous small-caliber, primary afferent axons are present. These smaller fibers represent around 25% of those present in either fasciculus and are similar in size to fibers found in Lissauer's tract.[1] Thus, the dorsal columns could also carry information concerning noxious stimuli.

At the cervicomedullary boundary, ascending axons in the fasciculus gracilis form a cusp around the nucleus gracilis. This nucleus is an oblong mass of neurons receiving the synaptic terminals of the axons in the fasciculus gracilis. Because of its large size, it forms the gracile tubercle on the dorsolateral surface of the brain stem. At a slightly more rostral level, the fasciculus cuneatus engulfs its nucleus and terminates. As such, this large nucleus and its surrounding fiber tract form the cuneate tubercle on the dorsolateral surface of the brain stem.

The gracile and cuneate nuclei (dorsal column nuclei) give rise to axons that cross the midline forming the internal arcuate fibers (see Plate 7) and ascend through the brain stem in the medial lemniscus (see Plates 8 to 20). These axons terminate in the ventroposterior lateral thalamic nucleus (see Plate 21). Ultimately, the information that they carry is relayed to the somatic sensory portion of the cerebral cortex (Fig. 3-1).

The functions ascribed to the dorsal column system as well as the clinical presentation of lesions in this system have been discussed in Chapter 2.

SPINAL TRIGEMINAL NUCLEUS (SpTNu) AND TRACT (SpTT)

The spinal trigeminal nucleus is located in the lateral aspect of the medulla, surrounded dorsolaterally by its tract. This prominent nucleus is divided into an external marginal portion (labeled **g** in Plate 6) and an inner magnocellular portion (labeled **m** in Plate 6); these two regions are continuous with the substantia gelatinosa and nucleus proprius of the spinal cord, respectively. The spinal trigeminal tract is a direct continuation of Lissauer's tract in the spinal cord. Thus, the spinal trigeminal complex of the medulla replaces, in function, the dorsal horn of the cervical spinal cord.

Axons from neurons in the spinal trigeminal nucleus group together in scattered fascicles, cross the

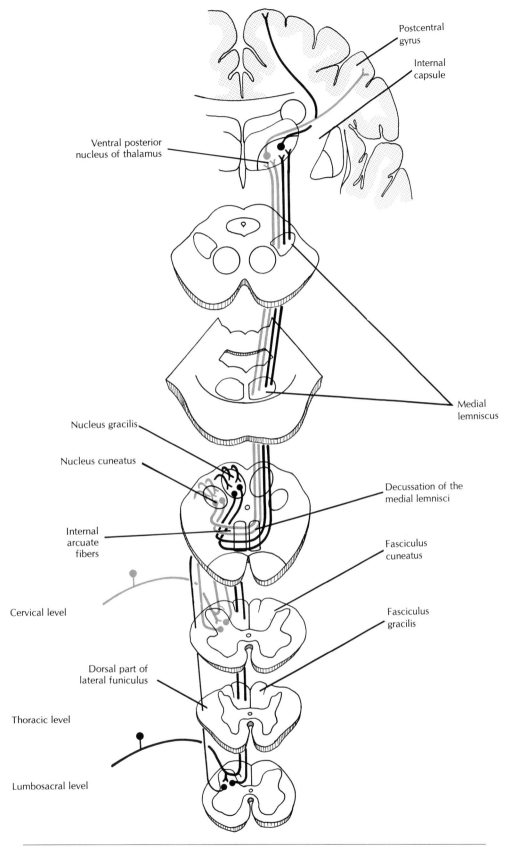

Figure 3-1. The dorsal column system and the origin of the medial lemniscus in the medulla. (Barr ML, Kiernan JA. The human nervous system; an anatomical viewpoint. 5th ed. Philadelphia: JB Lippincott, 1988:286)

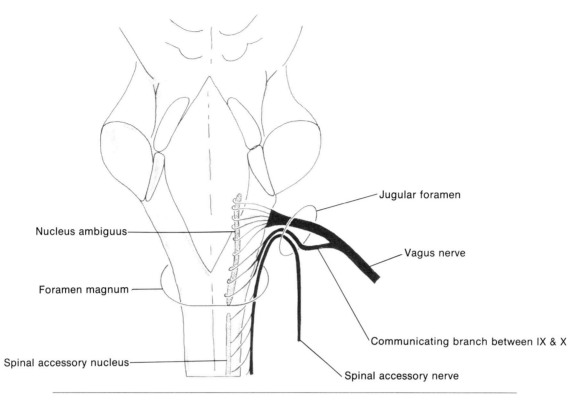

Figure 3-2. The origin of the spinal and cranial portions of the accessory nerve and portions of the vagus. Fibers arising in the nucleus ambiguus innervate the larynopharyngeal musculature while those arising in the spinal accessory nucleus innervate the sternomastoid and trapezoid muscles.

midline in the medulla, and form the ventral trigeminothalamic tract in the pons (see Plate 15). This tract follows the medial lemniscus into the thalamus (see Plates 16 to 20), where it terminates in the ventroposterior medial nucleus (see Plate 21).

The spinal trigeminal system, like its counterpart, the dorsal horn of the spinal cord, processes pain, thermal sense, and crude touch. It receives primary afferent fibers from the trigeminal nerve, carrying sensory information from the face, scalp, oral cavity, ear, mastoid air cells, and sinuses as well as dura matter of the anterior and middle cranial fossae.

CLINICAL DEFICIT

Damage to the spinal trigeminal system results in loss of pain and thermal sensation from the ipsilateral face. Irritation of the spinal trigeminal complex in the medulla can present as hyperalgesia, taking the form of sharp, stabbing pains in the ipsilateral eye and face.[2,3]

ACCESSORY NUCLEUS (AccNu)

A column of motoneurons is present lateral to the pyramidal decussation (Fig. 3-2). These neurons, forming the spinal accessory nucleus of cranial nerve

XI, represent a rostral continuation of the ventral horn of the cervical spinal cord. Their axons give rise to the spinal portion of the accessory cranial nerve, innervating the ipsilateral sternomastoid and trapezoid muscles. The cranial portion of the accessory nerve arises from the nucleus ambiguus (Figs. 3-2 and 3-3).

The accessory nucleus receives an innervation from corticonuclear fibers. The suprasegmental control of the trapezoid muscle arises from the contralateral cerebral cortex, whereas that for the sternomastoid muscle has a strong component from the ipsilateral cerebral cortex. There is clinical evidence that these latter connections are quite complex, possibly involving a double crossing of the corticonuclear axons.[4]

CLINICAL DEFICIT

Damage to the accessory nucleus or its nerve results in flaccid paralysis of the ipsilateral trapezoid and sternomastoid muscles. Clinically, paralysis of the trapezius presents as an inability to elevate the ipsilateral shoulder and as downward and lateral displacement of the scapula.[5] Paralysis of the sternomastoid muscle presents as weakness in rotating the head to the side contralateral to the lesion. On attempted flexion of the neck, the chin deviates slightly to the

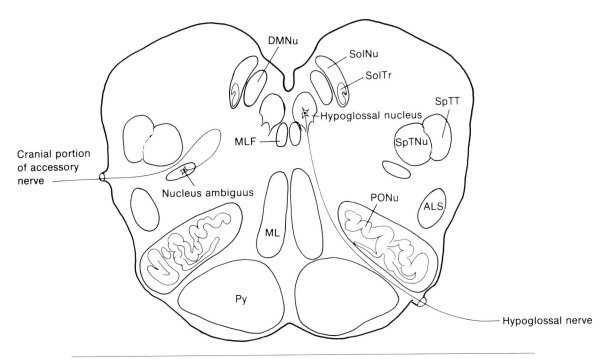

Figure 3-3. The origin of the hypoglossal nerve and cranial portion of the accessory nerve from the caudal medulla.

lesioned side because of the unopposed actions of the contralateral muscle. Fasciculations and atrophy can be seen in both of these muscles when damage is done to the accessory nucleus or its nerve.

Suprasegmental lesions (cerebral cortex or descending corticonuclear fibers in the upper brain stem) can result in spastic paresis of the contralateral trapezoid and the ipsilateral sternomastoid muscles.[4] The patient can present with weakness in the shoulder contralateral to the lesion (trapezoid muscle) and with weakness when turning the head away from the lesion (ipsilateral sternomastoid muscle).

PYRAMIDAL DECUSSATION (decPy)

The corticospinal axons arise in cerebral cortex and descend past the thalamus in the internal capsule (see Plates 22 to 25) to enter the brain stem. At the level of the medulla (see Plates 7 to 13), these axons are coursing in the medullary pyramids, from which they emerge to cross the midline and form the lateral corticospinal tract. Pyramidal decussation (decPy) is a salient feature of Plate 6, with crossing fibers distributed from the central gray area (CeGy) dorsally to the ventral border of the brain stem. A caudal portion of the decussation can also be seen in Plate 5. Within the decussation, fibers controlling upper-extremity musculature cross rostrally at the level of the hypoglossal

nerve; those controlling lower-extremity musculature decussate more caudally at the level of C_{1-2}. Corticospinal tract axons arise in motor portions of cerebral cortex and function to control fine, discriminative movements of the extremities, particularly of the distal musculature.

CLINICAL DEFICIT

Destruction of the pyramidal decussation is similar to section of both pyramidal tracts and leads to hyperreflexia and spastic paralysis in all four extremities. However, experimentally placed lesions of pyramidal tract in monkeys led to hypotonia and flaccid paralysis of the distal-extremity muscles.[6] The possible distinctions between the result of pyramidal tract section in monkeys and the clinically observable results in humans are discussed in Jagiella and Sung.[7]

Rostrally positioned lesions of the decussation, restricted to the midline, can section the crossing fibers related to the upper extremity. The result is bilateral spastic paralysis of the upper extremities and normally functioning lower extremities, a syndrome known as *cruciate paralysis*.[8]

DORSAL SPINOCEREBELLAR TRACT (DSCT)

The dorsal spinocerebellar tract (DSCT) is a thin band of fibers along the lateral border of the medulla. It contains axons from cells in the dorsal nucleus of

Clarke (see Chap. 2); these axons carry proprioceptive information to the cerebellum. At the level of the inferior olive (see Plate 8), this tract separates from its position close to the ventral spinocerebellar tract and begins rapidly increasing in size as it receives olivocerebellar fibers from the contralateral inferior olivary nucleus (see Plates 8 to 12). Collectively, these axons contribute to the inferior cerebellar peduncle (restiform body of old terminology), which curves superiorly to enter the cerebellum (see Plates 8 to 14).

CLINICAL DEFICIT

Lesions in the spinal cord that have involved the dorsal spinocerebellar tract, but not the dorsal column system, have presented with diminished position and vibratory sense[9] and ataxia.[10,11] Damage to the lateral aspect of the brain stem or the inferior cerebellar peduncle can also present with ataxia in the ipsilateral lower extremity.[3,12] The ataxia from medullary lesions presumably results from destruction of dorsal spinocerebellar fibers in the inferior cerebellar peduncle, thus depriving the cerebellum of its proprioceptive input from the lower extremity.

VENTRAL SPINOCEREBELLAR TRACT (VSCT)

The ventral spinocerebellar tract is a thin band of fibers wrapping around the lateral aspect of the medulla, ventral to dorsal spinocerebellar tract. These fibers originate from neurons in the contralateral dorsal horn, cross the midline, and ascend to the superior cerebellar peduncle (see Plates 3 to 15), eventually terminating in the cerebellum. Upon entering the cerebellum, many of the spinocerebellar fibers cross back to the opposite side. Thus, functionally the tract influences the cerebellum bilaterally. The ventral spinocerebellar tract carries information concerning the activity of ventral horn motor circuits.

ANTEROLATERAL SYSTEM (ALS)

Fibers of the anterolateral system (ALS) are found in the lateral aspect of the medulla, ventral to the spinal trigeminal complex and rubrospinal tract (Fig. 3-4). These axons originate from cells in laminae I, IV, and V of the contralateral dorsal horn, coccygeal through cervical segments. At each segmental level, axons cross the midline in the anterior white commissure, join the anterolateral system, and ascend through the brain stem (see Plates 6 to 20) to the ventroposterior lateral nucleus and interlaminar nuclei of the thalamus (see Plate 21). This system contains fibers carrying pain, thermal sense, and crude touch from the contralateral side of the body.

CLINICAL DEFICIT

Damage to the anterolateral system results in a diminution of pain and thermal sense from the contralateral body. Given the tract's close proximity to the spinal trigeminal complex, vascular lesions can affect both structures; in such cases, the presentation involves decrease of pain and thermal sense from the ipsilateral face (spinal trigeminal system) and contralateral body (anterolateral system), a constellation of signs termed **alternating analgesia.**

RUBROSPINAL TRACT (RuSp)

The rubrospinal tract (RuSp) is located between the spinal trigeminal complex and the anterolateral system. It contains fibers from the contralateral red nucleus (see Plates 20 and 21) traveling to the ventral horn of the cervical and thoracic spinal cord. This tract is involved in controlling flexor muscle tone in the proximal portion of the upper extremity.

CLINICAL DEFICIT

The loss of the rubrospinal tract in humans is masked in large part by the function of the corticospinal tract[13]; in other primates its isolated destruction results in some proximal limb weakness that eventually resolves.[6] Combined lesions of the corticospinal axons and rubrospinal tract in nonhuman primates result in a more severe weakness and spastic paralysis.

VESTIBULOSPINAL AND RETICULOSPINAL TRACTS (VesSp and RetSp)

The vestibulospinal and reticulospinal tracts (VesSp and RetSp) are closely associated in the ventral aspect of the medulla, where they are located between the pyramidal tract and the anterolateral system. The vestibulospinal tract arises in the lateral vestibular nucleus (see Plates 12 to 15), whereas the reticulospinal tract arises in the pontine and medullary reticular formation (see Plates 6 to 16). These tracts innervate the medial aspect of the ventral horn of the spinal cord and modulate tone and posture in axial and proximal limb musculature; thus, they regulate body–limb movements. As such, they represent components of the medial motor system.[14]

CLINICAL DEFICIT

Isolated lesions of these tracts have not been reported in humans; however, their destruction in monkeys leads to decomposition of body posture.[15] Although

Figure 3-4. The course of the anterolateral (spinothalamic) system in the brain stem. (Barr ML, Kiernan JA. The human nervous system; an anatomical viewpoint. 5th ed. Philadelphia: JB Lippincott, 1988:280)

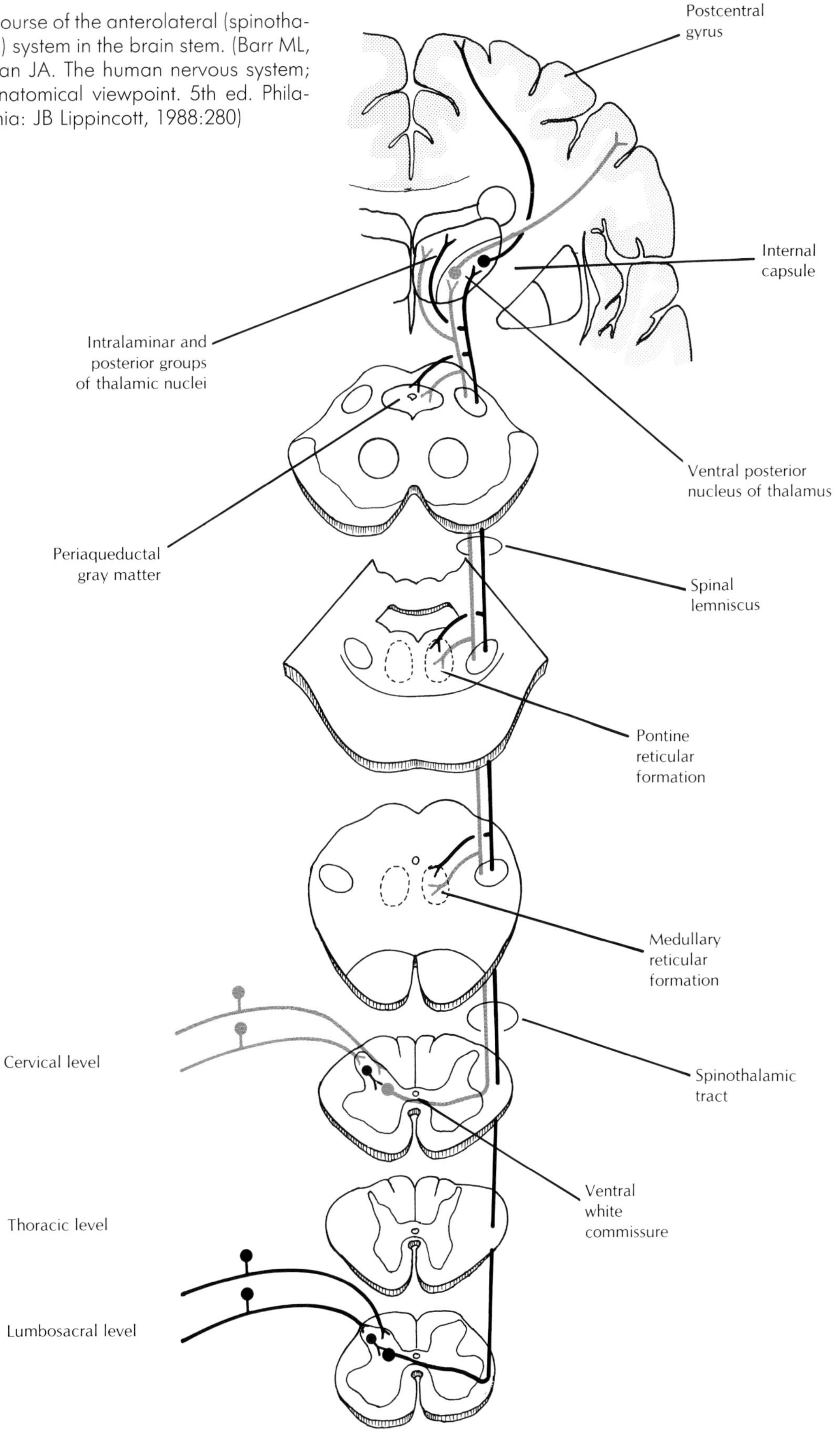

Postcentral gyrus

Internal capsule

Ventral posterior nucleus of thalamus

Intralaminar and posterior groups of thalamic nuclei

Spinal lemniscus

Periaqueductal gray matter

Pontine reticular formation

Medullary reticular formation

Cervical level

Spinothalamic tract

Ventral white commissure

Thoracic level

Lumbosacral level

these primates could still use their arms and hands, they were lacking a righting reflex and had few orientating reflexes.

MEDIAL LONGITUDINAL FASCICULUS (MLF)

The medial longitudinal fasciculus (MLF) extends from the level of the oculomotor nucleus in the midbrain (see Plate 20) into the cervical spinal cord. It serves to interconnect the vestibular nuclei with the oculomotor, trochlear, abducens nuclei as well as motoneurons controlling the cervical musculature. Along its route through the brain stem, the fasciculus is located close to the midline; however, at the cervicomedullary junction (see Plate 6), it is pushed laterally by the pyramidal decussation. As the medial longitudinal fasciculus enters the cord, its name is often changed to the medial vestibulospinal tract. (In this atlas the term *medial longitudinal fasciculus* is used throughout the length of this tract, instead of changing nomenclature as the tract enters the spinal cord.)

In the caudal medulla, the medial longitudinal fasciculus contains axons from the medial vestibular nucleus that are destined to innervate the medial aspect of the ventral horn of the ipsilateral cervical spinal cord. Thus, this portion of the tract is a component of the medial motor system controlling axial musculature.

CLINICAL DEFICIT

Isolated section of the medial longitudinal fasciculus in the brain stem below the abducens nucleus has not been reported in humans. Section of this tract above the level of the abducens nucleus can result in disassociated movements of the eyes, called *intranuclear ophthalmoplegia*. This will be discussed in Chapter 4.

TECTOSPINAL TRACT (TecSp)

A small cluster of axons close to the medial longitudinal fasciculus represents the tectospinal tract (TecSp). These axons arise from neurons in the deep layers of the contralateral superior colliculus of the midbrain (see Plate 19), cross the midline, and descend through the brain stem into the cervical spinal cord. The tectospinal tract is involved in mediating head and neck reflexes to unexpected stimuli.

CENTRAL GRAY (CeGy)

The area surrounding the central canal of the spinal cord expands at the level of the caudal medulla to form the central gray (CeGy). At slightly more rostral levels the hypoglossal and vagal nuclei will be contained within this region (see Plates 7 to 9).

MEDULLARY RETICULAR FORMATION (MRetF)

The medullary reticular formation (MRetF) is a centrally located collection of cells and fibers lacking distinct nuclear borders. It extends throughout the rostrocaudal length of the medulla (see Plates 6 to 11), continuing through the pons (see Chap. 4), and into the midbrain (see Chap. 6). Clusters of neurons in the reticular formation are involved in regulating cardiovascular and pulmonary functions as well as other autonomic processes. Descending autonomic fibers are found coursing along the dorsolateral aspect of the reticular formation, in close juxtaposition with the spinal trigeminal complex and the rubrospinal fibers. These fibers originate in the hypothalamus (see Plate 22) and brain stem and terminate in the nucleus intermediolateralis of the thoracic (see Plate 3) and upper lumbar spinal cord. They provide central control over spinally mediated autonomic functions.

CLINICAL DEFICIT

Lesions of the reticular formation can present with dysautonomia, such as tachycardia and nonrhythmic respiration rates.[3] Lesions of the descending autonomic fibers can present as Horner's syndrome—ptosis, miosis, and anhidrosis—on the ipsilateral face.[2] Unilateral lesions in the medullary reticular formation, positioned between the inferior olive medially and the inferior cerebellar peduncle laterally at the pontomedullary junction, can interrupt autonomic breathing.[16]

▷ **Atlas Plate 7**

Atlas Plate 7 is positioned between the pyramidal decussation caudally and the obex (the opening of the central canal into the fourth ventricle) rostrally. The prominent features of this section are three large sensory nuclei located dorsally (nucleus gracilis and cuneatus and the spinal trigeminal nucleus), decussation of the medial lemniscus centrally, and the medullary pyramidal tract ventrally.

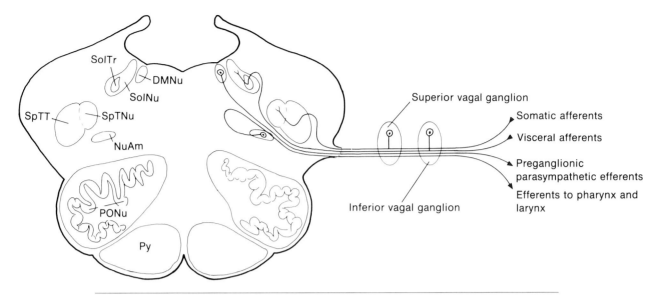

Figure 3-5. A medullary section (similar to Plate 10) illustrates the origin of motor and sensory conponents of the vagus nerve in the medulla. (Modified from Barr ML, Kiernan JA. The human nervous system; an anatomical viewpoint. 5th ed. Philadelphia: JB Lippincott, 1988:140)

NUCLEUS AMBIGUUS (NuAm)

The nucleus ambiguus, a long, thin column of motoneurons in the lateral medulla, is associated with the vagal complex (Figs. 3-2, 3-3, 3-5, and 3-6). It extends from the level of the decussation of the medial lemniscus (see Plate 7) to the rostral portion of the inferior olive (see Plate 11). Motoneurons in this nucleus provide innervation to muscles in the pharynx and larynx via the ipsilateral vagus (Fig. 3-5) and glossopharyngeal nerves (see Fig. 3-6) and contribute to the cranial portion of the ipsilateral spinal accessory nerve (see Figs. 3-2 and 3-3). The nucleus ambiguus and the dorsal motor nucleus of the vagus supply parasympathetic innervation to the heart.[17]

CLINICAL DEFICIT
A unilateral lesion of the vagal complex (including the nucleus ambiguus) or its efferent fibers results in hoarseness, dysphonia ("nasal twang"), difficulty swallowing (aphagopraxia), diminished gag reflex, and perhaps hiccups.[2] The palatine arch is flattened ipsilateral to the lesion and fails to elevate on that side. A bilateral lesion of the vagal nerve can produce bilateral palatine droop and profound dysphagia and dyspnea to the point of respiratory embarrassment.[16,18]

SOLITARY NUCLEUS (SolNu)

The **solitary nucleus** (SolNu) is a long column of cells located in the dorsocentral medulla (see Figs. 3-5 and 3-6), extending from the level of the decussation of the medial lemniscus (see Plate 7) to that of the rostral portion of the inferior olivary nucleus (see Plate 11). In all but the extreme caudal portion of the solitary nucleus, it surrounds the solitary tract. It is through this tract that the solitary nucleus receives afferent fibers carrying visceral sensory information from the facial, glossopharyngeal, and vagus nerves. The rostral pole of the solitary complex, called gustatory nucleus, receives afferent fibers from taste buds in the tongue through cranial nerves VII, IX, and X. The more caudal portions of the nucleus receive visceral afferent fibers from the pharyngeal and laryngeal walls, as well as from the cardiovascular and gastrointestinal systems. Closely related to the solitary complex are the chemical trigger zone and vomit center.

Cells in the solitary nucleus send axons to many regions of the surrounding brain stem, such as the nucleus ambiguus, dorsal motor nucleus of the vagus, and hypoglossal nucleus, as well as ascending projections to the hypothalamus and thalamus.

Rostrally in the medulla, the **solitary tract** (see Plates 8 to 11) is seen as a compact fiber bundle sur-

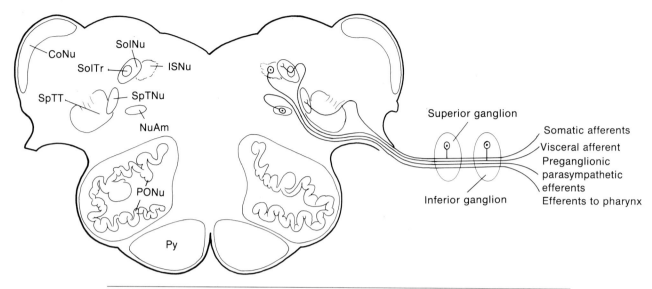

Figure 3-6. A medullary section (similar to Plate 11) illustrates the origin of motor and sensory components of the glossopharyngeal nerve in the medulla. (Modified from Barr ML, Kiernan JA. The human nervous system; an anatomical viewpoint. 5th ed. Philadelphia: JB Lippincott, 1988:139)

rounded by solitary nucleus; caudally, the tract diminishes and the nucleus approaches the midline to fuse with its counterpart from the opposite side (see Plate 7), forming the commissural nucleus of the vagus. The solitary tract is composed of primary afferent fibers from the facial, glossopharyngeal, and vagal nerves.

CLINICAL DEFICIT

Dyspnea, pseudoasthma, vomiting, and possibly coughing due to interruption of the vagal reflex arcs are signs of damage in the vicinity of the solitary nucleus or its connections. Diminution or loss of the gag reflex can result from lesions of the vagal afferent fibers or the solitary nucleus or tract. Loss of taste can result from damage to the gustatory component of the solitary nucleus.

DORSAL MOTOR NUCLEUS OF THE VAGUS (DMNu)

The dorsal motor nucleus (DMNu) is a long column of cells located in the central gray area between the solitary complex and the hypoglossal nucleus (see Fig. 3-5). It extends from the caudal medulla (see Plate 7) to the level of the rostral portion of the inferior olivary nucleus (see Plate 10). The dorsal motor nucleus is composed of preganglionic, parasympa-

thetic neurons of the vagus nerve and provides innervation to the viscera of the thoracic and abdominal cavities. It receives afferent fibers from the solitary nucleus as well as descending fibers from the hypothalamus.

CLINICAL DEFICIT

Bilateral lesions involving the dorsal motor nucleus can result in loss of parasympathetic outflow to the viscera. Clinical indications of this are tachycardia and dilation of the stomach.

HYPOGLOSSAL NUCLEUS (HyNu)

The hypoglossal nucleus (HyNu) is a long column of motoneurons located in the ventral aspect of the central gray and extending from the caudal border of the medulla (see Plate 7) to the midpoint on the long axis of the inferior olivary nucleus (see Plate 9 and Fig. 3-3). Its cells constitute the motoneurons of cranial nerve XII, providing innervation to the intrinsic muscles of the tongue. Portions of this nucleus receive a bilateral innervation from corticonuclear fibers; however, those motoneurons controlling the genioglossus muscle are predominantly innervated by the contralateral cerebral cortex.

CLINICAL DEFICIT

Damage to the hypoglossal nucleus (or the radiations of its nerve) results in denervation of the tongue. Clinically, the tongue deviates toward the side of the lesion on attempted protrusion. In addition, atrophy and fasciculations are present in the muscles of the tongue on the side of the lesion.[5]

Lesions of the cerebral cortex or corticonuclear fibers can also cause dysfunction in the hypoglossal nucleus. The genioglossus muscle is mainly innervated by crossed corticonuclear fibers; it will weaken with supranuclear lesions. The tongue deviates to the side opposite the supranuclear lesion; however, fasciculations and atrophy are not present.[19]

PYRAMIDAL TRACT (Py)

The pyramidal tract (Py) is located in the ventro-medial aspect of the medulla next to the medial accessory olivary nucleus. Its fibers originate from neurons in the motor area of the cerebral cortex. These fibers control the mastery of fine, discriminative movements of the extremities, particularly the distal musculature.[13] At the cervicomedullary junction (see Plate 6), the pyramidal tract decussates to the contralateral side and divides to form the lateral and anterior corticospinal tracts (see Plate 5).

CLINICAL DEFICITS

A lesion of the pyramidal tract in humans can initially result in flaccid paralysis that eventually resolves into hypertonia and spastic paralysis[7,20,21] as well as the Babinski sign. The deficits appear in the limbs on the side contralateral to the lesion.

INTERNAL ARCUATE FIBERS (IAF)

The dorsal column nuclei (nucleus gracilis and cuneatus; Plates 6 to 8) project axons to the contralateral thalamus. As these axons leave the ventral surface of their nucleus, they swing medially in a prominent arc, forming the internal arcuate fibers (IAF), decussate over the midline, and gather into the medial lemniscus (see Plate 8). This latter tract ascends through the brain stem to reach the ventroposterior lateral nucleus of the thalamus (see Plate 21).

CLINICAL DEFICITS

Damage to the internal arcuate fibers can present with loss of discriminative touch and vibratory sense, similar to the results of damage involving the medial lem-niscus. The clinical signs appear ipsilateral to the lesion. Damage to the decussation of the medial lemniscus can result in deficits that present bilaterally.

MEDIAL LONGITUDINAL FASCICULUS (MLF)

The medial longitudinal fasciculus (MLF or medial vestibulospinal tract) has moved from its lateral position on the previous plate (see Plate 6) into its more typical position along the midline of the brain stem, dorsal to the tectospinal tract. For the remaining sections through the rostral medulla (see Plates 7 to 11), these two tracts, plus the medial lemniscus and pyramidal tract, form a midline column of white matter.

MEDIAL ACCESSORY INFERIOR OLIVE NUCLEUS (MAONu)

A thin, angular band of cells in the ventral medulla is the first indication of the large inferior olivary complex (see Plates 8 to 12). The medial accessory inferior olive nucleus (MAONu), visible in Plate 7, will be replaced laterally, at more rostral levels by the principal nucleus of the inferior olive. Like the principal nucleus, the medial accessory nucleus projects its axons to the cerebellum.

Review Structures From Preceding Plates

Identify the following structures from preceding sections:

Gracile fasciculus and nucleus (FGr and NuGr)

Cuneate fasciculus and nucleus (FCu and NuCu)

Spinal trigeminal nucleus (SpTNu) and tract (SpTT)

Anterolateral system (ALS)

Dorsal spinocerebellar tract (DSCT)

Ventral spinocerebellar tract (VSCT)

Rubrospinal tract (RuSp)

Tectospinal tract (TecSp)

Vestibulospinal and reticulospinal tracts (VesSp and RetSp)

▷ Atlas Plate 8

The section in Plate 8 is located in the caudal medulla, rostral to the obex and passing through the olivary tubercle. Its salient features are the opening of the fourth ventricle and the presence of the principal inferior olivary nucleus.

LATERAL (ACCESSORY OR EXTERNAL) CUNEATE NUCLEUS (LCNu)

The lateral cuneate nucleus appears as swirled masses of gray, embedded in the lateral portion of the fasciculus cuneatus. It receives large-caliber, primary afferent fibers from peripheral nerves in the ipsilateral upper extremity. These fibers convey proprioceptive information from individual muscles. Lateral cuneate neurons give rise to axons that join the ipsilateral inferior cerebellar peduncle (see Plates 8 to 14) and terminate in the cerebellum. The lateral cuneate nucleus performs a function similar to that of the dorsal nucleus of Clarke in the spinal cord (see Plate 3), with the exception that its source of proprioception is from the upper extremity. (The dorsal nucleus of Clarke receives its sensory information from the lower extremity.)

CLINICAL DEFICIT

Damage to the lateral aspect of the spinal cord or to the inferior cerebellar peduncle in which lateral cuneocerebellar fibers course can result in ataxia in the upper extremity on the side ipsilateral to the lesion.[12]

PRINCIPAL INFERIOR OLIVARY NUCLEUS (PONu)

The highly convoluted principal inferior olivary nucleus (PONu) extends throughout most of the ventrolateral medulla (see Plates 8 to 12). The massive expansion in size of this nucleus in primates has created an enlargement, the olivary tubercle, on the external surface of the medulla. Two additional structures are in close juxtaposition with the principal nucleus: the dorsal accessory nucleus and the medial accessory nucleus of the inferior olive.

The principal nucleus receives input ipsilaterally from the red nucleus, contralaterally from the spinal cord and dorsal column nuclei, and bilaterally from the cerebral cortex. Its axons, known as climbing fibers, have a powerful influence on the activity of Purkinje cells in all parts of the contralateral cerebellum. It is part of the cerebellar system of motor control and training.

CLINICAL DEFICIT

Clinical evaluation of the inferior olive in humans is not done routinely. Destruction of the inferior olivary nucleus in nonhuman primates diminishes the ability of the animal to learn new skilled motor activities.[22]

The concept that the inferior olive is involved in motor learning received additional support in recent studies where motor learning defects were described in patients with degenerative disease of the inferior olive.[23,24]

MEDIAL LEMNISCUS (ML)

Large myelinated axons from cells in the dorsal column nuclei cross the midline as the internal arcuate fibers and coalesce into a long, narrow bundle called the medial lemniscus (ML). These fibers are joined by axons from nucleus Z in the caudal medulla (Fig. 3-7). The fibers of the medial lemniscus proceed rostrally (see Plates 8 to 20) through the medulla, pons, and midbrain to terminate in the ventroposterior lateral nucleus of the thalamus (see Plate 21), contralateral to its origin. Throughout most of its course, the medial lemniscus occupies a position dorsal to the pyramidal tract and close to the midline. Since this tract is composed of output from the dorsal column nuclei and nucleus Z, it contains most of the ascending information on two-point discrimination as well as vibratory and position sense.

CLINICAL DEFICITS

The medial lemniscus contains the output from the dorsal column nuclei and nucleus Z. Thus, damaging this tract is similar to combined lesions of the dorsal columns of the spinal cord and the cuneo- and dorsal spinocerebellar tracts. The patient experiences loss of two-point discrimination, position, and vibratory sense. Since, however, the axons of the medial lemniscus have crossed the midline in the internal arcuate fibers, its clinical signs localize on the side of the body contralateral to the lesion.

CENTRAL TEGMENTAL TRACT (CTT)

The central tegmental tract (CTT) is a large bundle of fibers forming the major ascending and descending pathway for intrinsic structures of the brain stem. It links the rostral brain stem with the medulla. Among other things, the tract carries axons from the gustatory nuclei in the rostral portion of the solitary complex to the thalamus.

The caudal extreme of this tract surrounds the inferior olivary nucleus (see Plate 8); rostrally, it extends beyond the red nucleus of the midbrain to reach the intralaminar nuclei of the thalamus (see Plate 21). Throughout the brain stem, it courses approximately in the center of the reticular formation.

CLINICAL DEFICIT
Destruction of the central tegmental tract is reported to result in palatal myoclonus, which presents as rhythmic contractions of the palate.

INFERIOR CEREBELLAR PEDUNCLE (ICP)

The inferior cerebellar peduncle (ICP) is a massive fiber bundle, formed by the union of the dorsal spinocerebellar tract and the olivocerebellar fibers from the contralateral inferior olive, that passes upward from the dorsolateral surface of the medulla to enter the cerebellum (see Plates 8 to 14). In its ascent it is joined by cuneocerebellar axons from the accessory cuneate nucleus. These fiber tracts carry proprioceptive information from the musculoskeletal system and terminate primarily in the anterior lobe of the cerebellum.

CLINICAL DEFICIT
Destruction of the inferior cerebellar peduncle results in ataxia of the extremities on the ipsilateral side of the body.[25] Clinically, this presents as veering or leaning to the side of the lesion and clumsiness with the ipsilateral hand.[2]

DORSAL LONGITUDINAL FASCICULUS (DLF)

A small fiber bundle located in the dorsal and medial portion of the medulla represents the dorsal longitudinal fasciculus (DLF). This composite tract extends from the hypothalamus (see Plate 22) to the caudal aspect of the medulla. Fibers from the hypothalamus, descending in this fasciculus, influence the brain stem nuclei involved in regulating the autonomic nervous system.

Review Structures From Preceding Plates
Identify the following structures from preceding sections:

Cuneate nucleus (NuCu) and fasciculus (FCu)

Nucleus ambiguus (NuAm)

Hypoglossal nucleus (HyNu)

Spinal trigeminal nucleus (SpTNu) and tract (SpTT)

Pyramidal tract (Py)

Internal arcuate fibers (IAF)

Anterolateral system (ALS)

Rubrospinal tract (RuSp)

Vestibulospinal and reticulospinal tracts (VesSp and RetSp)

Medial longitudinal fasciculus (MLF)

Tectospinal tract (TecSp)

Dorsal motor nucleus of the vagus (DMNu)

Medial accessory nucleus of the inferior olive (MAONu)

Ventral spinocerebellar tract (VSCT)

▷ Atlas Plates 9 and 10

Atlas Plates 9 and 10 are taken from the central portion of the medulla. The salient features of these sections are the expanded size of the inferior cerebellar peduncle and the prominent inferior olive.

MEDIAL VESTIBULAR NUCLEUS (MVNu)

The medial vestibular nucleus (MVNu) is located dorsolateral to the dorsal motor nucleus and solitary complex of the vagus. It is involved in coordinating head, neck, and eye movements. The nucleus receives primary afferent fibers from the semicircular canals of the ipsilateral vestibular apparatus and projects ascending and descending fibers into the medial longitudinal fasciculus. The descending fibers are distributed bilaterally to the spinal cord. At the cervicomedullary junction, this fiber tract is often renamed the medial vestibulospinal tract (see discussion on p.

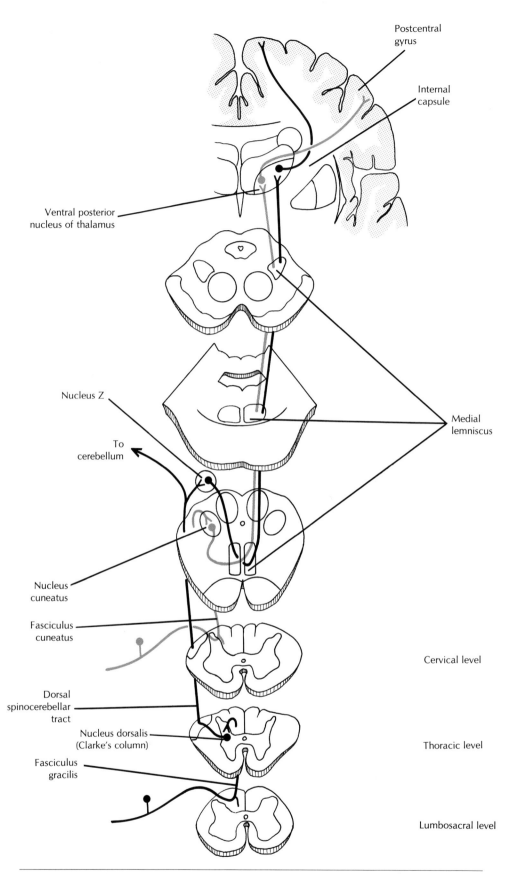

Figure 3-7. The spinocerebellar systems and the origin of projection of proprioceptive information to the cerebral cortex. (Barr ML, Kiernan JA. The human nervous system; an anatomical viewpoint. 5th ed. Philadelphia: JB Lippincott, 1988:288)

62). Some of the ascending fibers from the medial vestibular nucleus reach the contralateral abducens nucleus; this connection is a major component of vestibular control over horizontal gaze (see Chap. 4).

SPINAL VESTIBULAR NUCLEUS (SpVNu)

The spinal (or inferior) vestibular nucleus (SpVNu) is located between the medial vestibular and the lateral cuneate nuclei. It is the most caudal nucleus of the vestibular complex. Primary afferent fibers to the spinal vestibular nucleus arise in the saccule and utricle of the ipsilateral vestibular apparatus; the efferent fibers of this nucleus enter the inferior cerebellar peduncle and terminate in the ipsilateral cerebellum. It also innervates the ipsilateral inferior olivary nucleus.

CLINICAL DEFICIT

Damage to the vestibular nuclei or their tracts in the medulla can result in the **central vestibular syndrome.** The three signs are nystagmus, vertigo, and a Romberg fall. Unlike the peripheral vestibular syndrome (see p. 67), the central vestibular syndrome is said to be more permanent in nature. It also differs in the consistency of its presentation. The nystagmus can be of multiple different types: unilateral, bilateral, horizontal, rotary, or vertical. Nystagmus of central vestibular origin usually is not altered by visual fixation. The vertigo experienced in central vestibular syndrome can be ill defined and continuous, and the Romberg sign, elicited by closing the eyes while standing, can be to either side.[26]

LATERAL RETICULAR NUCLEUS (LRNu)

The lateral reticular nucleus (LRNu) is found in the ventrolateral medulla, positioned between the rubrospinal tract (dorsally) and the anterolateral system (ventrally). It receives fibers from a variety of sources (*e.g.,* the spinal cord, cerebral cortex, and red nucleus) and projects its axons, via the inferior cerebellar peduncle, to the ipsilateral cerebellum.

PREPOSITUS HYPOGLOSSAL NUCLEUS (NuPP)

The nucleus prepositus hypoglossi (NuPP) (see Plates 10 and 11) is located in the dorsal medulla, between the hypoglossal (see Plate 9) and abducens nuclei (see Plate 12). It receives information from the cerebellum, accessory optic nuclei in the midbrain, and vestibular nuclei. It projects to all the extraocular eye muscle motor nuclei: abducens, trochlear, and oculomotor, as well as to the paramedian pontine reticular formation, a region that controls conjugate horizontal eye movements (see Chap. 4). The prepositus hypoglossal nucleus participates in controlling eye movements, possibly by stabilizing the eyes in their new position following a saccade. Electrical stimulation of the nucleus results in ipsilateral conjugate horizontal movement of the eyes.

CLINICAL DEFICIT

Lesions in this area of the brain stem, of nonhuman primates, disturb optokinetic eye movements.[27]

DORSAL ACCESSORY INFERIOR OLIVARY NUCLEUS (DAONu)

The dorsal inferior accessory nucleus is a narrow band of olivary neurons on the dorsomedial border of the inferior olive. Like the principal nucleus of the olive, it projects its axons to the cerebellum.

Review Structures From Preceding Plates
Identify the following structures from preceding sections:

Lateral cuneate nucleus (LCNu)

Solitary nucleus (SolNu) and tract (SolTr)

Dorsal motor nucleus of the vagus (DMNu)

Nucleus ambiguus (NuAm)

Hypoglossal nucleus (HyNu)

Spinal trigeminal nucleus (SpTNu) and tract (SpTT)

Principal olivary nuclei (PONu)

Inferior cerebellar peduncle (ICP)

Central tegmental tract (CTT)

Pyramidal tract (Py)

Medial lemniscus (ML)

Anterolateral system (ALS)

Rubrospinal tract (RuSp)

Vestibulospinal and reticulospinal tracts (VesSp and RetSp)

Medial longitudinal fasciculus (MLF)

Dorsal longitudinal fasciculus (DLF)

Tectospinal tract (TecSp)

▷ Atlas Plate 11

Atlas Plate 11 passes through the medulla as the inferior cerebellar peduncle begins its ascent into the cerebellum. The cochlear nucleus, overhanging the inferior cerebellar peduncle, is a prominent feature of this section.

COCHLEAR NUCLEUS (CoNu)

The cochlear nucleus (CoNu) is the first nucleus in the central auditory pathways. It receives primary afferent fibers from the ipsilateral auditory nerve and its projections reach the superior olivary nuclei bilaterally (see Plate 14) as well as the contralateral inferior colliculus (see Plate 17).

CLINICAL DEFICIT
Destruction of the cochlear nucleus on one side results in unilateral sensorineural deafness.

SUPERIOR VESTIBULAR NUCLEUS (SVNu)

The superior vestibular nucleus (SVNu) is a small cluster of neurons positioned dorsal to the lateral vestibular nucleus along the lateral wall of the fourth ventricle. The superior vestibular nucleus receives primary afferent fibers from the semicircular canals of the ipsilateral vestibular apparatus as well as axons from the cerebellum. It projects ascending axons into the medial longitudinal fasciculus to innervate the extraocular eye muscle motor nuclei. This nucleus and its connections are a part of the vestibular system involved in coordinating head and eye movements. The clinical aspects of damage to the vestibular nuclei or their central connections have been presented on page 65.

INFERIOR SALIVATORY NUCLEUS (ISNu)

The inferior salivatory nucleus (ISNu) is located at the rostral end of the dorsal motor nucleus of the vagus and ventral to the medial vestibular nucleus. It contains preganglionic, parasympathetic neurons that innervate the otic ganglion and control secretions of the parotid gland.

CLINICAL DEFICIT
Lesion of the inferior salivatory nucleus or of its efferent fibers in the glossopharyngeal nerve results in loss of salivary release from the ipsilateral parotid gland.

RAPHE NUCLEI (RaNu)

The raphe nuclei (RaNu) are located along the midline of the medulla, sandwiched between the two fiber bundles of the medial lemnisci. Many cells in this complex produce the neuromodulator serotonin. Their fibers form diffuse tracts that descend in the dorsolateral funiculus of the spinal cord and innervate the dorsal and ventral horns. One function of the raphe-spinal system is to modulate the processing of pain in the dorsal horns. Appropriate production of serotonin also seems to be necessary for the onset of sleep.

CLINICAL DEFICIT
Information on isolated lesions of the raphe nuclei or raphe-spinal system in humans is unavailable; however, chemically blocking this system with naloxone in humans subjects can decrease their threshold of pain.[28]

Review Structures from Preceding Plates
Identify the following structures from preceding sections:

Nucleus ambiguus (NuAm)

Principal olivary nucleus (PONu)

Solitary nucleus (SolNu) and tract (SolTr)

Spinal trigeminal nucleus (SpTNu) and tract (SpTT)

Spinal vestibular nucleus (SpVNu)

Medial vestibular nucleus (MVNu)

Prepositus hypoglossal nucleus (NuPP)

Inferior cerebellar peduncle (ICP)

Central tegmental tract (CTT)

Medial lemniscus (ML)

Anterolateral system (ALS)

Pyramidal tract (Py)

Rubrospinal tract (RuSp)

Medial longitudinal fasciculus (MLF)

Dorsal longitudinal fasciculus (DLF)

Dorsal accessory olivary nucleus (DAONu)

▷ **Atlas Plate 12**

Atlas Plate 12 straddles the pontomedullary junction. The dorsal portion of the section, containing the abducens motor nucleus and facial motor nucleus, enters the pons; the ventral portion passes through the olivary tubercle and pyramids of the medulla. The pontine portion will be examined in Chapter 4.

VESTIBULOCOCHLEAR NERVE ROOT (VCNr)

The vestibulocochlear nerve (VCNr) can be seen entering the brain stem laterally, ventral to the middle cerebellar peduncle and in close juxtaposition with the pontobulbar nucleus. This nerve carries primary afferent fibers from the cochlea and the vestibular apparatus (utricle, sacculus, and three ampullae of the semicircular canals) to the brain stem. The cell bodies of origin for axons in this composite nerve are found in the spiral ganglion (cochlear portion of the nerve) and Scarpa's ganglion (vestibular portion of the nerve).

CLINICAL DEFICIT
Damaging the vestibulocochlear nerve can result in unilateral deafness sometimes accompanied by tinnitus; it also can result in the **peripheral vestibular syndrome** featuring nystagmus, vertigo, limb drift, and a Romberg sign. Unlike the central vestibular syndrome (p. 65), that arising from peripheral damage is usually short-lived but can be accompanied by a severe, paroxysmal vertigo. Also, all its signs tend to

be aligned in one direction. The slow component of the ocular drift in nystagmus, the fall in the Romberg test, and the drift in the outstretched arm are to the side of the lesioned nerve.[26]

LATERAL VESTIBULAR NUCLEUS (LVNu)

The lateral vestibular nucleus (LVNu) is wedged between the medial vestibular nucleus and the inferior cerebellar peduncle. It is penetrated by myelinated fibers and hence appears darkened in myelin-stained preparations. This nucleus receives primary afferent fibers from the utricle of the ipsilateral vestibular apparatus; it also receives a significant projection from the Purkinje cells in the ipsilateral cerebellum. Its axons innervate motoneurons in the limb portions of the ventral horn of the spinal cord via the lateral vestibulospinal tract. These fibers convey information with regard to posture and gravity to the motoneurons of the limb extensor muscles.

CLINICAL DEFICIT
Isolated lesions of the lateral vestibular nucleus or its tract in humans have not been reported. However, damage done to this system in experimental situations with nonhuman mammals decreases the tone in the extensor muscles of the extremities.[15]

PONTOBULBAR NUCLEI (PBNu)

A thin band of cells under the inferior cerebellar peduncle is seen at the pontomedullary border. These cells form the pontobulbar nucleus (PBNu) and represent the caudal extension of the pontine nuclei. The nucleus receives axons from the contralateral cerebral cortex and forms projections to the contralateral cerebellum.[29] Its function is similar to that of the pontine nuclei and will be discussed in Chapter 4.

Review Structures From Preceding Plates
Identify the following structures from preceding sections:

Principal olivary nuclei (PONu)

Spinal trigeminal nucleus (SpTNu) and tract (SpTT)

Cochlear nucleus (CoNu)

Medial vestibular nucleus (MVNu)

Superior vestibular nucleus (SVNu)

Prepositus hypoglossal nucleus (NuPP)

Inferior cerebellar peduncle (ICP)

Central tegmental tract (CTT)

Medial lemniscus (ML)

Anterolateral system (ALS)

Pyramidal tract (Py)

Rubrospinal tract (RuSp)

Medial longitudinal fasciculus (MLF)

Dorsal longitudinal fasciculus (DLF)

Medial accessory inferior olivary nucleus (MAONu)

UNIT B

Case Study 3-2

A 43-year-old man with weakness in his tongue and right limbs

This was a 43-year-old, right-handed man with a chief complaint of headaches, dysarthria, and weakness in his right arm and leg. The headaches began 3 weeks ago, and 2 weeks ago he noticed the onset of limb weakness and slurred speech. Currently, headaches have abated, but the weakness and dysarthria remain. His family physician has referred him for neurologic consultation.

Past Medical History

The patient was an accountant in a large business firm and regularly worked 60 to 70 hours per week. He was being treated for hypertension but admitted to recently decreasing his medications without the consent of his physician. He had a 30-pack-year history of smoking and consumed several ounces of alcohol daily. He denied the use of alcohol during the past 24 hours.

General Physical Examination

This was a well-nourished, alert, oriented man who appeared his stated age. He could comprehend spoken and written language but had dysarthria. His speech was thickened, as if his tongue was swollen. Heart sounds were normal, blood pressure was high (150/99), pulse rate and respirations were normal; chest was clear to auscultation and percussion. Abdomen was soft with no lumps, masses, or tenderness.

Neurologic Examination

Mental Status. He was alert and oriented with respect to time and place. His speech was dysarthric; however, word-finding ability, comprehension, and repetition were all normal. His reading and writing were appropriate.

Cranial Nerves. His tongue deviated to the left on attempted protrusion. The surface of the tongue on the left side was wrinkled, and muscular fasciculations were present. All other cranial nerves were intact.

Motor Systems. His right upper and lower limbs were noticeably weaker than those on the left. He had elevated deep tendon reflexes in the right limbs and increased muscle tone in both right limbs. A Babinski reflex was present on the right. All other regions were intact.

Sensation. All sensory systems were intact. There was no loss of pinprick or thermal sensation, no loss of vibratory, discriminative sensation, and no loss of proprioception throughout his body.

QUESTIONS

1. Does the patient exhibit a language or memory deficit or an alteration in consciousness or cognition?

2. Are signs of cranial nerve dysfunction present?

3. Are there any changes in motor functions, such as reflexes, muscle tone, movement, or coordination?

4. Are any changes in sensory functions detectable?

5. At what level in the central neuraxis is this lesion most likely located?

6. Is the pathology focal, multifocal, or diffuse in its distribution within the nervous system?

7. What is the clinical–temporal profile of this pathology: acute or chronic; progressive or stable?

8. Based on your answers to the previous two questions, decide whether the symptoms in this patient are most likely caused by a vascular accident, a tumor, or a degenerative or inflammatory process.

9. If you feel this is the result of a vascular accident, what vessels are most likely involved?

10. Explain the expression of a cranial nerve palsy on the left side while extremity palsies were expressed on the right.

► DISCUSSION
Medullary Vasculature

The medullary vasculature is derived from the vertebral and spinal arteries. These two sources represent the posterior circulatory contributions to the circle of Willis. Plates 6 through 12 illustrate the general distribution of these vessels in the medulla. Each vessel has perforating branches that perfuse a longitudinal zone of tissue. Although the spinal cord has only two vascular zones—anterior and posterior—supplied by separate arteries, a third or lateral zone has developed in the medulla.[30] Although sharp boundaries have been depicted for these zones in the atlas plates, it should be understood that considerable overlap and anastomosis can exist in vivo.

The *anterior zone* (fine screen shading, Plates 6 to 12) is perfused by medial branches of the anterior spinal artery caudally and medial branches of the basilar artery rostrally. This zone can be partitioned into anteromedial and anterolateral bundles of penetrating arteries. In total, the anterior zone supplies the midline structures, including the pyramidal tract, medial lemniscus, medial longitudinal fasciculus, and hypoglossal nucleus and its radiations.

The *lateral zone* (no shading, Plates 6 to 12) is perfused by the lateral branches from the vertebral and posterior inferior cerebellar artery, particularly at its caudal levels. At more rostral levels this zone is perfused by the lateral branches of the basilar artery and from the anterior inferior cerebellar artery. The lateral circulation supplies the nucleus ambiguus of the vagus, portions of the spinal trigeminal nucleus and tract, ventral portions of the inferior cerebellar peduncle, the anterolateral system, and portions of the medullary reticular formation, including the descending fibers modulating the autonomic nervous system of the spinal cord.

The *posterior zone* (small crosses, Plates 6 to 12) is perfused by the posterior spinal artery and by posterior branches of the posterior inferior cerebellar artery caudally. Rostrally this zone is absent (Plate 13). The posterior circulation supplies the dorsal columns and their nuclei (gracilis and cuneatus), the caudal portion of the vestibular nuclei, the dorsal motor nucleus of the vagus, the inferior cerebellar peduncle, and portions of the spinal trigeminal nucleus and its tract.

MEDULLARY VASCULAR SYNDROMES

Infarction or occlusion of a specific artery can lead to loss of function in the zone serviced by the damaged vessel and its branches. When this occurs in a penetrating vessel in a noncortical portion of the cerebrum or brain stem, it is called a *lacunar infarction*.[31] There are numerous constellations of presenting neurologic signs and symptoms that can be related to lacunar infarctions in the distribution of specific arteries. Such constellations are referred to as arterial syndromes. (Adams and Victor present a detailed review of brain stem arterial [or neurovascular] syndromes.[25]) Four vascular-related sets of neurologic constellations are described in the clinical literature for the medulla: the medial, lateral, and unilateral medullary syndromes plus a lateral pontomedullary syndrome.

Medial medullary syndrome (Table 3-1) involves reduced perfusion in the anterior zone of the medulla. It can result from damage to the vertebral or anterior spinal artery or their medial branches. Tissue destruction centers on midline structures. The neurologic presentation can involve spastic paralysis, weak-

Table 3-1.
Possible Origins of Neurologic Signs in the Medial Medullary Syndrome

NEUROLOGIC SIGN	ANATOMIC SOURCE
ON CONTRALATERAL SIDE	
Spastic paralysis	Pyramidal tract
Diminished tactile and proprioceptive sense	Medial lemniscus
ON IPSILATERAL SIDE	
Paralysis with atrophy of muscles in half of the tongue	Radiations of twelfth cranial nerve

(Adapted from Caplan LR, Stein RW, Stroke: a clinical approach. Boston: Butterworths 1986:343; and Adams RD, Victor M. Principles of neurology. New York: McGraw-Hill 1989; Chap. 34)

ness, and elevated tendon reflexes in the extremities on the contralateral side; flaccid paralysis, weakness, and fasciculations in the ipsilateral musculature of the tongue; and loss of primary sensory systems (tactile and proprioceptive sense) from the contralateral side of the body (see Table 3-1).[25] The combination of ipsilateral tongue paralysis and contralateral limb paralysis is referred to as **inferior alternating hemiplegia.** Presentation of the medial medullary syndrome is rare; however, when it does occur it can be bilateral in distribution.[32] It also has been observed to occur consequent to intervenous injection of nonprescription drugs.[33]

Lateral medullary syndrome (Table 3-2) involves reduction in perfusion to the lateral and/or posterior zones in the medulla. It can result from damage to the vertebral artery or its lateral branches, such as the posterior inferior cerebellar artery. The focus of tissue destruction lies in the upper lateral quadrant of the medulla.[34] The neurologic presentation can involve numerous structures in the upper lateral quadrant of the medulla (see Table 3-2).[12,35] The patient can present with any or all of the following: loss of pain and temperature sensation from the ipsilateral face and contralateral body, Horner's syndrome, hoarseness and dysphagia, ataxia of the ipsilateral limbs, vertigo, diplopia, nausea and vomiting, and nystagmus. The initial presentation may also include sharp, burning pains from the face presumably due to irritation of the spinal trigeminal complex.[36] The loss of pain and temperature sensation from the ipsilateral face and contralateral body is called **alternating analgesia.**

The **unilateral medullary syndrome** can result

Table 3-2.
Possible Origins of Neurologic Signs in the Lateral Medullary Syndrome

NEUROLOGIC SIGN	ANATOMIC SOURCE
ON CONTRALATERAL SIDE	
Loss of pain and temperature sensation and paresthesis on half of body	Anterolateral system
ON IPSILATERAL SIDE	
Hypalgesia, impaired sensation over half of the face	Spinal trigeminal nucleus or tract
Ataxia of limbs	Most likely the inferior cerebellar peduncle and spinocerebellar fibers
Vertigo, nausea and vomiting	Vestibular system
Nystagmus and diplopia	Vestibular system
Horner's syndrome	Descending fibers controlling the sympathetic nervous system
Hiccups	Medullary respiratory centers (?)
Dysphagia, dysphonia and dyspnea	Vagal and glossopharyngeal structures
Paresthesis from half of body	Irritation of dorsal column nuclei
Headache in the upper cervical region	Arterial irritation

(Adapted from Caplan LR, Stein RW. Stroke: a clinical approach. Boston: Butterworths 1986:343; and Adams RD, Victor M. Principles of neurology. New York: McGraw-Hill 1989; Chap. 34)

from complete occlusion of a vertebral artery. A caudal hemisection of the medulla is involved in the lesion, with restricted perfusion to all three zones: anterior, lateral, and medial. The neurologic presentation combines part or all of the medial and lateral medullary syndromes.

The **lateral pontomedullary syndrome** can result from occlusion of the lateral perfusion branches of the basilar artery rostrally, at the pontomedullary junction. It presents with many of the same signs as seen in the lateral medullary syndrome: alternating analgesia, appendicular ataxia, and dysarthria; however, an ipsilateral facial paresis (facial nerve or nucleus) as well as vestibular dysfunction such as nystagmus[37] and/or diminished hearing functions (cochlear nucleus and its efferent fiber tracts) can also occur.[38]

► Bibliography

Barr ML, Kiernan JA. External anatomy. In: The human nervous system: an anatomical viewpoint. Philadelphia: JB Lippincott, 1988; Chap. 6:84–91.

Barr ML, Kiernan JA. Brain stem: Nuclei and tracts. In: The human nervous system: an anatomical viewpoint. Philadelphia: JB Lippincott, 1988; Chap. 7:92–120.

Barr ML, Kiernan JA. Cranial nerves. In: The human nervous system: an anatomical viewpoint. Philadelphia: JB Lippincott, 1988; Chap. 8:121–147.

Barr ML, Kiernan JA. Reticular formation. In: The human nervous system: an anatomical viewpoint. Philadelphia: JB Lippincott, 1988; Chap. 9:148–159.

Brazis PW, Masdeu JC, Biller J. Localization in clinical neurology. Boston: Little, Brown, 1990; Chaps. 10–14.

Daube JR, Ragan TJ, Sandok BA, Westmoreland BF. The posterior cranial fossa level. In: Medical neurosciences. Boston: Little, Brown, 1986; Chap. 14:324–373.

Haines DE. Neuroanatomy: an atlas of structures, sections, and systems. Baltimore: Urban & Schwarzenberg, 1987 *(see especially Figs. 5-7 to 5-13)*.

Nieuwenhuys R, Voogd J, van Huijzen C. The human central nervous system. Berlin: Springer-Verlag, 1988:144–220.

► References

1. Briner RP, Carlton SM, Coggeshall RE, Chung K. Evidence for unmyelinated sensory fibers in the posterior columns in man. Brain 1988;111:999.
2. Caplan LR, Stein RW. Stroke: a clinical approach. Boston: Butterworths, 1986:343.
3. Caplan LR. Intracranial branch atheromatous disease: a neglected, understudied, and underused concept. Neurology 1989;39:1246.
4. Brazis PW. The localization of lesions affecting cranial nerve XI (the spinal accessory nerve). In: Brazis PW, Masdeu JC, Biller J, eds. Localization in clinical neurology. Boston: Little, Brown, 1990a:249–257.
5. Haymaker W, Kulhlenbeck H. Disorders of the brainstem and its cranial nerves. Clin Neurol 1976;3:1.
6. Lawrence DG, Kuypers HGJM. The functional organization of the motor system in the monkey. I. The effects of bilateral pyramidal lesions. Brain 1968;91:1.
7. Jagiella WM, Sung JH. Bilateral infarction of the medullary pyramids in humans. Neurology 1989;39:21.
8. Dumitru D, Lang JE. Cruciate paralysis. J Neurosurg 1986;65:108.
9. Ross ED, Kirkpatrick JB, Lastimosa ACB. Position and vibration sensations: functions of the dorsal spinocerebellar tracts? Ann Neurol 1978;5:171.
10. Gudesblatt M, Cohn J, Gerber O, Sacher M. Truncal ataxia presumably due to malignant spinal cord compression. Ann Neurol 1987;21:511.
11. Biller J, Brazis PW. The localization of lesions affecting the spinal cord. In: Brazis PW, Masdeu JC, Biller J, eds. Localization in clinical neurology. Boston: Little, Brown, 1990a:69–92.
12. Peterman AF, Siekert RG. The lateral medullary (Wallenberg) syndrome: clinical features and prognosis. Med Clin North Am 1960;44:887.
13. Kennedy PR. Corticospinal, rubrospinal, and rubro-olivary projections: a unifying hypothesis. Trends Neurosci 1990;13:474.
14. Kuypers HGJM. Anatomy of the descending pathways. In: Brookhart JM, Mountcastle VB, Brooks VB, eds. Handbook of

physiology. The nervous system, Vol II: Motor control. Bethesda, MD: American Physiology Society, 1981:597–666.

15. Lawrence DG, Kuypers HGJM. The functional organization of the motor system in the monkey. II. The effects of lesions of the descending brain-stem pathways. Brain 1968;91:15.

16. Bogousslavsky J, Khurana R, Deruaz JP, Hornung JP, Regli F, Janzer R, Perret C. Respiratory failure and unilateral caudal brainstem infarction. Ann Neurol 1990;28:668.

17. Natelson, BH. Neurocardiology: an interdisciplinary area for the 80s. Arch Neurol 1985;42:178.

18. Brazis PW. The location of lesions affecting cranial nerves IX and X (the glossopharyngeal and vagus nerves). In: Brazis PW, Masdeu JC, Biller J, eds. Localization in clinical neurology. Boston: Little, Brown, 1990.

19. Brazis PW. The localization of lesions affecting cranial nerve XII (the hypoglossal nerve). In: Brazis PW, Masdeu JC, Biller J, eds. Localization in clinical neurology. Boston: Little, Brown, 1990:259–267.

20. Paulson GW, Yates AJ, Paltan-Oritz JD. Does infarction of the medullary pyramid lead to spasticity? Arch Neurol 1986;43(1):93.

21. Milandre L, Habib M, Hassoun J, Khalil, R. Bilateral infarction of the medullary pyramids. Neurology 1990;40:556.

22. Ito M. The cerebellum and neural control. New York: Raven, 1984:580.

23. Sanes JN, Dimitrov B, Hallett M. Motor learning in patients with cerebellar dysfunction. Brain 1990;113:103.

24. Thach WT, Goodkin HP, Keating JG. The cerebellum and adaptive coordination of movement. Ann Rev Neurosci 1992;15:403.

25. Adams RD, Victor M. Principles of neurology. New York: McGraw-Hill, 1989.

26. Biller J, Brazis PW. The localization of lesions affecting cranial nerve VIII (the vestibulocochlear nerve). In: Brazis PW, Masdeu JC, Biller J, eds. Localization in clinical neurology. Boston: Little, Brown, 1990:219–237.

27. Bender MB. Brain control of conjugate horizontal and vertical eye movements. A survey of the structural and function correlates. Brain 1980;103:23.

28. Basbaum AI, Fields HL. Endogenous pain control mechanisms: review and hypothesis. Ann Neurol 1978;4:451.

29. Olszewski J, Baxter D. Cytoarchitecture of the human brain stem, 2nd ed. Basel: S Karger, 1982.

30. Duvernoy HM. Human brainstem vessels. Berlin: Springer-Verlag, 1978.

31. Fisher CM. Lacunar strokes and infarcts: a review. Neurology 1982;32:871.

32. Ho K-L, Meyer KR. The medial medullary syndrome. Arch Neurol 1981;38:385.

33. Mizutani T, Lewis RA, Gonatas NK. Medial medullary syndrome in a drug abuser. Arch Neurol 1980;37:425.

34. Baker AB. The medullary blood supply and the lateral medullary syndrome. Neurology 1961;11:853.

35. Currier RD, Giles CL, DeJong RN. Some comments on Wallenberg's lateral medullary syndrome. Neurology 1961;11:779.

36. Caplan L, Gorelick P. "Salt and pepper on the face" pain in acute brainstem ischemia. Ann Neurol 1983;13:344.

37. Fisher CM. Lacunar infarct of the tegmentum of the lower lateral pons. Arch Neurol 1989;46:566.

38. Brazis PW. The localization of lesions affecting the brainstem. In: Brazis PW, Masdeu JC, Biller J, eds. Localization in clinical neurology. Boston: Little, Brown, 1990:269–285.

4 PONS

► Introduction

The word *pons* means "bridge," an image evoked in reference to the middle cerebellar peduncle, which forms a prominent span across the ventral aspect of this portion of the brain stem. Within the pons are longitudinal fiber tracts connecting the spinal cord with midbrain and thalamus as well as the nuclei and radiations for four cranial nerves: trigeminal, abducens, facial, and portions of the vestibulocochlear. Pontine functions include the control of horizontal eye movements and participation in the ascending activation system, which controls cerebral cortical neural activity.

The major blood supply to the pons arises from branches of the basilar artery and creates a series of perfusion zones similar to those present in the medulla. Cerebrovascular accidents in specific perfusion zones of the basilar arterial branches can present as recognized pontine syndromes.

73

In this chapter the nucleus and tracts of the pons will be examined, its blood supply will be studied, and several clinicopathologic cases related to the pons will be considered.

GENERAL OBJECTIVES

1. To learn the location and function of major ascending and descending fiber tracts in the pons
2. To learn the location and function of the cranial nerves and their nuclei in the pons
3. To learn the presenting signs and symptoms consequent with lesions involving major tracts and cranial nuclei in the pons
4. To apply the preceding knowledge to an understanding of the clinical manifestations of major pontine vascular lesions

INSTRUCTIONS

In this chapter you will be presented with one or more clinical case studies. *Each study will be followed by a list of questions that can best be answered by using a knowledge of regional and functional neuroanatomy and by referring to outside reading material.* Following the questions will be a section devoted to structures from a specific region of the central nervous system. Before attempting to answer the questions, compile a list of the patient's neurologic signs and symptoms; then examine the structures and their functions and study their known clinical deficits. After becoming familiar with the material, reexamine the list of neurologic signs and symptoms and formulate answers to the questions. Be aware that some of the questions can have multiple responses or require information beyond the scope of this manual. It may be necessary to obtain material or advice from additional resources, such as specialty texts, a medical dictionary, or clinical personnel.

MATERIALS

1. A human brain stem or model
2. An atlas of the human brain stem
3. A medical dictionary

UNIT A

Case Study 4-1

A 55-year-old man with left-sided facial paralysis and right-sided limb paralysis

A 55-year-old right-handed man was brought to the emergency room by his wife because of the sudden onset of neurologic symptoms. Earlier that morning he had fallen in the bathroom while trying to shave. He was unable to get up without his wife's assistance. Once he got up, he found that his right leg felt weak and stiff and dragged slightly as he attempted to walk from the bathroom. He also found that his right arm would not support him as he attempted to lean on the walls. His wife stated that the left side of his face looked different and that he was drooling from the left side of his mouth.

Past Medical History

The patient was a professional accountant involved in management. He was married, with three children, one of whom was still living with him. He had enjoyed good health except for a mildly elevated blood pressure since turning 45 years of age. He had a 10-pack-year history of smoking but quit all smoking at age 53.

General Physical Examination

This was an alert, oriented, cooperative, and appropriately concerned male with an asymmetric facial expression who appeared his stated age. His eyes were clear with no papilledema; his chest was clear to auscultation and percussion; his pulse, respirations, and temperature were normal. He had an elevated blood pressure (193/98). His abdomen was soft with no signs of tenderness or masses; a large scar in the lower right quadrant of the abdomen was residual from an old appendectomy. His skin was soft and warm, with normal turgor.

Neurologic Examination

Mental Status. The patient was alert, oriented for time and place, and cooperative. His speech was dysarthric but fluent. Memory, language, and comprehension were intact. He could follow three- and four-step commands. He gave a coherent history.

Cranial Nerves. He denied any double vision, and his visual fields were intact to confrontation. His pupils were 3 to 4 mm in diameter and reactive to light, both direct and consensual. The patient had volitional conjugate vision vertically in both directions and to the right, but not to the left. Both eyes could be deflected to the left with the doll's head maneuver or by placing warm water in the left ear (caloric test). Convergence movements in both eyes were intact. He had normal hearing (tested to finger rub) in both ears. His corneal reflex was present on the right but diminished on the left; however, brushing the left cornea was painful to him. His facial expression was asymmetric. The left side of his mouth was open slightly and did not move when he spoke, his left eyelid would not shut as tightly as the right, and the wrinkles of the left side of the forehead were less pronounced than those on the right. When he attempted to puff out his cheeks, air escaped from the left side of his mouth. The jaw-jerk and gag reflexes were intact. His palate elevated along the midline and his tongue protruded on the midline.

Motor Systems. Strength was reduced in both extremities on the right compared to those on the left. Tendon reflexes were elevated at the wrist, elbow, knee, and ankle on the right (+3/5) and were normal in all places in the left extremities. Plantar reflexes were extensor on the right and flexor on the left. No past pointing was present on the left, and finger-to-nose and heel-to-shin tests were normal for that extremity. He was unable to execute these tests with the right extremities. His right upper extremity was flexed at the elbow and resisted passive movement; his right lower extremity was extended and resisted flexion, even as he attempted to walk. Normal tone and station were present in the left limbs.

Sensation. Pinprick, light touch, and position and vibratory senses were intact throughout body and face.

QUESTIONS

1. Does the patient exhibit a language or memory deficit or an alteration in consciousness or cognition?

2. Are signs of cranial nerve dysfunction present?

3. Are there any changes in motor functions, such as reflexes, muscle tone, movement, or coordination?

4. Are any changes in sensory functions detectable?

5. At what level in the central neuraxis is this lesion most likely located?

6. Is the pathology focal, multifocal, or diffuse in its distribution within the nervous system?

7. What is the clinical–temporal profile of this pathology: acute or chronic; progressive or stable?

8. Based on your answers to the previous two questions, decide whether the symptoms in this patient are most likely caused by a vascular accident, a tumor, or a degenerative or inflammatory process.

9. If you feel this is the result of a vascular accident, what vessels are most likely involved?

10. Damage to what fiber tracts could produce right-sided weakness and hyperreflexia?

11. Damage to what structure(s) could cause loss of volitional conjugate vision to the left without diplopia?

12. Damage to what structure could cause drooling from the left side of the mouth, left facial weakness, and inability to close the left eye completely?

13. What are the possible explanations for the patient's failure to perform the finger-to-nose test on the right?

► DISCUSSION
Pontine Structures

The pons is traversed by several of the long ascending and descending tracts. In addition, there are numerous intrinsic nuclei related to the cranial nerves and the surrounding reticular formation. These items are listed on the slides described later; the abbreviation following the name of each item corresponds to that used to identify the structure on the atlas plate. The first time you encounter a given structure, its description will be provided along with comments on function and any clinical deficit consequent to its destruction. For subsequent sections, the structure will be mentioned by name only unless significant changes have occurred in its location or composition.

▷ Atlas Plate 12

Atlas Plate 12 straddles the pontomedullary junction. The dorsal portion of the section, containing the abducens and facial nuclei, has passed through the pons. The ventral portion of the section, containing the olivary tubercle and pyramidal tract, has remained in the medulla. The medullary portion has been examined in Chapter 3.

MIDDLE CEREBELLAR PEDUNCLE (MCP)

The middle cerebellar peduncle (MCP) is a thick band of fibers visible on the external surface of the pons. It is composed of axons that arise in the pontine nuclei (see Plates 14 to 20) and innervate the contralat-

eral cerebellar hemisphere. As these fibers cross the midline they are called the pontocerebellar or transverse pontine fibers. Laterally, they coalesce to form the middle cerebellar peduncle (as seen on this plate). The transverse pontine fibers are intersected at right angles by bundles of the descending corticospinal and corticonuclear axons (see Plates 14 to 20). The ventral portion of the pons, containing the pontine nuclei, pontocerebellar fibers, and corticospinal fibers, is referred to as the **basis pontis** or **basilar pons.**

Information from the cerebral cortex passes through corticopontine axons to reach the pontine nuclei. From here it is projected across the midline and into the cerebellar hemispheres through the middle cerebellar peduncle. This circuit is referred to as the cortico-ponto-cerebellar pathway. It serves as a conduit through which the cerebral cortex instructs the cerebellum of impending movements.

CLINICAL DEFICIT
Damage to the middle cerebellar peduncle is similar to that of the cerebellar hemisphere and presents with limb ataxia on the side ipsilateral to the lesion. Small lesions in the basis pontis, close to the midline, can produce a complicated syndrome of contralateral hemiparesis and hemiataxia[1] (also see p. 85). In such cases, the extremity contralateral to the lesion is both weakened and ataxic. Additional information on cerebellar dysfunction can be found in Chapter 5.

ABDUCENS NUCLEUS (AbNu)

The abducens nucleus (AbNu) is a short column of motoneurons in the dorsal pons, lying along the floor of the fourth ventricle, in close juxtaposition with the medial longitudinal fasciculus (Fig. 4-1). The abducens

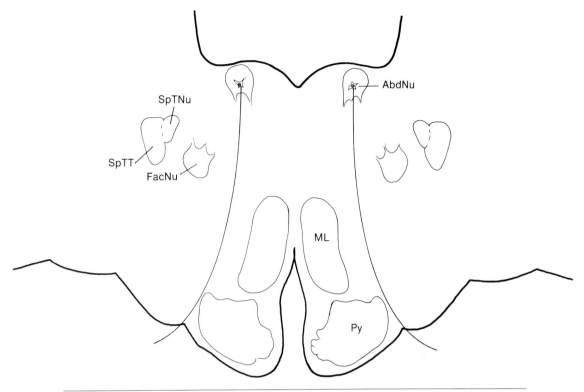

Figure 4-1. A caudal pontine section (similar to Plate 13) illustrates the origin of the abducens nerve.

nucleus receives bilateral projections from the medial vestibular nuclei and ipsilateral projections from the paramedian pontine reticular formation (see p. 87 and Plate 14). Primary afferent fibers to the medial vestibular nuclei arise in the ampulla of the ipsilateral horizontal semicircular canals. Motoneurons in the abducens nucleus innervate the lateral rectus muscle of the ipsilateral eye. Other neurons in abducens nucleus project axons via the medial longitudinal fasciculus to the contralateral oculomotor nucleus (Fig. 4-2), where they specifically target that portion of the nucleus controlling the medial rectus muscle.

The abducens nucleus serves to coordinate conjugate horizontal movements of the eyes (Fig. 4-2). Stimulation through vestibular input to the ipsilateral (right) abducens nucleus excites the right lateral rectus muscle and, through its projections to the contralateral oculomotor nucleus, the left medial rectus muscle. As both muscles contract, the eyes are deflected to the right, maintaining conjugate vision.

CLINICAL DEFICIT

Damage to the abducens nerve results in an infranuclear (segmental or lower motoneuron) form of paralysis of the lateral rectus muscle and failure of the ipsilateral globe to abduct on attempted lateral gaze to the side of the lesion (lesion 1, Fig. 4-2). Since the contralateral medial rectus is still receiving a signal from abducens nucleus via the oculomotor nucleus, it adducts on attempted lateral gaze, conjugate vision is compromised, and the patient reports diplopia on attempted lateral gaze.

Damage to the abducens nucleus is more complicated (lesion 2, Fig. 4-2). Such a lesion can remove control of the ipsilateral lateral rectus by denervation (segmental level). In addition, loss of the communication from abducens to contralateral oculomotor nucleus results in a supranuclear (suprasegmental level) form of paralysis expressed in the contralateral medial rectus muscle. The result is horizontal gaze paresis to the ipsilateral side, as both globes fail to move into that visual hemisphere. The patient experiences diminished ability to look into the field of vision ipsilateral to the damaged abducens nucleus but should not experience diplopia. This eye movement disorder is called **lateral gaze palsy.** Since the oculomotor nucleus itself is not damaged, the patient should be able to demonstrate convergence movements.

Finally, damage to the medial longitudinal fasciculus produces a third type of eye movement palsy (lesion 3; Fig. 4-2). If the lesion damages the medial longitudinal fasciculus on the left, axons from the right abducens nucleus to the left oculomotor nucleus are disrupted. The patient still has conjugate

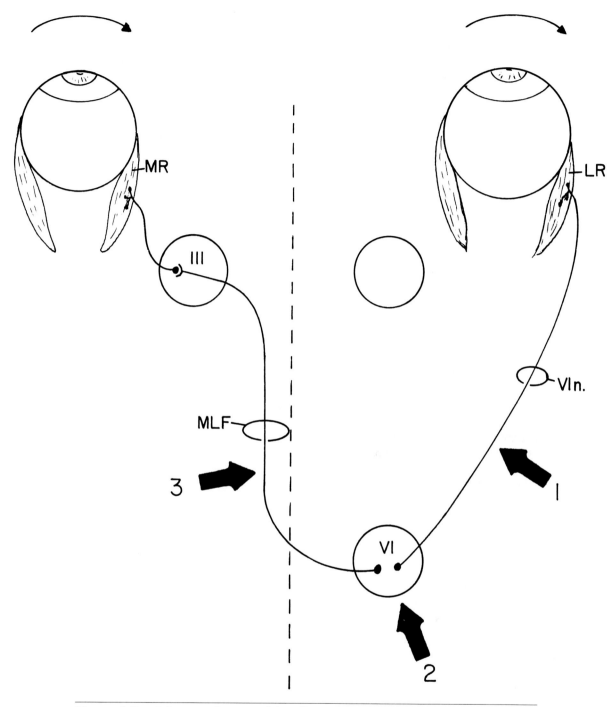

Figure 4-2. Schematic diagram of the efferent fibers from the abducens nucleus illustrates their control of conjugate lateral gaze. (See the text for explanation.)

gaze to the left; however, when attempting gaze to the right, the medial rectus on the left fails to respond, producing diplopia on attempted right lateral gaze. This type of supranuclear palsy of the oculomotor nucleus is called **intranuclear opthalmoplegia.**[2]

FACIAL NUCLEUS (FacNu) AND ITS RADIATIONS (FacNr)

A large cluster of motoneurons lying dorsomedial to the spinal trigeminal and anterolateral systems represents the facial nucleus (FacNu). These neurons innervate the muscles of facial expression as well as the stapedius, auricularis, and stylohyoid muscles and the posterior belly of the digastric muscle. Radiations of the facial nerve (FacNr) leave the nucleus and pass dorsally to reach the floor of the fourth ventricle (see Fig. 4-3 and Plate 13, from which they turn in a ventro-lateral direction (as the internal genu) to course diagonally across the pons and exit the brain stem in close juxtaposition with the acousticovestibular nerve (see Plate 14).

As the fibers of the facial nerve begin their ventral descent from the floor of the fourth ventricle they pass by the superior salvitory, gustatory, and spinal trigeminal nuclei. It is from these nuclei that the facial nerve acquires its additional components (Fig. 4-3).

The facial nucleus is innervated by corticonuclear fibers from frontal (motor) cortex (**A** in Fig. 4-4). Neurons controlling the musculature in the lower half of the face are innervated primarily by fibers from the contralateral cortex (**E** in Fig. 4-4). Those innervating muscles in the upper portion of the face receive a bilateral cortical innervation (**D** in Fig. 4-4).

CLINICAL DEFICIT

The most notable deficit in lesions of the facial nucleus, its radiations within the brain stem, or its nerve is paralysis of the ipsilateral muscles of facial expression, called peripheral type palsy.[3] Lesion of corticonuclear fibers to the facial nucleus produce paralysis of muscles in the lower half of the contralateral face, with much less involvement of the upper half of the face (see Fig. 4-4). Maintenance of muscle function in the upper portion of the face consequent to cortical destruction is due to the bilateral innervation of these motoneurons by corticonuclear fibers. Thus, hemifacial paralysis in a patient suggests a segmental-level lesion involving the ipsilateral facial nerve or nucleus, whereas lower-quadrant facial paralysis suggests a suprasegmental-level lesion of the contralateral cerebral cortex or its corticonuclear fibers to the facial nucleus.

COCHLEAR NUCLEUS (VCNu)

A small cluster of cells forming the rostral pole of the cochlear nucleus (VCNu) is embedded in the fibers of the vestibuloacoustic nerve. The cochlear nucleus receives primary afferent fibers from the auditory nerve and has efferent projections to the superior olivary nuclei (bilaterally) and the inferior colliculus (contralaterally; Fig. 4-5).

CLINICAL DEFICIT

Lesions of the lateral pons affecting the cochlear nucleus can result in ipsilateral diminution of hearing

functions.[4] This is referred to as **sensorineural hearing loss.**[5]

PONTINE RETICULAR FORMATION (PRetF)

The reticular formation (PRetF) of the medulla extends rostrally into the pons. It is composed of a collection of nuclei embedded in a dense matrix of fibers in the core of the brain stem. Descending pontine reticulospinal projections from these nuclei are involved in control of autonomic functions and motor activity. In addition, ascending efferent fibers from the rostral portion of the reticular formation participate in the **ascending reticular activating system**. This latter system serves to regulate neural activity in the thalamus and cerebral cortex; it also influences the sleep–wake cycle.

CLINICAL DEFICIT

Lesions of restricted size in the pontine reticular formation can present with disturbances in paradoxical (REM) sleep.[6] Large lesions of the pontine reticular formation, especially those disrupting the ascending reticular activating system, can result in coma often culminating in death.[7,8] Fatal outcome is more common for lesions occurring in the rostral portion of the pons.

Review Structures From Preceding Plates

Identify the following structures from previous sections:

Lateral vestibular nucleus (LVNu)

Medial vestibular nucleus (MVNu)

Superior vestibular nucleus (SrNu)

Medial longitudinal fasciculus (MLF)

Dorsal longitudinal fasciculus (DLF)

Spinal trigeminal nucleus and tract (SpTNu, SpTT)

▷ **Atlas Plate 13**

The dorsal portion of this section is midpontine in location, passing through the facial colliculus (a mound on the floor of the fourth ventricle for the abducens nucleus and the radiations of the facial nerve). The ventral portion of the section is located at the pontomedullary junction. Critical to recognizing

(*Text continues on page 83*)

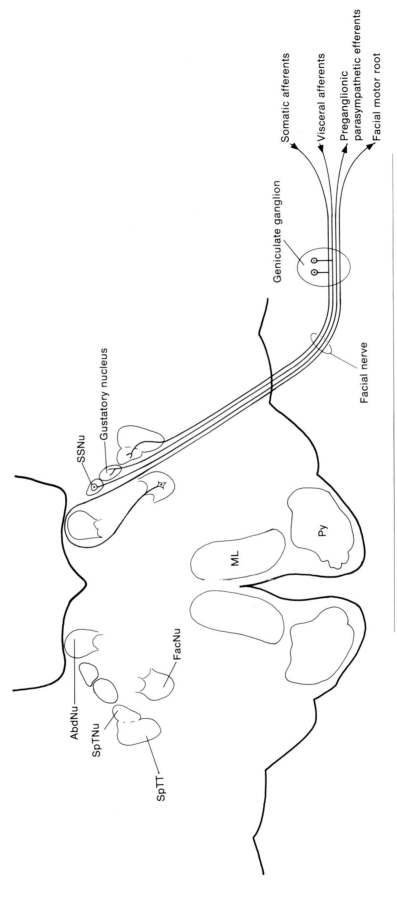

Figure 4-3. A pontine section (similar to Plate 13) illustrates the origin of the motor sensory components in facial nerve.

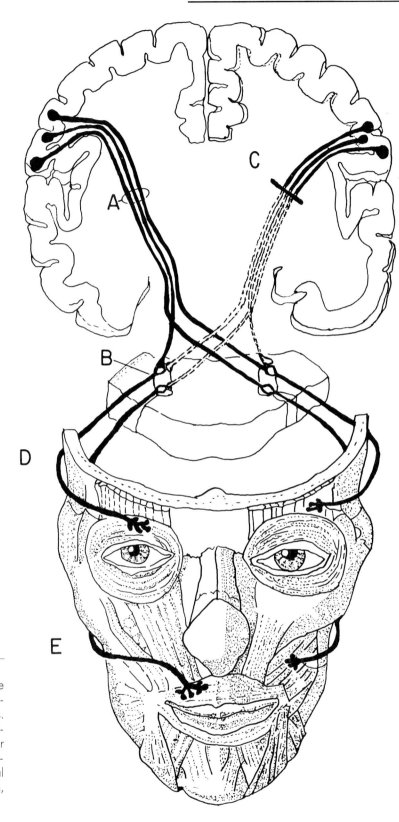

Figure 4-4.
Diagram illustrates the organization of the facial nerve and nucleus. **(A)** Corticonuclear fibers innervating the facial nucleus. **(B)** Facial nucleus. **(C)** Lesion of corticonuclear fibers. **(D)** Innervation of upper face. **(E)** Innervation of lower face. (Modified from Poritsky R. Neuroanatomical pathways. Philadelphia WB Saunders, 1984)

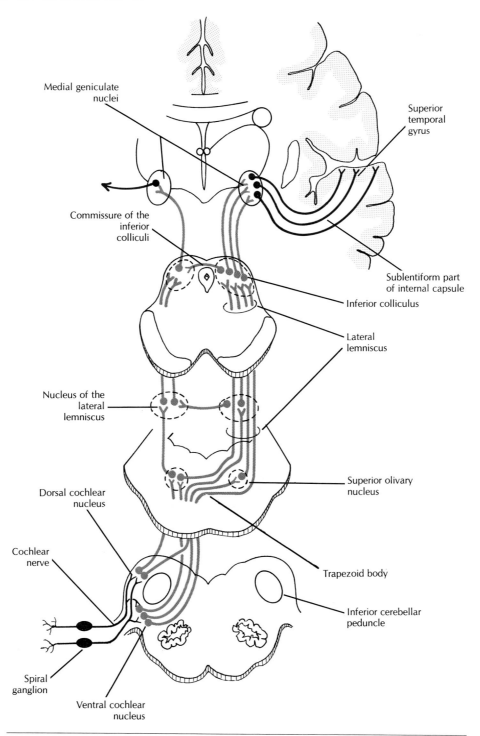

Medial geniculate
nuclei

Superior
temporal
gyrus

Commissure of the
inferior
colliculi

Sublentiform part
of internal capsule

Inferior colliculus

Lateral
lemniscus

Nucleus of the
lateral
lemniscus

Dorsal cochlear
nucleus

Superior olivary
nucleus

Cochlear
nerve

Trapezoid body

Inferior cerebellar
peduncle

Spiral
ganglion

Ventral cochlear
nucleus

Figure 4-5. The organization of the auditory pathways. (Barr ML, Kiernan JA. The human nervous system: An anatomical viewpoint. 5th ed. Philadelphia: JB Lippincott, 1988:320)

this section is the close juxtaposition of the radiation of the facial nerve and the abducens nucleus.

SUPERIOR SALIVATORY NUCLEUS (SSNu)

The superior salivatory nucleus (SSNu) is a small cluster of cells lying along the radiations of the facial nerve, just distal to its internal genu. This nucleus is considered a rostral extension of the dorsal motor nucleus of the vagus and is composed of preganglionic, parasympathetic neurons. Axons from this nucleus exit the brain stem in conjunction with the facial nerve (Fig. 4-3) and innervate the submandibular and pterygopalatine ganglia.

CLINICAL DEFICIT

Loss of the superior salivatory nucleus can result in diminished production of saliva in the oral cavity and reduced lacrimation in the ipsilateral eye. Aberrant regeneration of these autonomic systems can lead to fibers previously involved in salivation reinnervating postganglionic cells that control lacrimation. The result is the formation of "crocodile tears" in response to attempted salivation.

SUPERIOR OLIVARY NUCLEI (SONu)

Ventral to the facial nucleus are several clusters of cells called the superior olivary nuclei (SONu) (see Fig. 4-5), which are involved in the process of sound localization. Afferent fibers to the superior olive come from the cochlear nuclei bilaterally; efferent projections from these nuclei innervate primarily the contralateral superior olive and the inferior colliculus of the midbrain.

CLINICAL DEFICIT

Pontine lesions involving the superior olivary nuclei in humans diminish hearing functions in the ipsilateral ear[4]; in cats, lesions of the superior olive produce a deficit in the ability to localize sound.[9]

TRAPEZOID BODY (TrapB)

The trapezoid body (TrapB) is located between the two superior olivary nuclei, dorsal to the basilar pons. It is composed of decussating auditory fibers from the cochlear and superior olivary nuclei (see Fig. 4-5).

CLINICAL DEFICIT

Section of the trapezoid body interrupts the ascending fibers of the auditory pathways and results in bilateral diminution of hearing functions.[4] Lesions caudal to the trapezoid body present as diminished hearing in the ipsilateral ear, whereas those rostral to the trapezoid fibers present as diminished hearing in the contralateral ear. Thus, the trapezoid body is described as functioning somewhat similar to the optic chiasm of the visual system or the decussation of the medial lemniscus in the somatic sensory system.[9] Lesions in the pontine tegmentum, near or involving trapezoid body fibers from the cochlear nuclei, can present with unilateral auditory hallucinations.[10]

MESENCEPHALIC TRIGEMINAL NUCLEUS AND TRACT (MesNu and Tr)

The mesencephalic trigeminal nucleus (MesNu) is a thin column of cells, extending rostrally along the lateral wall of the fourth ventricle from the pons (Fig. 4-6 and Plate 13) into the midbrain (see Plate 16). This nucleus is surrounded by primary afferent axons from the trigeminal nerve, which form the tract (MesTr) of the mesencephalic trigeminal nucleus. The neurons of the mesencephalic trigeminal nucleus represent displaced trigeminal ganglion cells (primary afferent neurons) with peripheral processes innervating mechanoreceptors in the periodontal tissue, teeth, hard palate, and joint capsules as well as the spindle-organs in the muscles of mastication. Their central processes innervate the trigeminal motor nucleus. Thus, the neurons of the mesencephalic trigeminal nucleus form a monosynaptic reflex arc controlling the force exerted by the jaw during chewing.

CLINICAL DEFICIT

Damage to the mesencephalic trigeminal nucleus or its tract results in a diminished jaw-jerk reflex ipsilateral to the lesion.[11]

SUPERIOR CEREBELLAR PEDUNCLES (SCP)

The superior cerebellar peduncle (SCP) forms the major output pathway for the cerebellum. It arises in the dentate nucleus of the cerebellum (see Chap. 5), courses along the roof of the fourth ventricle through the pons (see Plates 13 to 16), and descends into the reticular formation of the midbrain to decussate (see Plates 17 to 19) before extending into the thalamus as the cerebellothalamic fibers (CThF), which contribute to the thalamic fasciculus (ThaFas) (see Plates 20 to 22).

CLINICAL DEFICIT

Lesions of the superior cerebellar peduncles produce neurologic sequelae similar to those of the cerebellar hemisphere: ataxia and clumsiness expressed in the

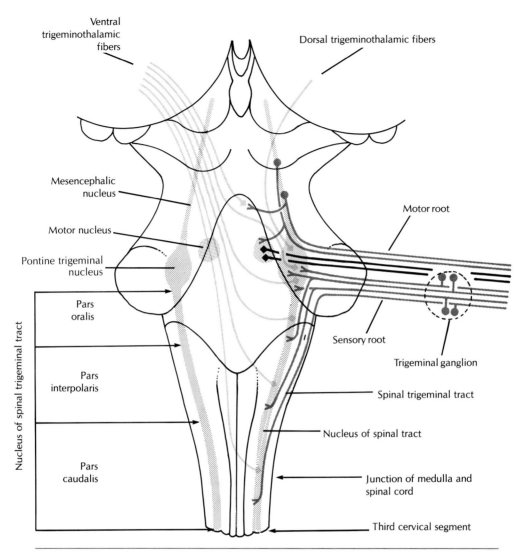

Ventral trigeminothalamic fibers

Dorsal trigeminothalamic fibers

Mesencephalic nucleus

Motor root

Motor nucleus

Pontine trigeminal nucleus

Pars oralis

Sensory root

Trigeminal ganglion

Pars interpolaris

Spinal trigeminal tract

Nucleus of spinal tract

Nucleus of spinal trigeminal tract

Pars caudalis

Junction of medulla and spinal cord

Third cervical segment

Figure 4-6. Origin of the trigeminal nerve and the trigeminal nuclei in the pons. (Barr ML, Kiernan JA. The human nervous system: An anatomical viewpoint. 5th ed. Philadelphia: JB Lippincott, 1988:131)

extremities. Deficits from lesions in the portions of the peduncle caudal to the decussation (nearest the cerebellum) present on the ipsilateral side; conversely, lesions rostral to the decussation of the peduncle (closest to the thalamus, Plates 18 to 21) present on the contralateral side of the body.

ARCUATE NUCLEUS (ArcNu)

The arcuate nucleus (ArcNu) is located at the caudal end of the pons and extends around the medial aspect of the pyramidal tract. It represents displaced cells from the pontine nuclei[12] and shares similar connections to those of the pontine nuclei (see p. 85).

CENTRAL TEGMENTAL TRACT (CTT)

At this level, the central tegmental tract (CTT) is a diffuse bundle of fibers, positioned lateral to the medial lemniscus and coursing along the long axis of the brain stem. It extends from the inferior olivary nuclei (see Plate 8) to the red nucleus of the midbrain (see Plate 20). Its connections and functions are discussed in Chapter 3.

INFERIOR CEREBELLAR PEDUNCLE (ICP)

The inferior cerebellar peduncle (ICP) has passed dorsally into the cerebellum. At this level, it is located lateral to the walls of the fourth ventricle. It will terminate in the anterior lobe of the cerebellum. Its connections and functions are discussed in Chapter 3.

Review Structures From Preceding Plates

Identify the following structures from previous sections:

Lateral vestibular nucleus (LVNu)

Medial vestibular nucleus (MVNu)

Superior vestibular nucleus (SvNu)

Inferior olivary nucleus (IONu)

Pyramidal tract (Py)

Medial lemniscus (ML)

Medial longitudinal fasciculus (MLF)

Anterolateral system (ALS)

Rubrospinal tract (RuSp)

Ventral spinocerebellar tract (VSCT)

Middle cerebellar peduncle (MCP)

Dorsal longitudinal fasciculus (DLF)

Spinal trigeminal nucleus and tract (SpTNu, SpTT)

▷ **Atlas Plate 14**

This section is taken through the caudal portion of the pons. Distinguishing features of the section are the rearrangement of the medial lemniscus from its vertical orientation in the previous section to a horizontal disposition, and the appearance of pontocerebellar fibers.

PONTINE NUCLEI (PonNu)

The pontine nuclei (PonNu) form the large mass of gray surrounding the pontocerebellar and corticospinal fibers in the basilar pons. Pontine neurons receive projections (corticopontine fibers) from most regions of neocortex. Their axons form the pontocerebellar (transverse pontine) fibers that cross the midline, traverse the contralateral pontine nuclei, and at the lateral border of the pons, coalesce to form the middle

cerebellar peduncle. The cortico-ponto-cerebellar pathway has been discussed on p. 76.

CLINICAL DEFICIT

Section of the middle cerebellar peduncles (which contain pontocerebellar fibers from the contralateral pontine nuclei) results in ataxia of the limbs ipsilateral to the lesion, similar to the situation when the cerebellar hemisphere is damaged (see Chap. 5). Lesions involving the pontine nuclei are more complex in their clinical presentation. Unilateral lesions involving cell bodies in the pontine nuclei should result in contralateral limb ataxia, because these axons will cross the midline to affect the opposite cerebellar hemisphere. However, such a lesion can also damage the descending corticospinal tract in the pons, with the resulting contralateral hemiparalysis masking any expression of ataxia in the affected limb.

In a few cases small lacunar infarcts have occurred in the dorsolateral basilar pons, neurons of the pontine nuclei were destroyed, but the underlying corticospinal fibers, although compromised, were not completely destroyed. These patients presented with a mild, contralateral *pure motor hemiparesis* because of the partially damaged corticospinal axons, and accompanying *hemiataxia* in the paretic limb due to the damaged pontine nuclei.[1,13,14] This presentation of hemiparesis and hemiataxia in the same extremities is called **ataxic hemiparesis.**[1]

PONTOCEREBELLAR FIBERS (PCeF)

The neurons of the pontine nuclei give rise to the pontocerebellar fibers (PCeF), which cross the midline of the brain stem and pass laterally to form the middle cerebellar peduncle. These fibers, also called the transverse pontine fibers, constitute the large mass of the pons.

CLINICAL DEFICIT

The complex presentations that accompany lesions in and around the pontocerebellar fibers have been discussed with the pontine nuclei (p. 85).

RADIATIONS OF THE ABDUCENS NERVE (AbNr)

Axons from motoneurons in the abducens nucleus form the radiations of the abducens nerve (AbNr). These axons pass ventrally from the nucleus along the lateral border of the medial lemniscus and corticospinal fibers to exit the brain stem at the pontomedullary junction (see Fig. 4–1).

CLINICAL DEFICIT

Lesions affecting the abducens radiations result in paresis of the lateral rectus muscle on the same side.

The patient complains of diplopia on attempted lateral gaze to the lesioned side. Unlike damage to the abducens nucleus, pure involvement of the nerve does not affect adduction of the contralateral eye (see pp. 76–77 and Fig. 4-2). Bilateral abducens nerve palsies are possible and can occur with mass-occupying lesions (tumors), degenerative–demyelinating diseases, subarachnoid hemorrhage, or infection.[15]

CHIEF SENSORY NUCLEUS OF THE TRIGEMINAL NERVE (CSNu)

The chief sensory nucleus (CSNu), located at the rostral end of the spinal trigeminal nucleus (see Fig. 4-6), receives group **II,** primary afferent fibers from mechanoreceptors in the tissues of the ipsilateral face. This nucleus is analogous in function to the dorsal column nuclei of the medulla. Axons from neurons in the chief trigeminal nucleus cross the midline to join the ventral trigeminothalamic tract and terminate in the contralateral thalamus. A few ascending trigeminal axons remain uncrossed and travel in the dorsal trigeminothalamic tract to reach the ipsilateral thalamus; they represent the region around the mouth that receives bilateral representation in each thalamic hemisphere. The segregation of function between the chief sensory and spinal trigeminal nuclei is incomplete; the chief sensory nucleus, along with the spinal trigeminal nucleus, processes some information from group **IV** (pain) afferent fibers.

CLINICAL DEFICIT

Lesion of the chief sensory nucleus can result in loss of discriminatory touch, vibratory sense, two-point discrimination, and stereognosis in the ipsilateral face; however, these lesions can also produce some analgesia. An extremely restricted hemorrhage in the dorsolateral pons in the area of the chief trigeminal sensory nucleus has been reported and documented with CT scan.[16] The patient presented with facial numbness featuring analgesia and hypoesthesia in the V^2 and V^3 dermatomes.

TRIGEMINAL MOTOR NUCLEUS (TriMoNu)

The trigeminal motor nucleus (TriMoNu) is a cluster of large neurons medial to the chief sensory nucleus (see Fig. 4-6). This motor nucleus receives primary afferent fibers from the ipsilateral mesencephalic trigeminal nucleus and bilateral input from the

cerebral cortex (corticonuclear fibers). The axons of these motoneurons leave the pons in the trigeminal nerve and innervate the ipsilateral muscles of mastication.

CLINICAL DEFICIT

Destruction of this nucleus or its radiations causes paralysis of the ipsilateral muscles of mastication. This is seen clinically as deviation of the jaw to the weakened side with attempted opening under resistance. Bilateral supranuclear lesions of the corticonuclear fibers can result in paresis of the jaw with hyperactive jaw-jerk reflex[11] (an example being pseudobulbar palsy where bilateral degeneration of the corticonuclear fibers can result in elevation of the jaw-jerk reflex).

SUPERIOR OLIVE (MSO, LSO)

The superior olive can be resolved into several nuclei, two of which are illustrated on this plate: the medial (MSO) and lateral (LSO) superior olivary nuclei (also see Fig. 4-5). The medial superior olivary nucleus is most responsive to low-frequency sounds and is involved in localizing sound at the low end of the frequency spectrum. Conversely, the lateral superior olive is more responsive to the higher frequencies and is involved in localizing sound at the high end of the acoustic spectrum.[17] The results of damage in and around the area of the superior olivary nuclei have been discussed (see p. 83).

LATERAL LEMNISCUS (TRACT AND NUCLEI) (LL)

The lateral lemniscus (LL) is a prominent fiber bundle passing rostrally from the superior olivary complex, along the lateral aspect of the brain stem, into the inferior colliculus (see Plate 17 and Fig. 4-5). This fiber tract represents a major ascending pathway in the auditory system. Embedded in the fiber tract are the nuclei of the lateral lemniscus (see Plate 16), which act as a relay for some of the ascending auditory fibers in passage to the midbrain and thalamus.

CLINICAL DEFICIT

Unilateral section of lateral lemniscus diminishes hearing bilaterally; however, the loss is greatest from the contralateral ear. Lesions in the pons in close juxtaposition with the lateral lemniscus can produce auditory hallucinations.[10]

PARAMEDIAN PONTINE RETICULAR FORMATION (PPRF)

The paramedian pontine reticular formation (PPRF) is a specialized region of the pontine reticular formation defined more by function than by cytology. It is an elongated cluster of cells located ventral to the medial longitudinal fasciculus and extending between the oculomotor–trochlear complex and the abducens nucleus; its exact boundaries have not been determined. It receives bilateral afferent projections from the cerebral cortex (frontal eye fields), from the contralateral superior colliculus, and from the ipsilateral vestibular nuclei. Its efferent connections control the ipsilateral abducens nucleus and the rostral interstitial nucleus of the medial longitudinal fasciculus in the midbrain (see Plate 20). The paramedian pontine reticular formation coordinates conjugate horizontal eye movements.[18]

CLINICAL DEFICIT

Damage to the paramedian pontine reticular formation presents as loss of ipsilateral conjugate horizontal gaze, called **horizontal gaze paresis** or lateral gaze palsy.[19] The patient can look into the contralateral hemisphere but cannot volitionally deviate the globes into the ipsilateral visual hemisphere. Since gaze remains conjugate, the patient should not experience diplopia. Horizontal gaze paresis can also result from damage of the contralateral corticonuclear fibers to the paramedian pontine reticular formation.

CORTICOSPINAL TRACT (CST)

The corticospinal tract (CST) originates the cerebral cortex and projects through the internal capsule (see Plates 21 to 25), crus cerebri (see Plates 19 and 20), and brain stem to decussate at the cervicomedullary junction (see Plate 6) and enter the spinal cord, terminating in the ventral horn (see Plates 1 to 4). Throughout its brain stem course it is topographically arranged with the upper-extremity representation located nearest the midline. As the tract passes through the basilar pons, it separates into numerous, small fascicles, which rejoin in the pyramidal tract of the medulla. The corticospinal tract is involved with volitional control of fine motor behavior, especially with respect to novel movements.[20]

CLINICAL DEFICIT

According to classic neurology, lesions affecting the corticospinal tracts in the human brain stem can present initially with contralateral flaccidity, mainly affecting the muscles of the distal portions of the extremities. With time, the affected limbs resolve into a spastic condition. There is considerable confusion concerning this concept in the literature. An opposing view claims that lesions truly confined to the corticospinal tract will present with mild hypotonia (reviewed in Davidoff[21]). Chapter 3 discusses the clinical presentation subsequent to corticospinal tract sections further.

Review Structures From Preceding Plates

Identify the following structures from previous sections:

Lateral vestibular nucleus (LVNu)

Medial vestibular nucleus (MVNu)

Superior vestibular nucleus (SVNu)

Spinal trigeminal nucleus and tract (SpTNu, SpTT)

Trapezoid body and nucleus (TrapB)

Medial lemniscus (ML)

Medial longitudinal fasciculus (MLF)

Anterolateral system (ALS)

Rubrospinal tract (RuSp)

Ventral spinocerebellar tract (VSCT)

Middle cerebellar peduncle (MCP)

Inferior cerebellar peduncle (ICP)

Superior cerebellar peduncle (SCP)

Central tegmental tract (CTT)

Radiations of the facial nerve (FacNr)

Dorsal longitudinal fasciculus (DLF)

▷ **Atlas Plate 15**

The dorsal portion of this section transects the pontomesencephalic border, whereas the ventral portion passes through the basilar pons. Prominent features of this section are the well-developed pontocerebellar fibers and middle cerebellar peduncle, the shift in position of the superior cerebellar peduncles to form the walls of the fourth ventricle, and the tapering of these walls to form the cerebral aqueduct.

CENTRAL GRAY (CeGy)

The central, or periaqueductal, gray (CeGy) extends out of the pons along the cerebral aqueduct to reach the caudal thalamus (see Plates 16 to 20). This is a continuation of the band of gray matter that surrounds the rostral end of the central canal of the spinal cord (see Plate 6) and that is extended around the obex along the floor of the fourth ventral. Numerous structures are embedded in the central gray, such as the vagal nuclei, locus coeruleus, and vestibular nuclei. Rostral portions of the central gray are known to contain neurons with opiate receptors and axons that innervate the raphe nuclei of the brain stem. In turn, raphe nuclei give rise to the raphe-spinal tract, which can modulate the activity of the anterolateral system in the dorsal horn of the spinal cord. This network of descending projections mediates opiate-dependent control of pain input through the spinal cord.[22]

Portions of the central gray may also play a role in the motor system, especially control over vocalizations and certain types of eye movements. Other studies suggest additional functions in the limbic system involving sexual behavior, rage, and fear reactions. Finally, the central gray also appears to have a role in the control of the autonomic nervous system (reviewed in Beitz[23]).

CLINICAL DEFICIT

Although there is not yet a well-accepted clinical sign related to lesions of the central gray, its destruction in monkeys can increase their sensitivity to painful stimuli. Depression of the chemical systems in the central gray decreases the threshold of pain in volunteer human subjects.[22]

LOCUS COERULEUS (LoCer)

The locus coeruleus (LoCer) is a small cluster of cells on the inferiolateral angle of the central gray, extending from the pontomesencephalic border, rostrally into the midbrain (see Plate 16). Its neurons produce norepinephrine, and their axons have wide-ranging projections reaching most portions of the central neuraxis.

The locus coeruleus is involved in learning and reinforcement processes, the sleep–wake cycle, and nociception,[24] as well as in influencing such emotional states as anxiety and depression by altering endocrine functions.[25] As such, this nucleus has been implicated in a "behavioral inhibition system" that offers protection by using anxiety to inhibit specific behaviors while increasing arousal and attention (reviewed in Gray[26]).

CLINICAL DEFICIT

Small lesions of the locus coeruleus in primates can reduce their anxietylike behavior. Pharmaceutical suppression of neural activity in the locus coeruleus is used to modify anxiety in humans (reviewed by Aston-Jones[24]).

Recently, the neurons of the locus coeruleus have been demonstrated to undergo age-related changes in number and morphology. These alterations can be greatly exacerbated in neurodegenerative diseases such as Alzheimer-type senile dementia and Parkinson's disease.[27,28]

RAPHE COMPLEX (RaNu)

The raphe complex (RaNu) extends along the midline of the brain stem from medulla (see Plate 11), through pons to midbrain (see Plate 18). It is composed of a cluster of nuclei related to each other in their production of the neurotransmitter serotonin. The pontine raphe nuclei project serotonergic axons to the dorsal horn of the spinal cord and the spinal trigeminal nucleus of the caudal brain stem. In both targets, raphe axons terminate on enkephalinergic cells that can inhibit transmission in the pain pathways. Through these projections, the raphe nuclei play a role in mediating opiate-dependent control over nociception.[22]

CLINICAL DEFICIT

Specific lesions of the raphe system have not been documented in the clinical literature. However, pharmaceutical suppression of the raphe-spinal and trigeminal systems will decrease the threshold of pain in volunteer subjects.[22]

VENTRAL TRIGEMINOTHALAMIC TRACT (VTTr)

The ventral trigeminothalamic tract (VTTr) contains ascending fibers from the contralateral spinal trigeminal nucleus (Fig. 4-6). The tract courses in close juxtaposition with the medial lemniscus to reach the thalamus, where it terminates in the ventroposterior medial nucleus (see Plate 21). It contains fibers carrying the modalities of crude touch, pain, and thermal sense from the face.

CLINICAL DEFICIT

Section of the ventral trigeminothalamic tract can result in the loss of crude touch, pain, and thermal sensation from the contralateral face. Note that since the tract has crossed the midline before reaching the pons, its deficit is now in register with that of damage to the anterolateral system (loss of crude touch, pain, and thermal sensation from the contralateral body). Consequently, unilateral pontine lesions affecting both tracts present with diminished sensation across the contralateral face and body.[7] This is in contrast to laterally placed lesions in the medulla that affect the spinal trigeminal nucleus (ipsilateral deficit) and anterolateral tract (contralateral deficit), producing alternating analgesia (see Chap. 3)

VENTROSPINOCEREBELLAR TRACT (VSCT)

The ventral spinocerebellar tract (VSCT) has shifted from its ventrolateral position on previous sections (see Plates 3 to 14) and is rising toward the superior cerebellar peduncle. In the caudal midbrain, it joins the peduncle and passes into the cerebellum.

RADIATIONS OF THE TRIGEMINAL NERVE (TriNr)

Fibers of the trigeminal nerve (TriNr) pass through the middle cerebellar peduncle to reach the trigeminal nuclei in the pontine tegmentum (see Fig. 4-6). This nerve contains primary afferent fibers from sensory receptors in the ipsilateral face as well as efferent axons from the trigeminal motor nucleus to the ipsilateral muscles of mastication. Additional information concerning this structure and its dysfunction is presented on pp. 83, 86, and 90 (see Chap. 3).

Review Structures From Preceding Plates
Identify the following structures from previous sections:

Trigeminal motor nucleus (TriMoNu)

Trigeminal sensory nucleus (CSNu)

Pontine nuclei (PonNu)

Corticospinal tract (CST)

Medial lemniscus (ML)

Medial longitudinal fasciculus (MLF)

Anterolateral system (ALS)

Rubrospinal tract (RuSp)

Middle cerebellar peduncle (MCP)

Superior cerebellar peduncle (SCP)

Central tegmental tract (CTT)

Pontocerebellar fibers (PCeF)

Dorsal longitudinal fasciculus (DLF)

▷ Atlas Plate 16

The ventral portion of this section passes through the midpons; the dorsal portion passes through the caudal midbrain. Its salient features are the exit of the trigeminal nerve from the lateral aspect of the basilar pons and the reduction in size of the fourth ventricle as it tapers to form the cerebral aqueduct. The midbrain structures will be discussed in Chapter 6.

SUPERIOR CEREBELLAR PEDUNCLE (SCP)

The ventral border of the superior cerebellar peduncle (SCP) has begun to curl medialward; this is the first sign of the impending decussation of the superior cerebellar peduncle that will occur in the midbrain (see Plate 18; additional information concerning this structure is presented on p. 83).

LATERAL LEMNISCUS AND NUCLEI (LL, LLNu)

The lateral lemniscus (LL) and its associated nuclei (LLNu) have shifted dorsally into a position lateral to the superior cerebellar peduncle. Here it will remain until reaching the base of the inferior colliculus in the midbrain (see Plate 17; additional information concerning this structures is presented on p. 86).

TRIGEMINAL NERVE (TriNr)

The root of the trigeminal nerve (TriNr) is seen exiting the ventrolateral aspect of the basilar pons (see Fig. 4-6). Contained within these fibers are the ophthalmic, maxillary, and mandibular divisions of the sensory root and the motor root to the muscles of mastication.

CLINICAL DEFICIT

Damage to the radiations of the trigeminal nerve or to the trigeminal root in its preganglionic course can result in the loss of sensation, paresthesia, or numbness from the ipsilateral face, loss of the corneal reflex, and flaccid paralysis of the ipsilateral muscles of mastication. This presentation can be accompanied by signs of damage to surrounding structures, such as ataxia (middle cerebellar peduncle), nystagmus (cerebellum), vertigo (vestibular system), tinnitus (auditory system), and facial palsy (facial nerve).[11]

CORTICONUCLEAR FIBERS (CoNF)

Axons from the cerebral cortex innervate most of the brain stem nuclei. Collectively, these axons are called the **corticonuclear fibers (CoNF)** and mediate cerebral control over the brain stem functions. Corticonuclear fibers begin leaving the crus cerebri medially as this massive fiber bundle enters the midbrain (see Plate 19). Specific names are given to these corticonuclear fibers contingent on their brain stem targets: Corticomesencephalic fibers innervate the midbrain, corticopontine fibers innervate the pons, and corticomedullary fibers innervate the medulla (Fig. 4-7).

CLINICAL DEFICIT

The results of a lesion in the corticonuclear fibers are complex because of the varying innervation patterns that these fibers establish. The portions of the brain stem controlling horizontal eye movements (paramedian pontine reticular formation) receive a contralateral corticonuclear input; hence, unilateral lesions can result in horizontal gaze palsies involving the side opposite the lesion. The trigeminal motor nucleus and nucleus ambiguus, as well as structures controlling the oculomotor nucleus, receive bilateral corticonuclear innervation. Hence, they experience more subtle deficits in unilateral lesions of these fibers. The neurons of the hypoglossal nucleus innervating the genioglossus muscle of the tongue receive a contralateral cortical input. Consequently, the tongue can exhibit weakness following unilateral corticonuclear lesions. The corticonuclear innervation of the facial nucleus has already been presented (pp. 78–79).

Extensive vascular damage to the ventral pons, interrupting the corticospinal and corticonuclear tracts bilaterally, can produce the "locked-in syndrome."[8,29] The patient is unable to move extremities or truncal musculature due to the loss of the corticospinal fibers and cannot control muscles innervated by the trigeminal or facial nerves because of loss of the corticonuclear fibers. Communication with such an akinetic and mute patient can be obtained through the only remaining muscles they can move, those controlled by the oculomotor nucleus. As such, these vertical eye movements have been used to establish that the patient is not unconscious.

Review Structures From Preceding Plates

Identify the following structures from previous sections:

Locus coeruleus (LoCer)

Raphe complex (central superior) (RaNu)

Pontine reticular formation (PRetF)

Pontine nuclei (PonNu)

Corticospinal tract (CST)

Medial lemniscus (ML)

Medial longitudinal fasciculus (MLF)

Anterolateral system (ALS)

Rubrospinal tract (RuSp)

Middle cerebellar peduncle (MCP)

Superior cerebellar peduncle (SCP)

Central tegmental tract (CTT)

Dorsal longitudinal fasciculus (DLF)

Pontocerebellar fibers (PCeF)

Ventral trigeminothalamic fibers (VTTr)

▷ Atlas Plates 17 to 20

Although Atlas Plates 17 to 20 mainly concern the midbrain, portions of the ventral pons are also represented. The prominent features are the massive ponto-

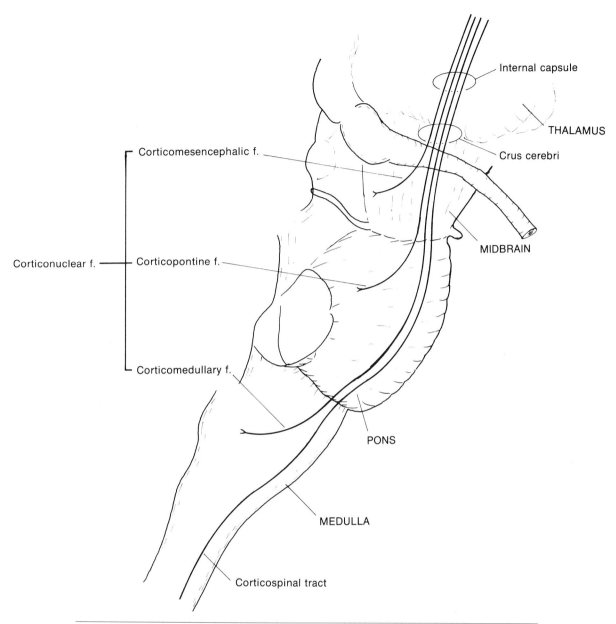

Figure 4-7. This diagram illustrates the corticonuclear fibers overlaid on a lateral view of the brain stem.

cerebellar fibers, the pontine nuclei, and the condensation of the corticospinal and corticonuclear fibers to form the crus cerebri. The midbrain structures will be considered in Chapter 6.

CORTICOPONTINE FIBERS (CoPF)

The pontine nuclei receive input from many areas of the ipsilateral cerebral cortex. Specific components of these corticopontine fibers (CoPF) are named based on their origin in the cortex: frontopontine, occipitopontine, parietopontine, and temporopontine. The frontopontine fibers travel in the ventral-most portion of the crus cerebri and are the first to innervate the pontine nuclei. The projections from other regions of the cortex are contained in the dorsal portion of the crus cerebri (see Chap. 6).

CLINICAL DEFICIT
Lesions of the corticopontine fibers in the pons as well as in the internal capsule have presented with

contralateral ataxia.[30] Accompanying damage to the corticospinal axons can result in a spastic hemiparesis expressed in the ataxic limb; this is called *ataxic hemiparesis*.[1] If the locus of damage is above the corticospinal fibers in the paramedian basilar pons, the resulting loss of corticopontine fibers can be expressed as dysarthria with an accompanying clumsy (ataxic) hand but with no observable paresis.[31]

Review Structures From Preceding Plates

Identify the following structures from previous sections:

Pontine nuclei (PonNu)

Corticospinal tract (CST)

Middle cerebellar peduncle (MCP)

UNIT B

Case Study 4-2

A 49-year-old with facial paralysis, limb ataxia, and sensory loss

A 49-year-old, right-handed hypertensive patient called his physician after experiencing a brief loss of consciousness while taking his morning shower. He reported that he had suffered severe headaches over the prior 24-hour period and now finds it difficult to walk because his left leg is clumsy. He is also complaining of dizziness and a loud, roaring sound in his left ear. After arranging for his transportation, the physician met him at the emergency room in the community hospital.

Past Medical History

The patient is married, with two children, and works as a salesman for a large pharmaceutical company. He has been diagnosed as hypertensive for 10 years and has been controlled under a physician's care for much of the time. He is a heavy smoker (25-pack-year history) and consumes 2 to 3 ounces of alcohol daily.

General Physical Examination

He was awake, oriented, communicative, and concerned with his problem. He was well nourished, well hydrated, and appeared the stated age. Small hemorrhages were present on the retinal discs. The external auditory canal was patent and clear. Pharynx and larynx were nonreddened. The chest was clear to auscultation, blood pressure was elevated (163/102), and pulse rate and respirations were normal. Peripheral pulses were intact at the ankles and wrists; normal tissue turgor was present. Abdomen was soft, with no masses or tenderness. No lymphadenopathy was detected in the cervical, axillary, or inguinal regions.

Neurologic Examination

Mental Status.   He was oriented to time and place, with no defect in memory, reading, or writing. Speech was dysarthric but fluent and meaningful. Word comprehension was good, and he could follow three- and four-step commands.

Cranial Nerves.   His visual fields are complete, and he has a full range of eye movements. Horizontal nystagmus was present bilaterally. His pupils were symmetric and reactive to light, both direct and consensual. Convergence movements in both eyes were intact. Hearing was markedly reduced in the left ear, and he had poor word discrimination ability in the left ear compared to that in the right. He complained of a vertiginous sensation of the world drifting around him. He had a dense analgesia for pinprick over most of his face on the left. Some loss of sensation for pinprick was also present on the right, but it was less dense than that on the left. Corneal reflex was absent on the left and weak on the right. Jaw-jerk was normal. Two-point discrimination and vibratory sense were normal throughout the face bilaterally. He had no tone in the facial muscles above or below the eye on the left. Creases in his forehead were asymmetric, and the right side wrinkled on an attempted smile. The left corner of his mouth was open 0.5 cm at rest, and the left eye would not shut completely on attempted blink or squint. Gag reflex was normal, and he denied any dysphagia. Although his speech was slurred, his voice had normal tone, volume, and emotion. His tongue protruded on the midline and appeared normal.

Motor Systems. Strength and reflexes were normal and symmetric in all four limbs, and plantar responses were flexor in both lower limbs. Finger-to-nose and heel-to-shin testing were normal on the right but grossly abnormal on the left side. Past pointing and dysmetria was present in the left limbs. A left drift was seen when the arms were outstretched.

Sensation. Two-point discrimination, vibratory sense, and proprioception were normal throughout the body. Pinprick and thermal sensations were normal on the left but absent on the right side of the face, arm, trunk, and leg.

QUESTIONS

1. Does the patient exhibit a language or memory deficit or an alteration in consciousness or cognition?

2. Are signs of cranial nerve dysfunction present?

3. Are there any changes in motor functions, such as reflexes, muscle tone, movement, or coordination?

4. Are any changes in sensory functions detectable?

5. At what level in the central neuraxis is this lesion most likely located?

6. Is the pathology focal, multifocal, or diffuse in its distribution within the nervous system?

7. What is the clinical–temporal profile of this pathology: acute or chronic; progressive or stable?

8. Based on your answers to the previous two questions, decide whether the symptoms in this patient are most likely caused by a vascular accident, a tumor, or a degenerative or inflammatory process.

9. If you feel this is the result of a vascular accident, what vessels are most likely involved?

► DISCUSSION
Pontine Vasculature

ARTERIAL DISTRIBUTION

The pons can be divided into three vascular perfusion zones: anterior, lateral, and posterior.[32] Each of these zones is serviced by branches of the basilar artery.

Anterior Zone

The anterior vascular zone is perfused by small branches of the basilar artery that quickly penetrate the basilar pons and extend upward along the midline. Two groups of anterior branches are recognized. The *anteromedial* (or paramedian) branches extend posteriorly to reach the floor of the fourth ventricle, thus supplying the corticospinal tract, medial lemniscus, medial longitudinal fasciculus, and abducens nucleus. The *anterolateral* (or short circumferential) branches penetrate through the corticospinal tract, ending in the pontine nuclei and pontocerebellar fibers.

Lateral Zone

The lateral vascular zone is perfused by penetrating branches from two groups of vessels: the pontine arteries (or long circumferential arteries) and the anterior inferior cerebellar artery. These are branches from the basilar artery and supply the lateral half of the pons, including the lateral lemniscus; anterolateral system; the trigeminal, fascial, and vestibular nuclei; and the middle cerebellar peduncles. Some of the penetrating branches of the lateral zone also service the lateral aspect of the corticospinal tract.

A small infarction in the lateral vascular zone at the pontomedullary junction was recently reported.[33] The extent of the infarction was confirmed with magnetic resonance imaging. The patient presented with dysarthria, staggering gait, diminished handwriting capability, and ipsilateral appendicular ataxia, all of which could result from damage to the inferior (or caudal portion of the middle) cerebellar peduncle. In addition, the patient displayed ipsilateral facial weakness from damage to the radiations of the facial nerve, nystagmus and ocular overshoot from damage to the vestibular structures, and sensory dissociation of pain and temperature over the contralateral hemibody from damage to the anterolateral system. Since the anterior vascular zone was not involved, there was **no** paresis (corticospinal tract) and **no** loss of discriminative sensory capabilities (medial lemniscus).

Posterior Zone

The posterior vascular zone is small and restricted to the rostral end of the pons. It is supplied by penetrating branches of the superior cerebellar artery and perfuses the tissue surrounding the superior cerebellar peduncle.

ANASTOMOSIS

The basilar artery, which arises from the fusion of the two vertebral arteries, plays a key role in the circulation of the pons; however, it is not the sole source of ascending perfusion in all cases. Anastomosis of the posterior and anterior cerebellar arteries with the superior cerebellar artery can, in some individuals, sup-

ply blood to the rostral end of the basilar artery when occlusion has occurred in its middle segment.[34]

ARTERIAL SYNDROMES

Most cerebrovascular accidents in the pons are large and devastating in their presentation. Significant occlusion of the basilar artery or a large hemorrhage into the central portion of the pons results in bilateral damage and presents with a triad of neurologic signs: *coma, quadriplegia,* and *ocular paresis* followed by lethal demise.[35] Unilateral hemorrhage into the pons has been documented, and survival in this situation is much greater than that in the bilateral hemorrhages.[7] The hemipontine syndromes present with hemiparesis, hemisensory loss, and signs of unilateral involvement of cranial nerves V through VIII, but consciousness can be preserved.

Small lacunar infarctions, although rare can be restricted to the anterior or lateral vascular zones of the pons, thus creating *medial* and *lateral pontine syndromes.* Although usually not lethal, these syndromes can contain a myriad of neurologic deficits (Tables 4-1 and 4-2).

Table 4-1.
Possible Origins of Neurologic Signs in the Medial Medullary Syndrome

NEUROLOGIC SIGN	ANATOMIC SOURCE
ON CONTRALATERAL SIDE	
Spastic paralysis	Pontine corticospinal tract
Limb ataxia	Pontine nuclei or transverse pontine fibers
Hypoesthesia in arm	Medial border of medial lemniscus
ON IPSILATERAL SIDE	
Diplopia on lateral gaze	Abducens nerve
Horizontal gaze palsy (involuntary)	Abducens nucleus or paramedian pontine reticular formation
Horizontal gaze palsy (voluntary)	Paramedian pontine reticular formation
Intranuclear ophthalmoplegia	Medial longitudinal fasciculus

(*Adapted from Caplan LR, Posterior cerebral artery syndromes. Hdbk Clin Neurol 1988;53(9): 409; and Adams RD, Victor M. Principles of neurology. New York: McGraw-Hill 1989; Chap. 34*)

Table 4-2.
Possible Origins of Neurologic Signs in the Lateral Pontine Syndrome

NEUROLOGIC SIGN	ANATOMIC SOURCE
ON CONTRALATERAL SIDE	
Analgesia of body	Anterolateral tract
Analgesia of face	Ventral trigeminothalamic tract
Hypoesthesia of body	Medial lemniscus
ON IPSILATERAL SIDE	
Hypoesthesia of face	Chief sensory trigeminal nucleus
Horizontal gaze palsy	Paramedian pontine reticular formation
Paralysis of jaw	Trigeminal motor nucleus
Facial paralysis	Facial nucleus or nerve
Limb ataxia	Middle cerebellar peduncle
Vertigo/nystagmus	Vestibular nerve or nuceli
Deafness/tinnitus	Auditory nerve or nuclei

(Adapted from Caplan LR, Posterior cerebral artery syndromes. Hdbk Clin Neurol 1988;53(9):409; and Adams RD, Victor M. Principles of neurology. New York: McGraw-Hill 1989; Chap. 34)

The *medial pontine syndrome* results when disease occludes the paramedian branches of the basilar artery. Damage can be done to the corticospinal tract, transverse pontine fibers, abducens nerve or nucleus, medial longitudinal fasciculus, and portions of the medial lemniscus, particularly the region of arm representation. The patient presentation can involve any or all of the signs listed in Table 4–1.

The *lateral pontine syndrome* results when a vascular accident occurs in the lateral zone, usually perfused by the anterior inferior cerebellar artery. Damage can be done to the middle cerebellar peduncle, anterolateral tract, ventral trigeminothalamic tract, trigeminal nuclei or nerve, facial nerve, and vestibular and cochlear nuclei, as well as the paramedian pontine reticular formation.[36] The neurologic signs presented in this syndrome are listed in Table 4–2. Not all signs have to be present, since the size of the infarction may vary considerably; thus, partial syndromes can occur. Medial branches from this zone can also penetrate into the corticospinal tract; therefore, contralateral hemiparesis can accompany the neurologic sequelae listed in Table 4-2.

The salient signs of the lateral pontine syndrome are loss of nociception from hemiface and body, hemi-

ataxia, and cranial nerve palsies. This syndrome complex can be classified further along the rostral–caudal axis of the brain stem based on the cranial nerve structures involved. Lateral *inferior* pontine lesions involve the facial nucleus or nerve; the sensory loss is in the form of alternating analgesia. Lateral *midpontine* lesions involve the trigeminal motor nucleus or nerve, and the sensory loss can involve bilateral analgesia of the face, being more dense on the ipsilateral side. This is due to involvement of the spinal trigeminal system on the ipsilateral side and the ventral trigeminothalamic fibers from the contralateral side. Lateral *superior* pontine lesions can occur without involving a cranial motor nerve or nucleus, but they infringe on the lateral aspect of medial lemniscus (see Plate 15), thus producing loss of discriminative touch in the lower extremities. Since the lesion can affect the ventral trigeminothalamic fibers and the anterolateral system, analgesia presents contralateral to the lesion.

A specific subset of the lateral pontine lesion is called Foville's syndrome. It features facial palsy and lateral gaze palsy on the side of the lesion. This is accompanied by a mild, crossed hemiparesis but involves no overt loss of discriminative touch or vibratory sense. This occurs consequent to occlusion of a long circumferential branch from the basilar artery (see Plate 13). The branch supplies the lateral aspect of corticospinal tract before arching dorsally into the pontine tegmentum to end by perfusing the area around the facial nucleus and pontine reticular formation (including its paramedian region). Since these branches can pass lateral to the medial lemniscus, there can be no affect on discriminative touch.

Comparison of Tables 4-1 and 4-2 reveals that horizontal gaze palsies can appear in both medial and lateral pontine syndromes. This results from the fact that the paramedian pontine reticular formation and its corticonuclear fibers lie in the overlap between anterior and lateral perfusion zones.

COMPRESSION SYNDROMES

Cranial nerves span the subarachnoid space between the brain stem and the basicranium. They are accompanied in this space by cerebral vessels; specific relationships are of interest because of the possibility of compression lesions. The trigeminal nerve is in close juxtaposition with the superior cerebellar, anterior inferior cerebellar, and basilar arteries. The sixth, seventh, and eighth cranial nerves are closely related to the anterior inferior cerebellar artery and sometimes to the posterior inferior cerebellar artery. These vessels are capable of exerting pressure on the associated nerves. This situation is exacerbated as the vessel becomes more tortuous with age and as the aging brain stem sags along the clivus.[37] Pressure or irritation to these cranial nerves can present as trigeminal neuralgia, hemifacial spasm, deafness, vertigo, or facial paralysis.[38]

► Bibliography

Adams RD, Victor M. Disorders of ocular movement and pupillary function. In: Principles of neurology. New York: McGraw-Hill, 1989; Chap. 13:206–225.

Adams RD, Victor M. Deafness, dizziness and disorders of equilibrium. In: Disorders of ocular movement and pupillary function. In: Principles of neurology. New York: McGraw-Hill, 1989; Chap. 14:226–246.

Adams RD, Victor M. Cerebrovascular diseases. In: Disorders of ocular movement and pupillary function. In: Principles of neurology. New York: McGraw-Hill, 1989; Chap. 34:617–692.

Barr ML, Kiernan JA. Brain stem external anatomy. In: The human nervous system: an anatomical viewpoint. Philadelphia: JB Lippincott, 1988; Chap. 6:84–91.

Barr ML, Kiernan JA. Brain stem nuclei and tracts. In: The human nervous system: an anatomical viewpoint. Philadelphia: JB Lippincott, 1988; Chap. 7:92–120.

Barr ML, Kiernan JA. Cranial nerves. In: The human nervous system: an anatomical viewpoint. Philadelphia: JB Lippincott, 1988; Chap. 8:121–147.

Barr ML, Kiernan JA. Reticular formation. In: The human nervous system: an anatomical viewpoint. Philadelphia: JB Lippincott, 1988; Chap. 9:148–159.

Barr ML, Kiernan JA. Auditory system. In: The human nervous system: an anatomical viewpoint. Philadelphia: JB Lippincott, 1988; Chap. 21:312–324.

Barr ML, Kiernan JA. Vestibular system. In: The human nervous system: an anatomical viewpoint. Philadelphia: JB Lippincott, 1988; Chap. 22:325–333.

Brazis PW, Masdeu JC, Biller J. Localization in clinical neurology. Boston: Little, Brown, 1990.

Daube JR, Ragan TJ, Sandok BA, Westmoreland BF. The posterior cranial fossa level. In: Medical neurosciences. Boston: Little, Brown, 1986; Chap. 14:260–295.

Haines DE. Neuroanatomy: an atlas of structures, sections, and systems. Baltimore: Urban & Schwarzenberg, 1987 *(see especially Figs. 5-16 to 5-20).*

Nieuwenhuys R, Voogd J, van Huijzen, C. The human central nervous system. Berlin: Springer-Verlag, 1988:144–220.

► References

1. Fisher CM. Ataxic hemiparesis. Arch Neurol 1978;35:126.
2. Masdeu JC, Brazis PW. The localization of lesions in the ocular motor system. In: Brazis PW, Masdeu JC, Biller J, eds. Localization in clinical neurology. Boston: Little, Brown, 1990:127–187.
3. Brazis PW. The localization of lesions affecting cranial nerve VII (the facial nerve). In: Brazis PW, Masdeu JC, Biller J, eds. Localization in clinical neurology. Boston: Little, Brown, 1990:203–218.
4. Parker W, Decker R, Richards NG. Auditory function and lesions of the pons. Arch Otolaryngol 1968;87:26.
5. Biller J, Brazis PW. The localization of lesions affecting cranial nerve VIII (the vestibulocochlear nerve). In: Brazis PW, Masdeu JC, Biller J, eds. Localization in clinical neurology. Boston: Little, Brown, 1990:219–237.
6. Autret A, Laffont F, de Toffol B, Cathala HP. A syndrome of REM and non-REM sleep reduction and lateral gaze paresis after medial tegmental pontine stroke. Arch Neurol 1988;45:1236.
7. Kushner MJ, Bressman SB. The clinical manifestations of pontine hemorrhage. Neurology 1985;35(5):636.
8. Plum F, Posner JB. The diagnosis of stupor and coma. Philadelphia: FA Davis, 1982:377.
9. Jenkins WM, Masterton, RB. Sound localization: effects of unilateral lesions in central auditory system. J Neurophysiol 1982;47:987.
10. Cascino GD, Adams RD. Brainstem auditory hallucinosis. Neurology 1986;36:1042.
11. Brazis PW. The localization of lesions affecting cranial nerve V (the trigeminal nerve). In: Brazis PW, Masdeu JC, Biller J, eds. Localization in clinical neurology. Boston: Little, Brown, 1990:198–218.
12. Olszewski J, Baxter D. Cytoarchitecture of the human brain stem, 2nd ed. Basel: S Karger, 1982.
13. Fisher CM. Lacunar strokes and infarcts: a review. Neurology 1982;32:871.
14. Nabatame H, Fukuyama H, Akiguchi I, Kameyama M, Nishimura K, Torizuka K. Pontine ataxic hemiparesis studied by a high-resolution magnetic resonance imaging system. Ann Neurol 1987;21:204.
15. Keane J. Bilateral sixth nerve palsy. Arch Neurol 1976;33:681.
16. Holtzman RN, Zablozki V, Yang WC, Leeds NE. Lateral pontine tegmental hemorrhage presenting as isolated trigeminal sensory neuropathy. Neurology 1987;37(4):704.
17. Brugge JF, Geisler CD. Auditory mechanisms of the lower brainstem. Ann Rev Neurosci 1978;1:363.
18. Bender MB. Brain control of conjugate horizontal and vertical eye movements. A survey of the structural and function correlates. Brain 1980;103:23.
19. Goebel H, Komatsuzaki A, Bender M, Cohen B. Lesions of the pontine tegmentum and conjugate gaze paralysis. Arch Neurol 1971;24:431.
20. Kennedy PR. Corticospinal, rubrospinal, and rubro-olivary projections: a unifying hypothesis. Trends Neurosci 1990;13:474.
21. Davidoff RA. The pyramidal tract. Neurology 1990;40:332.
22. Basbaum AI, Fields HL. Endogenous pain control mechanisms: review and hypothesis. Ann Neurol 1978;4:451.
23. Beitz AL. Central gray. In: Paximos G, eds. The human nervous system. San Diego: Academic Press, 1990:307–329.
24. Aston-Jones G, Foote S, Bloom FE. Anatomy and physiology of locus coeruleus neurons: functional implications. In: Ziegler MG, Lake CR, eds. Norepinephrine. Baltimore: Williams & Wilkins, 1984.
25. Gold PW, Goodwin FK, Chrousos GP. Clinical and biochemical manifestations of depression: relation to the neurobiology of stress. N Engl J Med 1988;319:348.
26. Gray JA. The neuropsychology of anxiety. Oxford: Claredon Press, 1982.
27. Chan-Palay V, Asan E. Quantitation of catecholamine neurons in the locus coeruleus in human brains of normal young and older adults and in depression. J Comp Neurol 1989;287:357.

28. Chan-Palay V, Asan E. Alterations in catecholamine neurons of the locus coeruleus in senile dementia of the alzheimer type and in parkinson's disease with and without dementia and depression. J Comp Neurol 1989;287:373.

29. Kemper TL, Romanul FC. State resembling akinetic mutism in basilar artery occlusion. Neurology 1967;17(1):74.

30. Helweg-Larsen S, Larsson H, Henriksen O, Sorensen PS. Ataxic hemiparesis: three different locations of lesions studied by MRI. Neurology 1988;38:1322.

31. Glass JD, Levey AI, Rothstein JD. The dysarthria–clumsy hand syndrome: a distinct clinical entity related to pontine infarction. Ann Neurol 1990;27:487.

32. Duvernoy HM. Human brainstem vessels. Berlin: Springer-Verlag, 1978.

33. Fisher CM. Lacunar infarct of the tegmentum of the lower lateral pons. Arch Neurol 1989;46:566.

34. Caplan LR. Posterior cerebral artery syndromes. Handbook Clin Neurol 1988;53(9):409.

35. Fisher CM. Clinical syndromes in cerebral hemorrhage. In: Fields WS, ed. Pathogenesis and treatment of cerebrovascular disease. Springfield, IL: Charles C Thomas, 1961:318–342.

36. Amarenco P, Hauw J-J. Cerebellar infarction in the territory of the superior cerebellar artery: a clinicopathologic study of 33 cases. Neurology 1990;40:1383.

37. Jannetta PJ. Neurovascular compression in cranial nerve and systemic disease. Ann Surg 1980;192:518.

38. Escobedo F, Solis G. Vascular compression of cranial nerves at the posterior fossa. Adv Neurol 1979;25:243.

5 CEREBELLUM

► Introduction

The cerebellum is a large, foliated structure perched on the dorsal surface of the brain stem and forming the roof of the fourth ventricle. It is contained in the acute angle created by the brain stem and the ventral surface of the occipital lobes of the cerebrum. Since the cerebellum is located within the posterior cranial fossa and is separated from the occipital cortex by the tentorium cerebelli, it is by definition an infratentorial structure.

Three large-fiber bundles connect the cerebellum to the brain stem: the superior, middle, and inferior cerebellar peduncles. These peduncles contribute to the walls of the fourth ventricle. Blood supply to the cerebellum is derived from three branches of the vertebrobasilar system: superior, anterior inferior, and posterior inferior cerebellar arteries.

In this chapter the organization, connections, and cell structure of the cerebellum will be examined. The vasculature of the cerebellum will be studied and several clinicopathologic cases involving cerebellar lesions will be presented.

GENERAL OBJECTIVES

1. To define the main divisions of the cerebellum, relating them to specific patterns of afferent and efferent connections
2. To identify the functions of the main divisions of the cerebellum
3. To describe clinical signs and symptoms associated with disease in these cerebellar divisions

INSTRUCTIONS

In this chapter you will be presented with one or more clinical case studies. *Each study will be followed by a list of questions that can best be answered by using a knowledge of regional and functional neuroanatomy and by referring to outside reading material.* Following the questions will be a section devoted to structures from a specific region of the central nervous system. Before you attempt to answer the questions, compile a list of the patient's neurologic signs and symptoms; then examine the structures and their functions and study their known clinical deficits. After becoming familiar with the material, reexamine the list of neurologic signs and symptoms and formulate answers to the questions. Be aware that some of the questions can have multiple responses or require information beyond the scope of this manual. It may be necessary to obtain material or advice from additional resources, such as specialty texts, a medical dictionary, or clinical personnel.

MATERIALS

1. A model of the human brain stem
2. A whole human cerebellum and a cerebellum sectioned in the sagittal plane
3. A cerebellum and brain stem with intact vasculature

UNIT A

Case Study 5-1

A 36-year-old man with headaches and intention tremor

A 36-year-old attorney was referred with a chief complaint of headaches and vomiting. The patient had had frontal and biparietal headaches for approximately 1 month. These were precipitated by coughing, sneezing, or bending. On at least one occasion the patient had been awakened by a headache. He experienced nausea and vomiting independent of the headaches. At times, vomiting occurred suddenly without preceding nausea.

For several weeks prior to admission he had been unsteady on his feet with a tendency to fall to the right. He admitted to occasional clumsiness of his right hand. During the week prior to admission he had been excessively drowsy and constantly tired. The headaches had become more frequent, so that they were now occurring three to four times per day.

Past Medical History

His past medical history was unremarkable except for an episode of rheumatic fever at age 6.

Family and Social History

He was unmarried, lived alone, and was employed by a large law firm. His parents were alive and in good health; he had no siblings. He professed to be heterosexual and was involved in a monogamous relationship that had lasted for several years. He had a 10-pack-year history of smoking but had quit 6 years previously. He had been active in outdoor sports since age 31 and had been running up to 4 miles daily until 4 weeks before, when he had to quit because of an unsteady gait and headaches.

100

General Physical Examination

This was an awake, oriented, well-nourished, well-hydrated, and distressed man in considerable pain. He appeared the stated age and in otherwise good physical condition. His eyes had no cotton wool patches, but papilledema was evident. His chest was clear to auscultation and percussion; his abdomen was soft without lumps or masses. Blood pressure, pulse rate, temperature, and respirations were normal. Peripheral pulses were intact; no edema was present; and no cervical, axillary, or inguinal lymphadenopathy was detected.

Neurologic Examination

Mental Status.   He was awake and oriented with respect to person, place, and time. His memory and knowledge base were appropriate for his training. Speech was fluent and meaningful. He was a coherent historian.

Cranial Nerves.   His pupils were 3 to 4 mm in diameter and reactive to light, both direct and consensual. On funduscopic examination there was evidence of bilateral papilledema. Horizontal nystagmus in the direction of gaze was present on attempted lateral gaze to either side. He denied any double vision. Hearing was normal and equal in both ears. Corneal, jaw-jerk, and gag reflexes were intact. Facial expressions were full and symmetric. Uvula and tongue protruded on the midline. Shoulder shrug was symmetric.

Motor System.   His strength was intact in all extremities and his deep tendon reflexes were symmetric and physiologic. His plantar responses were flexor. The patient's gait was wide-based. When walking, he tended to veer to the right and was unable to stand on his right leg alone. Closing his eyes did not alter his instability on his right leg. He could stand comfortably on his left leg with his eyes open or shut. Significant intention tremor was present in the right upper extremity on finger-to-nose testing and in the right lower extremity on heel-to-shin testing. Alternating movements of the right hand were slow and disorganized (dysdiadochokinesia).

Sensory System.   Pinprick, two-point discrimination, vibratory sense, and proprioception were intact throughout body and face.

QUESTIONS

1. Does the patient exhibit a language or memory deficit or an alteration in consciousness or cognition?

2. Are signs of cranial nerve dysfunction present?

3. Are there any changes in motor functions, such as reflexes, muscle tone, movement, or coordination?

4. Are any changes in sensory functions detectable?

5. At what level in the central neuraxis is this lesion most likely located?

6. Is the pathology focal, multifocal, or diffuse in its distribution within the nervous system?

7. What is the clinical–temporal profile of this pathology: acute or chronic; progressive or stable?

8. Based on your answers to the previous two questions, decide whether the symptoms in this patient are most likely caused by a vascular accident, a tumor, or a degenerative or inflammatory process?

9. If you feel this is the result of a vascular accident, what vessels are most likely involved?

10. What events can cause papilledema?

11. What is the significance of the absence of Romberg's sign? Is it consistent with the rest of the motor tests?

Case Study 5-2

An 8-year-old girl with unsteady balance, nausea, and nystagmus

An 8-year-old girl was brought to the family physician by her mother because the child was "sick all the time" and had become "unsteady" when walking.

Past Medical History

The mother had had an uneventful pregnancy and delivery. At birth the child weighed 3.25 kg; by 5.5 months she could maintain a seated, upright posture, and she could roll over at 6 months of age. She could rise to a standing position and take several steps by 15 months and could climb stairs by 20 months. By 3 years of age she could stand on one foot, unassisted. For the next 4 years she was active in outdoor play. Seven months earlier, she had begun complaining of nausea frequently. She is still complaining of nausea, but she is also vomiting frequently. In the past 3 months, the child has begun walking unsteadily with a broad-based gait. When seated, she swayed from side to side and occasionally fell over. Her head rotated from side to side as her body swayed. The mother also noted that the child had recently become extremely irritable. No one else in her family had similar or related symptoms. All of her immunizations were current.

Family History

The mother was a social worker for the state and a single parent; the father has remarried. The child's maternal and paternal grandparents were in good health. The mother had a 12-pack-year history of smoking and smoked through the pregnancy; she denied any use of alcohol either at this time or during the pregnancy.

General Physical Examination

This was an awake, oriented child who was complaining of headaches and dizziness. Face and personality appeared the stated age, but she was underweight and lacked appropriate muscle mass. Edges of optic discs were blurred but lacked cotton wool patches or papilledema. Nystagmus was evident on lateral gaze to either side. Her chest and abdomen were normal; blood pressure, pulse rate, temperature, and respirations were physiologic. Peripheral pulses were intact, with normal tissue turgor, and no cervical, axillary, or inguinal lymphadenopathy was detected.

102

Neurologic Examination

Mental Status.   The child was awake and oriented with respect to time and place. Memory and knowledge were appropriate for her age. However, response time to questions was protracted and she appeared preoccupied with her headache pain.

Cranial Nerves.   She had a full range of eye and facial movements. However, nystagmus was present on horizontal gaze to either side. Hearing was normal in both ears. Corneal, jaw-jerk, and gag reflexes were normal. The facial expressions were complete, the eyes were closed tightly, and the forehead was wrinkled symmetrically when frowning. Uvula and tongue protruded on the midline.

Motor Systems.   Strength was normal in all extremities; deep tendon reflexes were physiologic in all extremities. Truncal ataxia was evident when the child was seated; she could not maintain her torso in a vertical position and swayed from side to side. Her gait was broad-based and reeling. However, finger-to-nose and heel-to-shin testing were normal if her torso was supported in a vertical position.

Sensation.   Pinprick, thermal, vibratory, two-point discrimination, and proprioceptive senses were normal throughout the body and face.

QUESTIONS

1. Does the patient exhibit a language or memory deficit or an alteration in consciousness or cognition?

2. Are signs of cranial nerve dysfunction present?

3. Are there any changes in motor functions, such as reflexes, muscle tone, movement, or coordination?

4. Are any changes in sensory functions detectable?

5. At what level in the central neuraxis is this lesion most likely located?

6. Is the pathology focal, multifocal, or diffuse in its distribution within the nervous system?

7. What is the clinical–temporal profile of this pathology: acute or chronic; progressive or stable?

8. Based on your answers to the previous two questions, decide whether the symptoms in this patient are most likely caused by a vascular accident, a tumor, or a degenerative or inflammatory process?

9. If you feel this is the result of a vascular accident, what vessels are most likely involved?

10. What are some of the criteria for differentiating between limb and truncal ataxia?

11. What are some the pathophysiologic mechanisms of nystagmus, and what is the diagnostic significance of nystagmus?

► DISCUSSION
Macrostructure of the Cerebellum

The cerebellum consists of a thin, outer veneer of cells called the **cortex,** wrapped around a large tuft of fibers or white matter that arise from three **peduncles** attached to the brain stem. At the base of the peduncles are several cell clusters called the **deep nuclei.** Cells in the cerebellar cortex receive afferent information from many sources. Axons from the cerebellar cortical neurons are mapped topographically onto the deep nuclei. These nuclei form the main outflow of the cerebellum.

There are several systems of nomenclature for subdividing the cerebellum (Figs. 5-1 and 5-2); these are based on gross anatomic features, afferent and efferent connections, and paleontology. At a gross anatomic level, three transversely oriented lobes can be defined. The **anterior** and **posterior lobes** are separated by the primary fissure. Inferior to the posterior lobe lies a small, **flocculonodular lobe** (see Fig. 5-1). These three lobes are transected by two longitudinally oriented structures, the midline **vermis** and the laterally positioned **hemispheres.** Thus, the vermis and both hemispheres are represented in the anterior, posterior, and flocculonodular lobes.

The vermis and hemispheres of the cerebellum can be further partitioned based on connectivity into three longitudinal zones (see Figs. 5-1 and 5-2). Each zone represents an area of the cortex directly related to a specific deep cerebellar nucleus (see p. 110). On the midline, completely contained within the vermis, is the **median zone;** its cells project to the fastigial nucleus. The lateral edge of the vermis and a narrow strip of adjacent hemisphere represent the **paramedian zone,** which projects to the interpositus nucleus. Finally, the remainder of the hemisphere is the **lateral zone,** directly connected to the underlying dentate nucleus.

The cerebellum can also be classified by the organization of its afferent fibers. The flocculonodular lobe receives a significant projection from the vestibular system and is called the **vestibulocerebellum.** Afferent fibers from the spinal cord (spinocerebellar tracts) terminate in the anterior lobe and in portions of the vermis. These regions are therefore called the **spinocerebellum.** Lateral portions of the posterior lobe receive a significant projection of fibers from the neocortex through the pontine nuclei; this area is called the **pontocerebellum.**

From an evolutionary perspective, the flocculonodular lobe represents the oldest part; it is therefore known as the **archicerebellum.** The anterior lobe and associated portions of the vermis represent the "not-so-old" cerebellum, or **paleocerebellum.** Finally, the enlarged hemispheres of the posterior lobe represent the phylogenetically newest part, or **neocerebellum** (see Fig. 5-1).

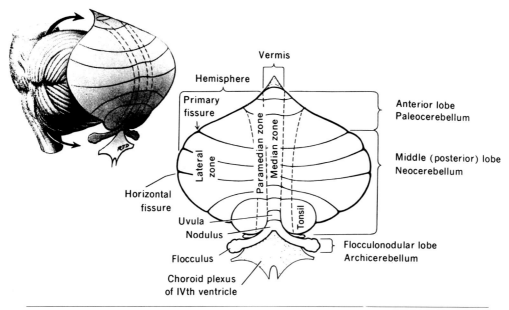

Figure 5-1. Diagram of the cerebellum demonstrates its various nomenclatures. (Noback CR, Demarest RJ. The human nervous system: basic principles of neurobiology. 3rd ed. New York: McGraw-Hill, 1981:323)

104

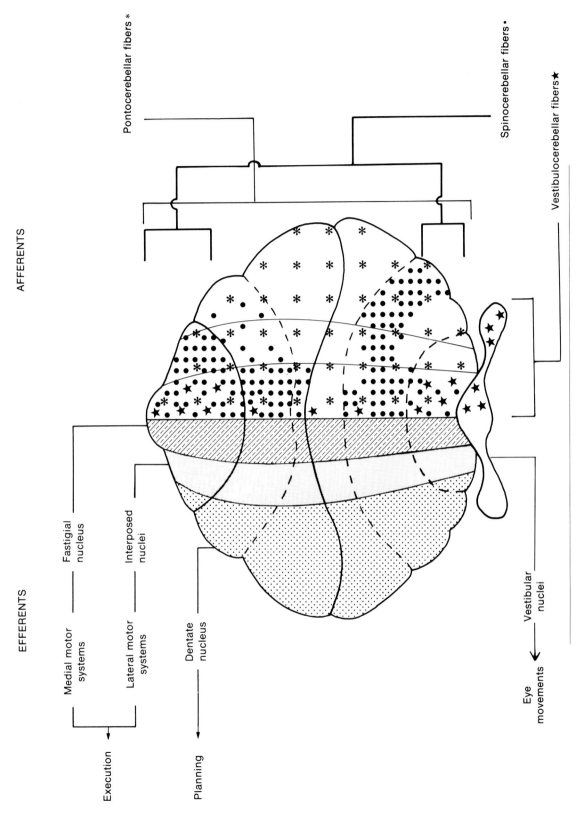

AFFERENTS

Pontocerebellar fibers *

Spinocerebellar fibers •

Vestibulocerebellar fibers ★

EFFERENTS

Medial motor systems —— Fastigial nucleus

Lateral motor systems —— Interposed nuclei

—— Dentate nucleus

Eye movements ←—— Vestibular nuclei

Execution

Planning

Figure 5-2. A diagram of the cerebellum indicates its input and output zones. These zones are positioned on the gross anatomic divisions of this structure.

CEREBELLAR REGIONS

Vestibulocerebellum

The vestibulocerebellum receives primary afferent fibers from the ipsilateral vestibular apparatus. These projections are directed mainly to the nodulus, whereas the flocculus receives input from visuomotor nuclei located along the medial longitudinal fasciculus. Efferent fibers from the vestibulocerebellum project directly to the ipsilateral vestibular nuclei (see Figs. 5-2 and 5-5). In turn, the vestibular nuclei influence axial musculature through the vestibulospinal tracts and extraocular eye muscles through the medial longitudinal fasciculus (see Fig. 5-5). The vestibulocerebellum uses information from the otolithic organ (gravity) to control posture, balance, and eye movements.

Spinocerebellum

The spinocerebellum consists of the median and intermediate zones. Geographically, these comprise most of the vermis and anterior lobe. Inputs to the median zone arise in the neck and trunk musculature and in the vestibular, auditory, and visual systems. Its output is directed to the fastigial nucleus (see p. 110), which then projects axons to the sources of the vestibulospinal and reticulospinal tracts. Through these connections, the median zone of the cerebellum coordinates muscle activity in the medial motor system, which regulates axial and proximal limb musculature.

The intermediate zone receives input from the spinocerebellar tracts carrying proprioceptive information from the limb musculature. Its output is directed through the interpositus nuclei (emboliformis and globose) to the red nucleus and ventrolateral thalamic nucleus. This output influences muscle coordination in the lateral motor system through the rubrospinal and corticospinal tracts (see Figs. 5-2 and 5-5). The lateral motor system functions to control the distal limb musculature.

Pontocerebellum

The lateral hemispheres of the posterior lobe consist of most of the pontocerebellum (see Fig. 5-2). Their major afferent connections arise in the contralateral pontine nuclei. These nuclei are innervated by neurons in the ipsilateral cerebral cortex. It is through this cortico-ponto-cerebellar pathway that cerebral cortex and cerebellum plan patterns for coordinated muscle activities in the distal portion of the extremities. Efferent fibers, which carry these motor patterns from the pontocerebellum, are relayed through the

dentate nucleus to contralateral thalamus and subsequently, to motor cortex.

The dentate nucleus also participates in a complex feedback circuit involving the red nucleus of the midbrain and the inferior olivary nucleus of the medulla. In this pathway, efferent projections from the dentate nucleus innervate the contralateral red nucleus, rubro-olivary axons course over the central tegmental tract to reach the inferior olive, and olivocerebellar fibers cross the midline to join the inferior cerebellar peduncle and innervate the cerebellar cortex. These olivocerebellar axons form climbing fibers in the cortex (see p. 108); each climbing fiber innervates the dendritic arbor of one Purkinje cell. This rubro-olivary feedback loop to the cerebellum is involved in learning new motor skills.[1]

CLINICAL DEFICIT

Damage to the cerebellum usually is caused by toxic substances, tumor, or infarction. It is possible to catalog some of the clinical cerebellar syndromes with respect to specific anatomic regions.[2–4] The cerebellum is composed of three zones: median, paramedian, and lateral, based on their connections. In the simplest schema of clinical cerebellar presentations, two general regional syndromes are recognized. The *median cerebellar syndrome* involves damage to the midline structures in the sagittal plane; the presentation can feature abnormalities in equilibrium, posture, gait, eye movements, and head position as well as truncal ataxia and vestibular nystagmus. The *lateral cerebellar syndrome* involves damage to the lateral zone and can present with signs of limb ataxia: hypotonia, dysmetria, decomposition of movement, past pointing, and impaired check. Since isolated lesions to the paramedian zone have not been reported, the clinical presentation of this zone has been linked to those of the lateral zone.[3]

A further classification breaks the midline syndrome into anterior and posterior components. The *anterior lobe* or *rostral vermis syndrome* features disturbed gait and postural reflexes such as those seen in chronic alcoholic degeneration (a process that attacks the anterior lobe. The *posterior lobe* or *caudal vermis syndrome* (also called basal or flocculonodular syndrome), results from damage to the flocculonodular lobe and the posterior portion of the median zone. It can present with disturbances of equilibrium, truncal ataxia, and vestibular nystagmus. Each of these syndromes will be discussed further.

Anterior Cerebellar or Rostral Vermis Syndrome. Lesions of the anterior spinocerebellum present as gait disturbances, usually involving the lower limbs, without changes in reflexes.[2] Outwardly, this is characterized by a wide-based stance and reeling gait. There can be little indication of ataxia in the limbs on heel-to-shin or finger-to-nose testing. Although infrequent, hypotonia, nystagmus, or dysarthria can be expressed as well. This presentation is called the anterior cerebellar or rostral vermis syndrome and can indicate a tumor in the anterior lobe or alcohol-induced degeneration.[4]

Basal Cerebellar or Caudal Vermis Syndrome. Damage to the vestibulocerebellum and lower portion of the posterior (spinocerebellum) lobe can result in the basal or caudal vermis cerebellar syndrome (truncal ataxia). The three signs are (1) gait disturbance and axial disequilibrium characterized by difficulty maintaining balance while walking (this is not considered limb ataxia) or while sitting, (2) head rotation, and (3) nystagmus. Signs of limb ataxia, such as past pointing and dysmetria, are usually not present. Because of its small size, pure lesions of the flocculonodular lobe are rare; damage to this structure usually occurs in concert with damage to other portions of the cerebellum or brain stem.[2,4]

Lateral Cerebellar Syndrome. The complex neurologic sequelae following lateral cerebellar hemisphere damage has various names: the lateral cerebellar syndrome, neocerebellar syndrome, limb ataxia, or hemisphere syndrome. This syndrome features defective postural fixation of the limbs as well as errors in rate, range, direction, timing, and force of skilled movements. All movements of the limb are slow. Past pointing, dysmetria, and movement (intention) tremor can be present. The affected limb is on the side of the lesion. Horizontal nystagmus, in the direction of gaze, can present with hemisphere lesions.[2,4]

Cerebellar Peduncles

Inferior Cerebellar Peduncle (ICP)

The spinocerebellar and olivocerebellar fibers enter the cerebellum through the inferior cerebellar peduncle (ICP) (the *restiform body* of old terminology). The medial border of this peduncle also contains projections from the vestibulocerebellum to the vestibular nuclei. The inferior cerebellar peduncle is first recognizable in the caudal medulla (see Plate 8) where it forms from the union of the dorsal spinocerebellar tract and the olivocerebellar fibers. It rises dorsally into the cerebellum at the pontomedullary border (see Plates 13 and 14). Olivocerebellar fibers are distributed throughout the cerebellar cortex, whereas the spinocerebellar fibers are targeted on the anterior lobe and on portions of the median and intermediate zones.

CLINICAL DEFICIT

Lesions of the inferior cerebellar peduncle can result in ataxia similar to that resulting from lesions of the spinocerebellum. The lateral medullary syndrome (see Chap. 3) features ataxia due to involvement of this peduncle (or in caudal medullary infarcts, the spinocerebellar tracts).

Middle Cerebellar Peduncle (MCP)

The middle cerebellar peduncle is the largest of the fiber tracts entering the cerebellum. It arises in the pontine nuclei (see Plates 14 to 19). The axons from pontine neurons, representing the transverse pontine fibers, cross the midline and coalesce along the lateral aspect of the brain stem to become the massive, middle cerebellar peduncle. These fibers terminate in the cortex of the cerebellum. The pontine cells receive input from the corticopontine fibers, thus establishing a cortico-ponto-cerebellar pathway.

CLINICAL DEFICIT

Lesions of the middle cerebellar peduncle can result in ipsilateral ataxia, often combined with signs of cranial nerve damage, such as that seen in the lateral pontine syndrome. Lesions involving the pontine nuclei (the source of the middle cerebellar peduncle) and adjacent corticospinal tract can result in complex presentations such as ataxic hemiparesis.[5] These are also discussed in Chapter 4.

Superior Cerebellar Peduncle (SCP)

The efferent pathway of the cerebellum is the superior cerebellar peduncle. Arising in the deep nuclei (see Fig. 5-4), this peduncle passes rostrally along the lateral walls of the fourth ventricle (see Plates 13 and 14). At the pontomesencephalic junction, it slips from under the rostral edge of the middle cerebellar peduncle (Plate 15) and enters the tegmentum of the brain stem (see Plates 16 and 17). Deep in the midbrain tegmentum, the superior cerebellar peduncle decussates (see Plates 18 and 19) and passes around the red nucleus (see Plates 20 and 21). Rostral to the red nucleus the fibers in the superior cerebellar peduncle are referred to as the cerebellothalamic tract (CThT, Plates 20 and 21). After entering the caudal thalamus, these fibers pass through the thalamic fasciculus (ThFas, Plate 22) to end in its ventrolateral nucleus (see Plates 22 and 23).

Although most of the fibers in the superior cerebellar peduncle are leaving the cerebellum, a small component is entering. The ventral spinocerebellar tract, which arises in the dorsal horn of the spinal cord, joins the ventral border of the superior cerebellar peduncle in the rostral pons (see Plate 15). After entering the cerebellum, the ventral spinocerebellar tract leaves the peduncle and proceeds into the anterior lobe (see Chap. 2).

CLINICAL DEFICIT

Lesions of the superior cerebellar peduncle can result in ataxia similar to lesions of the middle cerebellar peduncle and cerebellar hemispheres. If the lesion is caudal to the decussation of the superior cerebellar peduncle in the midbrain, the ataxia is expressed on the ipsilateral side. However, lesions rostral to the decussation are expressed contralaterally. Signs of midbrain dysfunction can accompany lesions involving the superior cerebellar peduncle (see Chap. 6).

► Microstructure of the Cerebellum

The cerebellum can be divided into two general regions based on cytology. The outermost, or **cortex,** contains several layers of cells, one of which is a monolayer of large Purkinje cell bodies. The innermost region is a massive zone of white matter. Embedded in the base of the white matter are the **deep cerebellar nuclei.** Afferent fibers to the cerebellum travel through its peduncles. They pass around the deep nuclei (often with collateral branches to these nuclei) and ascend through the white matter to the cortex, where they make connections with Purkinje cells or closely related interneurons. The axons of the Purkinje cells represent the efferent fibers of the cerebellar cortex. They descend through the white matter to terminate in the deep cerebellar nuclei. Finally, the deep nuclei give rise to fibers that enter the superior cerebellar peduncle, the major efferent pathway of the cerebellum.

CEREBELLAR CORTEX

A prominent feature of the cerebellar cortex is the monolayer of Purkinje cell bodies. These cells are the largest neurons of the cortex; their dendrites extend outward in elaborate arbors through the molecular or outer-most layer. Their axons enter the white matter, eventually reaching the deep nuclei. The dendritic tree of the Purkinje cell is flattened in the transverse plane (see Fig. 5-3). Passing through its dendrites are axons from granule cells. These axons are oriented parallel to the folia of the cerebellum. Their arrangement with the Purkinje cell dendrites is somewhat reminiscent of telegraph wires and poles; they are referred to as *parallel fibers,* a term reflecting their common orientation.

Also synapsing on Purkinje cell dendrites are climbing fibers that arise in the contralateral inferior olivary nuclei (see Plates 8 to 12). Each climbing fiber closely invests a Purkinje cell dendritic arbor. Thus, neurons in the inferior olive can have a profound effect on Purkinje cell activity.

The granule cells are located in a layer deep to the Purkinje cell bodies (granule cell layer; see Fig. 5-3); granule cell dendrites receive afferent fibers from the vestibular system, spinal cord, and pontine nuclei. Granule cell axons pass by the Purkinje cell body to enter the molecular layer, where they bifurcate to form parallel fibers. These fibers are strung through the Purkinje cell dendrites. Afferent stimuli activate the granule cell/parallel fiber system, which in turn, activates Purkinje cells.

Numerous stellate, basket, and Golgi cells are also found in the cerebellar cortex. Activated by mossy fi-

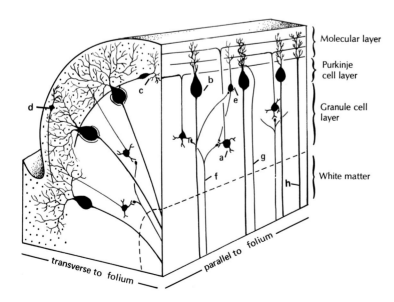

Molecular layer

Purkinje cell layer

Granule cell layer

White matter

transverse to folium

parallel to folium

Figure 5-3.
Cytoarchitecture of the cerebellar cortex. **(a)** Granule cell. **(b)** Purkinje cell. **(c)** Basket cell. **(d)** Stellate cell. **(e)** Golgi cell. **(f)** Mossy fiber. **(g)** Climbing fiber. **(h)** Catecholamine fiber. (Barr ML, Kiernan JA. The human nervous system: an anatomical viewpoint. 5th ed. Philadelphia: JB Lippincott, 1988:165)

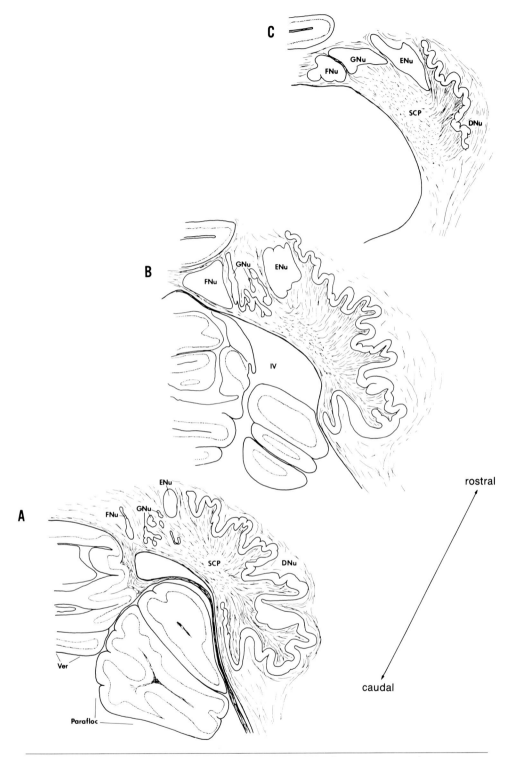

Figure 5-4. The deep or intracerebellar nuclei. This figure contains three sections throughout the deep cerebellar nuclei illustrating their position and surrounding fiber tracts.

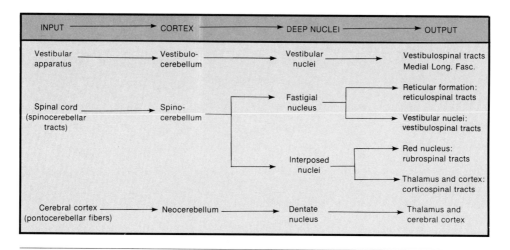

Figure 5-5. A diagram of the deep cerebellar nuclei and their major connections.

ber afferent stimuli similar to granule cells, these other interneurons have an inhibitory effect on Purkinje cells. Thus, the Purkinje cells integrate excitatory and inhibitory input from several different sources, and their output influences the activity of cells in the deep nuclei.

DEEP OR INTRACEREBELLAR NUCLEI

Embedded in the base of the white matter are the deep cerebellar nuclei. These structures represent the main source of efferent projections from the cerebellum. From medial to lateral, they are fastigial, interpositus (globose and emboliform), and dentate (see Fig. 5-4). Purkinje cell axons are a major source of input and have an inhibitory influence on these nuclei. Each nucleus receives its afferent fibers from a specific region of the cerebellar cortex and in turn, forms efferent projections to specific targets in the brain stem. Figure 5-5 illustrates the relationship between cerebellar cortex, deep nuclei, and specific cerebellar efferent projections.

Fastigial Nucleus (FNu)

Afferent fibers from Purkinje cells in the median zone (spinocerebellum) innervate the fastigial nucleus (FNu). The efferent connections of this nucleus are complex (see Fig. 5-5). Axons of neurons in the fastigial nucleus innervated the ipsilateral medial and lateral vestibular nuclei (source of the medial and lateral vestibulospinal tracts) as well as the pontine and medullary reticular formation (source of the pontine and medullary reticulospinal tracts). A small component of the fastigial nucleus projects to the accessory optic nuclei in the midbrain, and the intralaminar and ventrolateral nucleus of the thalamus. (These latter

projections are not shown in Fig. 5-5.) The fastigial nucleus is concerned with maintaining truncal posture and head and neck position, as well as influencing eye movements. These represent functions of the medial motor system.

Interpositus Nuclei

The intermediate zone of cerebellar cortex is the source of afferent fibers to the two interpositus nuclei: globose (GNu) and emboliform (ENu). Axons from these nuclei innervate the ipsilateral red nucleus of the midbrain and the contralateral ventrolateral nucleus of the thalamus (which then communicates with motor cortex). Through these connections, the intermediate zone of the cerebellum influences the rubrospinal and corticospinal tracts, coordinating movement of the musculature in the limbs. Thus, the intermediate zone regulates the lateral motor system.

Dentate Nucleus (DNu)

The prominent dentate nucleus (DNu) appears very similar to the inferior olive in appearance (see Fig. 5-4 and Plates 8 to 12). It receives Purkinje cell axons from the lateral zone, including the pontocerebellum. Its efferent fibers cross the midline in the decussation of the superior cerebellar peduncle and reach two major targets, the red nucleus (see Plates 20 and 21) and the ventrolateral nucleus of the thalamus (see Plates 22 to 24). In the red nucleus, dentate axons influence rubral neurons projecting to the inferior olive. The dento-rubro-olivo-cerebellar circuit is a complex feedback loop for the cerebellum and is involved in learning motor skills.[1,6] The dentothalamic axons form a portion of the dento-thalamo-cortical circuit, which is involved in the planning of and preparation for skilled movements by the distal limb musculature.

UNIT B

Case Study 5-3

A 49-year-old with acute onset headaches and ataxia

A 49-year-old man was admitted to the hospital after experiencing acute gait imbalance for 3 days. He tended to lean to the left on standing or walking. He had a mild headache but no vertigo. There was no history of neck trauma. Vomiting had occurred once or twice; whether it was related to postural change was unknown. No one else in his family had had similar complaints.

Family History

He was married, with two children, both of whom were in college. His mother was alive and in good health; his father had died from "heart disease" 10 years before, at the age of 60.

Past Medical History

He had had diabetes since childhood; control was maintained daily with insulin. He had recently experienced visual loss and numbness in his toes. He has a history of mild hypertension which has been controlled with pharmaceuticals for the past 3 years.

General Physical Examination

He was an awake, oriented, and afebrile male, appearing his stated age and of appropriate weight. He was well nourished; his skin had good color, texture, and temperature. He had several small bruises on his left foot. Optic discs had numerous microaneurysms, with several surrounding deep hemorrhages and scattered hard exudates. Chest was clear to auscultation and percussion; abdomen was soft with no masses or lumps. Blood pressure, pulse, temperature, and respirations were normal on the date of admission.

Neurologic Examination

Mental Status. He was awake and oriented to time and place. Memory and knowledge were appropriate. He was mildly dysarthric.

Cranial Nerves. Eye movements were full, with left-beating nystagmus on gaze to the left, more marked in the left than in the right eye. The left pupil was smaller than the right; both pupils reacted normally to light. The left palpebral fissure was greater than the right. Normal hearing to finger rub was present in both ears, and he denied tinnitus. He had diminished sensation to pinprick on the right side of his face, with slightly diminished corneal reflex on the right. Pinprick sensation and corneal reflex on the left were intact. His gag and jaw-jerk reflexes were intact. He had a mild paralysis of the facial muscles around the corner of his mouth on the right. Palate elevated on the midline and tongue protruded on the midline.

Motor Systems. Limb strength and reflexes were physiologic in all extremities. The left arm and leg were ataxic, with dysmetria and mild intention tremor. Left pronator drift was evident, and he deviated to the left on walking.

Sensation. Vibratory, two-point discrimination, and proprioceptive senses were intact throughout the body. Pinprick sensation was intact on the left side of his body but diminished in the upper and lower extremities on the right.

QUESTIONS

1. Does the patient exhibit a language or memory deficit or an alteration in consciousness or cognition?

111

2. Are signs of cranial nerve dysfunction present?

3. Are there any changes in motor functions, such as reflexes, muscle tone, movement, or coordination?

4. Are any changes in sensory functions detectable?

5. At what level in the central neuraxis is this lesion most likely located?

6. Is the pathology focal, multifocal, or diffuse in its distribution within the nervous system?

7. What is the clinical–temporal profile of this pathology: acute or chronic; progressive or stable?

8. Based on your answers to the previous two questions, decide whether the symptoms in this patient are most likely caused by a vascular accident, a tumor, or a degenerative or inflammatory process.

9. If you feel this is the result of a vascular accident, what vessels are most likely involved?

10. What are the major neurologic signs and symptoms that would help differentiate infarction in any of the three cerebellar arterial systems?

► DISCUSSION
Cerebellar Vasculature

The cerebellum is supplied by three major vessels: the *superior cerebellar* artery, the *anterior inferior cerebellar* artery, and the *posterior inferior cerebellar* artery (see Fig. 5-6) The distribution of these three arterial systems is not restricted to any specific geographic region of the cerebellum; consequently, the following vasculature syndromes are not identical to the regional syndromes presented on pp. 106–107.

Occlusion or infarction of the distal branches of any one of the cerebellar vessels will damage the hemispheres and peduncles of this structure. The resulting presentation usually involves ataxia, dizziness, vertigo, nausea and vomiting, and nystagmus.[7,8] However, the stems of these vessels also supply significant portions of the brain stem; consequently, cranial nerve and long tract signs often accompany stem infarctions of these arteries. The specific cranial nerves or long tracts involved differ with each arterial system. Therefore, these signs represent significant differentiating factors for distinguishing infarctions in each of the three cerebellar arterial territories.

SUPERIOR CEREBELLAR ARTERY (SCA)

The superior cerebellar artery (SCA) arises from the basilar artery near its point of bifurcation into the two posterior cerebral arteries (see Fig. 5-6). The superior cerebellar artery and the posterior cerebral artery sandwich the oculomotor nerve. The superior cerebellar artery passes caudal to the trochlear nerve and rostral to the trigeminal nerve as it winds around the cerebral peduncle to reach the superior surface of the cerebellum. (See the description of arteries in Chap. 6.) The penetrating branches of the superior cerebellar artery supply the dorsolateral quadrant of the caudal midbrain (see Plates 15 to 19), middle and superior cerebellar peduncles, deep cerebellar nuclei, and cerebellar white matter. Cortical branches supply the anterior vermis, anterior hemispheres, and lateral margins of the cerebellum.

CLINICAL DEFICIT
The major signs of infarction restricted to the cerebellar territory of superior cerebellar artery are limb and gait ataxia,[9] abnormal saccades,[10] and several forms of nystagmus

Brain stem signs of superior cerebellar artery pathology include transient chorea,[9] loss of pain and temperature sensation from the contralateral face and

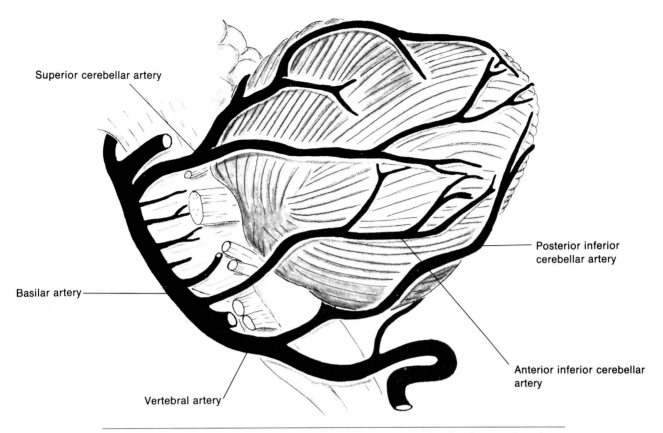

Superior cerebellar artery

Basilar artery

Vertebral artery

Posterior inferior cerebellar artery

Anterior inferior cerebellar artery

Figure 5-6. This lateral view of the cerebellum illustrates the distribution of its three major arteries. (Modified with permission from Melloni JL, Doxi I, Melloni HP, Melloni BJ. Melloni's illustrated review of human anatomy. Philadelphia: JB Lippincott, 1988:7)

body, ipsilateral Horner's syndrome, and contralateral supranuclear facial palsy.[7]

ANTERIOR INFERIOR CEREBELLAR ARTERY (AICA)

The anterior inferior cerebellar artery (AICA) arises from the basilar at the level of the caudal pons (see Fig. 5-6). It sweeps laterally, in close relationship to the facial and acousticovestibular cranial nerves. After passing through the cerebellopontine angle, the artery reaches the inferior surface of the cerebellum. Its penetrating branches supply the dorsolateral quadrant of the rostral medulla and caudal pons (see Plates 10 to 14), inferior portion of the middle cerebellar peduncle, and inferior cerebellar peduncle. Its cortical branches supply flocculus, part of vermis, and inferior portions of cerebellar cortex.

CLINICAL DEFICIT

Lesions restricted to the cerebellar distribution of the anterior inferior cerebellar artery are not well docu-

mented in the literature. Textbooks often include ataxia and dysmetria; however, these signs could also reflect involvement of the middle cerebellar peduncle.

Lesions involving the entire territory of this artery result in limb and gait ataxia caused by involvement of the middle cerebellar peduncle. Infarction in the brain stem territory of the anterior inferior cerebellar artery can present with hemifacial paralysis (nuclear or nerve lesion), Horner's syndrome, and lateral gaze palsy on the ipsilateral side, alternating analgesia involving the ipsilateral face and contralateral body, as well as deafness, tinnitus, vertigo, nausea, vomiting, and nystagmus.[11,12]

POSTERIOR INFERIOR CEREBELLAR ARTERY (PICA)

The posterior inferior cerebellar artery (PICA) arises from the vertebral at approximately the cervicomedullary junction (see Fig. 5-6). It is in close relationship with cranial nerves IX through XII as it winds its way around the brain stem to reach the posterior mar-

113

gin of the cerebellum. It supplies the dorsolateral quadrant of the medulla (see Plates 7 to 10), inferior and posterior vermis, tonsils, and inferolateral surface of the cerebellum. Its penetrating branches supply part of the dentate nucleus.

CLINICAL DEFICIT

The major signs of infarction restricted to the cerebellar territory of the posterior inferior cerebellar artery are rotatory dizziness, which is intensified by motion, nausea, vomiting, imbalance, and nystagmus.[13] The *nystagmus is often horizontal in both directions of gaze.*[14]

The neurologic signs resulting from infarction of the medullary distribution of this artery can represent the lateral medullary syndrome (see Chap. 3) dysphagia, dysphonia, hiccup, ipsilateral Horner's syndrome, paralysis of the soft palate and larynx, and alternating analgesia involving ipsilateral face and contralateral body.[7] Ipsilateral ataxia and dysmetria can result from damage to the inferior cerebellar peduncle in the brain stem.

► Bibliography

Adams RD, Victor M. Abnormalities of movement and posture due to disease in the extrapyramidal motor systems. In: Principles of neurology. New York: McGraw-Hill, 1989; Chap. 4:54–77.

Barr ML, Kiernan JA. Cerebellum. In: The human nervous system: an anatomical viewpoint. Philadelphia: JB Lippincott, 1988; Chap. 10:160–177.

Biller J, Brazis PW. The localization of lesions affecting the cerebellum. In: Brazis PW, Masdeu JC, Biller J, eds. Localization in clinical neurology. Boston: Little, Brown, 1990.

Haines DE. Neuroanatomy: an atlas of structures, sections, and systems. Baltimore: Urban & Schwarzenberg, 1987 *(see especially Figs. 2-26 through 2-28, 5-14, and 5-15).*

Ghez C. The cerebellum. In: Kandel ER, Schwartz JH, Jessell TM, eds.
Principles of neural science. New York: Elsevier, 1991; Chap. 41:626–646.

Nieuwenhuys R, Voogd J, van Huijzen C. The human central nervous system. Berlin: Springer-Verlag, 1988:221–236.

► References

1. Sanes JN, Dimitrov B, Hallett M. Motor learning in patients with cerebellar dysfunction. Brain 1990;113:103.
2. Brown JR. Diseases of the cerebellum. In: Joyny RJ, ed. Clinical neurology, Vol 4. Philadelphia: JB Lippincott, 1982.
3. Gilman S. Cerebellum and motor dysfunction. In: Asbury AK, McKhann GM, McDonald WI, eds. Diseases of the nervous system. Philadelphia: WB Saunders, 1986:401–422.
4. Biller J, Brazis PW. The localization of lesions affecting the cerebellum. In: Brazis PW, Masdeu JC, Biller J, eds. Localization in clinical neurology. Boston: Little, Brown, 1990.
5. Fisher CM. Ataxic hemiparesis. Arch Neurol 1978;35:126.
6. Thach WT, Goodkin HP, Keating JG. The cerebellum and adaptive coordination of movement. Ann Rev Neurosci 1992;15:403.
7. Marshall J. Cerebellar vascular syndromes. Hdbk Clin Neurol 1989;11(55):89.
8. Sypert GW, Alvord EC. Cerebellar infarction. Arch Neurol 1975;32(6):357.
9. Kase CS, White JL, Joslyn JN, Williams JP, Moher JP. Cerebellar infarction in the superior cerebellar artery distribution. Neurology 1985;35(5):705.
10. Ranalli PJ, Sharpe JA. Contrapulsion of saccades and ipsilateral ataxia: a unilateral disorder of the rostral cerebellum. Ann Neurol 1986;20:311.
11. Toole JF, Patel AN. Cerebrovascular disorders. New York: McGraw-Hill, 1974:412.
12. Amarenco P, Haaw JJ. Cerebellar infarction in the territory of the anterior and inferior cerebellar artery. Brain 1990; 113:139–155.
13. Duncan GW, Parker SW, Fisher CM. Acute cerebellar infarction in the PICA territory. Arch Neurol 1975;32(6):364.
14. Bogousslavsky J, Meienberg O. Eye-movement disorders in brain-stem and cerebellar stroke. Arch Neurol 1987;44:141.

6 MIDBRAIN

► Introduction

The midbrain, the narrowest portion of the brain stem, lies between supra- and infratentorial compartments, surrounded by the incisure of the tentorium cerebelli. This portion of the brain stem is characterized by the massive cerebral peduncles (legs) located ventrally and by the superior and inferior colliculi (little hills) dorsally. The neural circuits intrinsic to this region involve coordination of body and eye movements with respect to external stimuli and maintain consciousness by influencing the level of neural activity in the cerebral cortex. The midbrain contains the nuclei and radiations of oculomotor, trochlear, and portions of trigeminal cranial nerves. It receives its blood supply from penetrating branches of the basilar and posterior cerebral arteries.

In this chapter the nuclei and tracts of the midbrain will be examined. The vascular supply to the midbrain will be studied and several clinicopathologic cases will be presented.

115

GENERAL OBJECTIVES

1. To learn the location and function of the major tracts and cranial nuclei in the midbrain
2. To learn the presenting signs and symptoms consequent to lesions involving these tracts and nuclei
3. To apply the preceding knowledge to an understanding of the clinical manifestations of the major midbrain vascular lesions

INSTRUCTIONS

In this chapter you will be presented with one or more clinical case studies. *Each study will be followed by a list of questions that can best be answered by using knowledge of regional and functional neuroanatomy and by referring to outside reading material.* Following the questions will be a section devoted to structures from a specific region of the central nervous system. Before you attempt to answer the questions, compile a list of the patient's neurologic signs and symptoms; then examine the structures and their functions and study their known clinical deficits. After becoming familiar with the material, reexamine the list of neurologic signs and symptoms and formulate answers to the questions. Be aware that some of the questions can have multiple responses or require information beyond the scope of this manual. It may be necessary to obtain material or advice from additional resources, such as specialty texts, a medical dictionary, or clinical personnel.

MATERIALS

1. A human brain stem and brain stem model
2. A human brain stem with intact blood supply
3. A medical dictionary

UNIT A

Case Study 6-1

A 57-year-old woman with diplopia and paralysis of the lower extremity

This 57-year-old, right-handed housewife suddenly developed double vision and drooping of the right eyelid on the day prior to admission; in addition, she had had difficulty walking. The following morning her husband brought her to the emergency room for examination.

Past Medical History

This patient had had moderate hypertension for many years. She had also experienced several episodes suggesting cerebral vascular ischemia in the past 5 years.

Family History

The patient has been married for 35 years and has three children in college. Both parents are living; her father has had a long history of hypertension. She has a 25-pack-year history of smoking and claims to consume a moderate amount of alcohol each week.

Physical Examination

She was awake, oriented, and of anxious demeanor. The patient was well nourished, well hydrated, obese, and in poor physical condition; she appeared slightly older than her stated age. Optic discs had sharp edges. Her chest was clear to auscultation and percussion. Her blood pressure was 160/100; pulse, temperature, and respirations were physiologic. Abdomen was difficult to palpate because of her obesity; however, no tenderness was observed. Peripheral pulses were difficult to access; mild edema was present at the ankles but not at the wrists.

Neurologic Examination

Mental Status. The patient was alert and oriented to time and place. Speech was articulate and content was meaningful. Memory and knowledge were appropriate for her background. She could follow two- and three-step commands and was an adequate historian.

Cranial Nerves. Visual fields were full to confrontation. If asked to open her eyes, the right eyelid did not elevate beyond 2 mm; the left opened 10 to 12 mm. When the right eyelid was elevated by external force, the right eye was deviated to the right and down; she could effect no medial or upward movement of the right eye. The right eye did not respond to caloric testing, nor did it respond during attempted convergence. A full range of motion was present with the left eye. Pupillary responses were intact bilaterally. Although it did not move, the right eye would dilate with the left eye on attempted convergence. Hearing was normal in both ears. A minor weakness was noted in the left corner of her mouth when she attempted to grimace. Her palate elevated symmetrically, and corneal, jaw-jerk, and gag reflexes were intact. Her tongue protruded on the midline and her shoulder shrug was symmetric and of physiologic strength.

Motor System. Strength was intact in all limbs. Deep tendon reflexes were physiologic and symmetric in the upper extremities and increased in the left lower extremity compared with the right. There was a left Babinski response. The abdominal reflex was absent on the left.

Sensation. Pinprick, two-point discrimination, vibratory sense, and proprioception were present throughout face and body.

QUESTIONS

1. Does the patient exhibit a language or memory deficit or an alteration in consciousness or cognition?

2. Are signs of cranial nerve dysfunction present?

3. Are there any changes in motor functions such as reflexes, muscle tone, movement, or coordination?

4. Are any changes in sensory functions detectable?

5. At what level in the central neuraxis is this lesion most likely located?

6. Is the pathology focal, multifocal, or diffuse in its distribution within the nervous system?

7. What is the clinical–temporal profile of this pathology: acute or chronic; progressive or stable?

8. Based on your answers to the previous two questions, decide whether the symptoms in this patient are most likely caused by a vascular accident, a tumor, or a degenerative or inflammatory process.

9. If you feel this is the result of a vascular accident, what vessels are most likely involved?

10. What brain stem structures, when damaged, can cause ptosis in a patient?

11. Is the right eye paralysis consistent with the left-sided increase in deep tendon reflexes and Babinski sign?

12. Is the loss of motor function consistent with preservation of the sensorium?

► DISCUSSION
Mesencephalic Structures

The major ascending and descending tracts of the spinal cord pass through the midbrain. In addition, there are numerous intrinsic nuclei related to the cranial nerves and reticular formation with which you should become familiar. These items are listed on the following plates. The abbreviation following the structure corresponds to that used on the atlas plate. The first time you encounter a given structure, its description will be provided, along with comments on function and any clinical deficit consequent to its destruction. For subsequent sections, the structure will be mentioned by name only unless significant changes have occurred in its location or composition.

▷ Atlas Plates 16 and 17

The dorsal portions of these sections pass through the caudal midbrain; the ventral portions are located in the pons. The prominent feature of Plate 17 is the appearance of the inferior colliculus on the dorsal surface of the midbrain tegmentum. The pontine structures on this plate were presented in Chapter 4.

SUPERIOR CEREBELLAR PEDUNCLE (SCP)

The superior cerebellar peduncle (SCP) has a ventral tail that curves in a medial direction (more prominent on Plate 17), giving this fiber bundle a calycine profile. To the inside of the calyx lies the central tegmental tract; to the outside are the three sensory lemnisci: medial lemniscus, anterolateral tract (or spinal lemniscus), and lateral lemniscus. The composition of the superior cerebellar peduncle and the clinical deficits resulting from its destruction were discussed in Chapters 4 and 5.

RADIATION OF THE TROCHLEAR NERVE (TroNr)

The trochlear nucleus lies rostral to Plate 17 in the midbrain (see p. 121) however, the radiations of its nerve (TroNr) can be seen as small fiber bundles in the lateral aspect of the central gray (see Plate 17). These fascicles leave the nucleus and pass dorsally around the central gray to reach the tectum. They emerge from the brain stem and cross the midline posterior to the inferior colliculus (Fig. 6-1). After leaving the dorsal aspect of the midbrain, the trochlear nerve crosses the subarachnoid space to reach the inferior surface of the tentorium cerebelli. This nerve innervates the contralateral superior oblique muscle, which, if contracted, causes the globe to deflect downward from the adducted position, and to rotate inward from the abducted position. The trochlear nucleus and its nerve are further discussed on p. 121.

LATERAL LEMNISCUS AND ITS NUCLEI (LL, LLNu)

The lateral lemniscus (LL) has extended dorsally to enter the base of the inferior colliculus. This prominent fiber tract is carrying ascending axons from the cochlear nuclei and superior olive to the inferior colliculus. The nuclei of the lateral lemniscus (LLNu) can be seen embedded in the fibers of the lemniscus at its rostral end.

CLINICAL DEFICIT
Section of the lateral lemniscus will produce diminished hearing functions in the contralateral ear. Symmetric, bilateral lesions of the lateral lemniscus and inferior colliculus by contusion on the tentorial incisura in an automobile accident produced complete bilateral deafness.[1] Damage to the area around the base of the inferior colliculus and the tegmentum near the lateral lemniscus can produce "acoustic hallucinations."[2]

INFERIOR COLLICULUS (IC)

The two bilateral masses of the inferior colliculus (IC) in the posterior tectum are major relay centers for the auditory pathways. The inferior colliculus receives afferent projections from the contralateral cochlear nucleus and bilateral projections from the superior olivary nuclei and the nuclei of the lateral lemniscus. Combining these projections within the inferior collic-

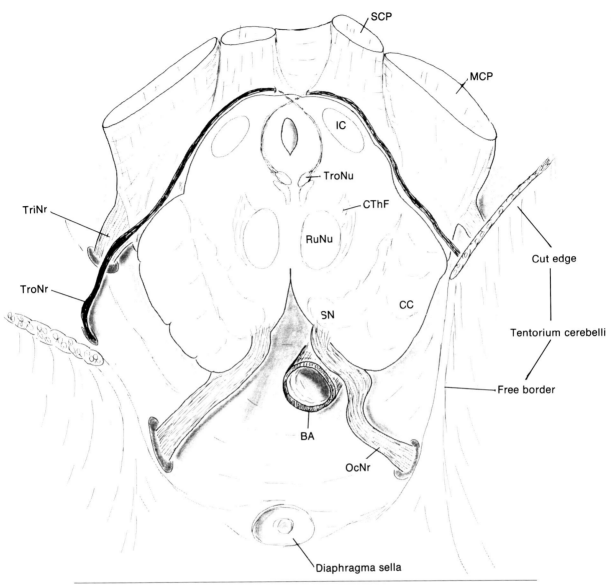

Figure 6-1. A drawing of the midbrain and its relationship to the tentorium cerebelli. The tentorium has been cut and the cerebellum removed to reveal the brain stem, which has been transected at the midbrain-thalamic border. The trochlear nerve is seen leaving the dorsal surface of the midbrain and penetrating the inferior surface of the tentorium. The oculomotor nerve is seen leaving the ventral surface of the midbrain and penetrating the dura.

ulus generates a map of acoustic space. The inferior colliculus uses this map in the process of sound localization[3] data and in generating reflex responses to unexpected stimuli. Ascending projections from the inferior colliculus are directed through its brachium (see p. 122) to the ipsilateral medial geniculate nuclei of the thalamus; descending projections travel through the lateral lemniscus to reach the superior olives and cochlear nucleus.

CLINICAL DEFICIT

Lesions of the inferior colliculus diminish hearing functions from the contralateral ear. Consequently, compression of the inferior colliculi by pineal tumors can result in loss of hearing. Distortions of acoustic perception can result from lesions around the margins of this structure. Damage to the ventromedial aspect of the inferior colliculus and the superior medullary vellum resulted in bilateral hyperacusis in a patient.[4]

MIDBRAIN RETICULAR FORMATION (MRetF)

Numerous groups of cells, serving differing functions, are present in the midbrain reticular formation (MRetF). Along the dorsal midline are those nuclei involved in control of conjugate eye movement: rostral interstitial nucleus of the medial longitudinal fasciculus, nucleus of Darkschewitschi, and interstitial nucleus of Cajal. Collectively, these nuclei are referred to as the **preoculomotor system,**[5] since many of their efferent fibers have a direct influence on the motor nuclei of the extraocular eye muscles (also see pp. 125–126). They are found embedded in the central gray of the midbrain, closely associated with the rostral end of the medial longitudinal fasciculus. Afferent projections to the preoculomotor nuclei originate in the paramedian pontine reticular formation (horizontal gaze center) as well as in the contralateral frontal cortex (eye fields, area 8), superior colliculus, pretectum, and vestibular nuclei. Efferent fibers from the preoculomotor nuclei innervate the oculomotor, trochlear, and vestibular nuclei. The preoculomotor system and the paramedian pontine reticular formation are involved in controlling vertical and horizontal eye movements.[6]

The midbrain reticular formation also gives rise to a diffuse projection of axons into the intralaminar nuclei of thalamus for eventual relay onto the cerebral cortex. These axons are part of the **ascending reticular activating system.** The cell bodies of origin for these projections are found in a portion of the reticular formation extending from the rostral pons through the midbrain. This diffuse system of fibers is involved in modulating the level of neural activity in the cerebral cortex.

Passing through the lateral midbrain reticular formation are the corticonuclear fibers that are involved with control of horizontal gaze. These fibers leave the internal capsule, descend through the posterior thalamus and midbrain, and cross the midline to innervate the paramedian pontine reticular formation.

CLINICAL DEFICIT

Damage to the ascending reticular activating system by lesions of the midbrain reticular formation can result in coma.[7] Unilateral damage to this system can diminish the input to one cerebral hemisphere, resulting in a profound, contralateral "neglect syndrome."[8]

Laterally placed lesions of the midbrain reticular formation can interrupt the descending corticonuclear fibers to the paramedian pontine reticular formation, resulting in loss of horizontal gaze. Since these fibers have not decussated at this point, the deficit is expressed on the contralateral side, and the patient is unable to gaze volitionally into the visual hemisphere opposite the lesion. However, the eyes can be deflected into this hemisphere using the oculocephalic reflex or caloric stimuli.

Ventrally positioned lesions of the midbrain or pons that leave the preoculomotor nuclei and the ascending reticular activating system intact but interrupt the descending corticospinal and corticonuclear fibers bilaterally can create a "locked-in" syndrome. Patients are conscious and aware of events in their surroundings, but because of the loss of the descending motor control systems they cannot respond except through the initiation of vertical eye movements.[7]

Review Structures From Preceding Plates

Identify the following structures from previous sections:

Central gray (CeGy)

Medial lemniscus (ML)

Anterolateral system (ALS)

Ventral trigeminothalamic tract (VTTr)

Central tegmental tract (CTT)

Rubrospinal tract (RuSp)

Midbrain reticular formation (MRetF)

Raphe complex (Central superior) (RaNu)

▷ **Atlas Plate 18**

The dorsal portion of this section passes through the inferior colliculus, crossing the extreme caudal border of the superior colliculus. The ventral portion is located in the pons. (The pontine structures are discussed in Chap. 4.)

SUPERIOR COLLICULUS (SC)

The superior colliculi (SC) form two mounds in the tectum at the rostral border of the midbrain. (They are best observed in Plate 19.) The cells and fibers of the superior colliculi are arranged in a series of horizontal layers. These layers receive input from the visual, auditory, and somatic sensory systems, as well as projections from frontal and parietal cortex. The deeper layers of the superior colliculus contain the efferent neurons of the tectobulbar and tectospinal tracts.

Projections from the superior colliculus are directed to numerous sites. The tectobulbar tract projects to the accessory optic nuclei of the midbrain and the reticular formation. The tectospinal tract reaches the cervical spinal cord, and the tectocortical fibers project to extrastriate visual cortex.

Using its visual, auditory, and somatic sensory inputs, the superior colliculus forms a map of the body and of external space. It uses this map to guide head, eye, and upper limb movements in tracking and responding to unexpected stimuli.[9] The superior colliculus is involved particularly in generating visually guided saccades.

The superior colliculus participates in the parallel processing of visual information. The retino-tecto-cortical fibers form a pathway to the visual cortex that runs parallel to the retino-geniculo-cortical projections passing through the thalamus. In humans this parallel pathway can still process visual stimuli when there is damage in the thalamic route. If forced to use the tectal pathway alone, the patient does not see recognizable images but can detect flashing light and moving targets.[10]

CLINICAL DEFICIT

Isolated lesions of the superior colliculus in monkeys interfere with the animal's ability to attend to novel stimuli, especially when they are unexpected. Collicular lesions in humans cause increased saccade latencies and a defect in saccade execution (hypometria), so that they fall short of the target.[11]

DECUSSATION OF THE SUPERIOR CEREBELLAR PEDUNCLE (dSCP)

The superior cerebellar peduncle contains fibers from the dentate nucleus of the cerebellum that will terminate in the contralateral red nucleus of the midbrain (see Plates 20 and 21) and ventrolateral thalamic nucleus (see Plate 21). The decussation of this large fiber tract in the midbrain marks the point where its axons cross the midline.

CLINICAL DEFICIT

Lesions that damage the central portion of the midbrain, including the decussation of the superior cerebellar peduncle, often produce coma,[12] thus masking any motor deficits. However, cases have been reported of small vascular lesions in the caudal tectal plate and midbrain tegmentum that produce unsteady gait and ataxia in all four limbs[4] as well as truncal ataxia.[13] These symptoms are presumably due to the involvement of the superior cerebellar peduncle.

TROCHLEAR NUCLEUS (TroNu)

The trochlear nucleus (TroNu) is located in the ventral portion of the central gray, indented into the dorsal border of the medial longitudinal fasciculus. Its axons form the radiations of the trochlear nerve that arch dorsally along the border of the central gray and cross the midline on the dorsal surface of the tectum before exiting the brain stem (see Fig. 6-1). This nucleus provides the motor innervation of the superior oblique muscle (see p. 118).

CLINICAL DEFICIT

An isolated lesion of the trochlear nucleus or nerve can result in paralysis of the superior oblique muscle; in such a case the affected eye may move slightly upward and outward (extortion). Diplopia may occur on attempted downward and inward vision. The patient's head is tipped to the opposite side in an effort to bring the visual fields of both eyes into alignment and reduce the diplopia.

Head trauma is the most common cause of trochlear nerve palsy.[14] Extracerebral damage to the nerve distal to the decussation results in paralysis of the ipsilateral superior oblique muscle. The trochlear nerve can be damaged by compression as it enters the incisure of the tentorium cerebelli (see Fig 6-1). In addition, traumatic head injuries that induce bleeding into the superior cerebellar cistern are a source of trochlear palsy. In bleeding accidents, the onset of the palsy can be hours after the injury.[15]

Trochlear palsy due to an intracranial lesion is very rare but has been reported.[16] Casual factors of such lesions are aneurysms and vascular malformations, usually positioned posterior to the inferior colliculus or in the superior medullary velum.[16]

CUNEIFORM NUCLEUS (CunNu)

The cuneiform nucleus (CunNu) is a small, wedge-shaped nucleus closely associated with the central gray of the midbrain. The nucleus is thought to be involved with the pathways processing pain.[17] It receives afferent fibers from the spinal cord and projects axons to the raphe nuclei of the medulla. The medullary raphe nucleus is the source of axons to the dorsal horn that modulate input from the nociceptive, primary afferent fibers.

Review Structures From Preceding Plates

Identify the following structures from previous sections:

Inferior colliculus (IC)

Lateral lemniscus (LL)

121

Central gray (CeGy)

Medial lemniscus (ML)

Anterolateral system (ALS)

Ventral trigeminothalamic tract (VTTr)

Central tegmental tract (CTT)

Rubrospinal tract (RuSp)

Midbrain reticular formation (MRetF)

Raphe complex (central superior) (RaNu)

Dorsal longitudinal fasciculus (DLF)

Medial longitudinal fasciculus (MLF)

▷ **Atlas Plate 19**

The dorsal portion of this section passes through the superior colliculus; the ventral portion transects the pontomesencephalic junction. (The pontine structures on this section have been discussed in Chap. 4.) Characteristic of this section is the merger of the cerebral peduncle into the basilar pons.

OCULOMOTOR NUCLEUS (OcNu)

The oculomotor nucleus is positioned along the midline, under the cerebral aqueduct (Fig. 6-2). It contains general somatic motoneurons that innervate four of the extraocular eye muscles: the medial, inferior, and superior rectus muscles and the inferior oblique muscle. These muscles function to move the globe on the vertical axis. With the eye in full abduction, the superior and inferior recti move the globe up and down on the vertical axis, respectively. With the eye in full adduction the inferior and superior oblique muscles move the globe up and down on the vertical axis, respectively (see Masdeu and Brazis[11] for further details). The oculomotor nucleus also innervates the levator palpebrae muscle, which elevates the eyelid.

The oculomotor nucleus is situated at the rostral end of the medial longitudinal fasciculus and receives projections from the vestibular nuclei, abducens nucleus, prepositus hypoglossal nucleus, and the paramedian pontine reticular formation (horizontal gaze center). Afferent projections to this nucleus also arise

from a cluster of small nuclei surrounding the rostral end of the median longitudinal fasciculus. Two nuclei in this region, the rostral interstitial nucleus of the medial longitudinal fasciculus and the interstitial nucleus of Cajal, as well as their surrounding neurons, are referred to as the vertical gaze center. Collectively, the nuclei at the rostral end of the median longitudinal fasciculus, which project axons into the oculomotor nucleus, are referred to as the *preoculomotor nuclei* (see p. 120).

On the rostrodorsal border of the oculomotor nucleus is the nucleus of Edinger-Wesphal containing general visceral efferent (preganglionic), parasympathetic neurons. These cells innervate the ciliary ganglion and control pupillary constriction.

CLINICAL DEFICIT

In total paralysis of the oculomotor nucleus or nerve, ptosis is present in the ipsilateral eye because of loss of the levator palpebrae muscle. When the lid is elevated forcefully, the globe is found fully abducted with little or no vertical movement and only slight medial movement due to relaxation of the lateral rectus muscle. The pupil is dilated and unresponsive to light. Partial paralysis, involving selected muscles in the oculomotor system, can occur; this event is discussed on p. 126.

BRACHIUM OF THE INFERIOR COLLICULUS (BrIC)

The brachium (arm) of the inferior colliculus (BrIC) contains axons from the inferior colliculus in the midbrain to the ipsilateral medial geniculate of the thalamus. This tract is the major auditory projection from the midbrain to the thalamus.

CLINICAL DEFICIT

Lesion of the brachium of the inferior colliculus in cats results in deficits similar to those associated with lesions of the inferior colliculus,[3] contralateral diminution of hearing functions (also see pp. 118–119).

INTERPEDUNCULAR NUCLEUS (IPNu)

The interpeduncular nucleus (IPNu) is a small cluster of neurons on the ventral surface of the midbrain nestled between the two massive cerebral peduncles. This nucleus is a relay station in the flow of information from the limbic forebrain to the brain stem serotonergic systems. It receives afferent fibers from the septal area of the forebrain through the habenulointerpeduncular tract (see Chap. 7). Efferent fi-

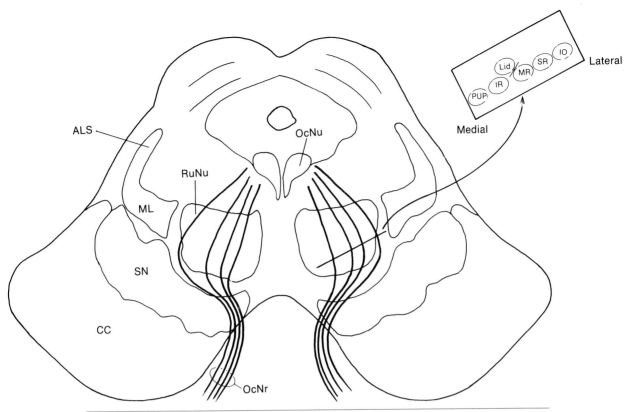

Figure 6-2. The course of the oculomotor nerve in the midbrain demonstrates the topography of fiber fascicles within the radiations of the oculomotor nerve. The inset is taken from the main section and illustrates the position the fascicles of the oculomotor nerve. Each oval represents a fascicle associated with a specific muscle (IO, inferior oblique; IR, inferior rectus; Lid, levator palpebrae; MR, medial rectus; PUP, pupillary fibers; SR, superior rectus. (Modified from Castro O, Johnson LN, Mamourian AC. Isolated inferior oblique paresis from brain-stem infarction. Arch Neurol 1990;47:235)

bers from the interpeduncular nucleus project to the raphe nuclei and central gray.[18]

SUBSTANTIA NIGRA (SN)

The substantia nigra (SN) is embedded in the dorsomedial surface of the cerebral peduncles. It receives a projection from the corpus striatum (caudate nucleus and putamen) called the striatonigral tract. The substantia nigra includes cell types producing dopamine. These axons form the nigrostriatal tract, which projects to the caudate nucleus and putamen. The substantia nigra plays a role in control of the motor system. The integration of this nucleus with the basal ganglia is further discussed in Chapter 10.

CLINICAL DEFICIT

Vascular lesions in the vicinity of the substantia nigra usually involve the cerebral peduncles as well; the paralysis resulting from the loss of the corticospinal fibers tends to mask any signs generated by the loss of the substantia nigra. Neurodegeneration of the dopamine-containing neurons in the substantia nigra results through a complicated pathway (Chap. 10) in a deregulation of the internal segment of the globus pallidus,[19] which can then increase its inhibition of the ventral lateral thalamic nucleus. The result is a diminished output from thalamus to motor cortex. The patient experiences hypokinesia, or decreased ability to initiate motion, and bradykinesia, a decreased speed of motion.[20] These two motor deficits are part of the Parkinson's syndrome.

VENTRAL TEGMENTAL AREA (VTA)

The ventral tegmental area (VTA) is a loose collection of dopaminergic cells located medial to the substantia nigra and continuous rostrally with the lateral hypothalamic area. Its ascending projections reach many of the limbic forebrain structures.[21]

CLINICAL DEFICIT

Dopaminergic neurons in the ventral tegmental area are depleted in Parkinson's disease. Just how much this contributes to the syndrome is unclear at this writing. Being connected to the limbic forebrain, it is conceivable that diminution in the function of these neurons plays a role in the personality changes seen in the parkinsonian patient. Excessive production of dopamine by these cells has been found in the postmortem brains of schizophrenic patients.[22]

CEREBRAL PEDUNCLE OR CRUS CEREBRI (CC)

The massive cerebral peduncles or crus cerebri (CC) are present in the ventrolateral quadrant of the midbrain. Rostrally, this fiber bundle represents a derivative of the internal capsule; caudally, it is continuous with the corticospinal tract in the pons and pyramidal tract in the medulla.

A topographic distribution of axons is present in the cerebral peduncles. The frontopontine fibers are located most ventrally; the corticonuclear, corticospinal, temporopontine, occipitopontine, and parietopontine fibers follow in order, progressing dorsally.

The fibers of the crus cerebri arise in large part from the cerebral cortex and pass through the internal capsule. Damage to either structure can result in degeneration of a portion of the crus and is expressed as hemiplegia in the patient. This reduction in mass of the crus is detectable by imaging and is proportional to the extent of the causal lesion in the forebrain.[23] In addition, the reduction in area of the crus is inversely proportional to the probability of recovery of function.[24]

CLINICAL DEFICIT

Vascular accidents involving the peduncles usually present with contralateral paresis of the limbs (involving the distal extremities more than the proximal), which is assumed to be due to the loss of the corticospinal fibers. In addition, contralateral facial paralysis in the lower quadrant of the face from the loss of the supranuclear innervation of these cranial motor nuclei and contralateral dystaxia from loss of the corticopontine fibers are present.[25,26]

The effects of small lesions in the cerebral peduncles are controversial. Surgical lesions, placed in the corticospinal portion of the human cerebral peduncles, produced only slight hypokinesia and very mild loss of function.[27] Based on these studies, it is proposed that section of the corticospinal portion of the peduncle alone will not result in spasticity. It is certainly possible that the vascular accidents observed clinically have damaged more than the corticospinal fibers, such as the corticonuclear fibers to the reticular formation, accounting for the spastic paralysis present in these patients.

Review Structures From Preceding Plates

Identify the following structures from previous sections:

Superior colliculus (SC)

Central gray (CeGy)

Medial lemniscus (ML)

Anterolateral system (ALS)

Ventral trigeminothalamic tract (VTTr)

Central tegmental tract (CTT)

Rubrospinal tract (RuSP)

Midbrain reticular formation (MidRetF)

Medial longitudinal fasciculus (MLF)

Dorsal longitudinal fasciculus (DLF)

▷ **Atlas Plate 20**

The dorsal portion of this section passes through the caudal thalamus; the ventral portion passes through the midbrain and an extreme rostral edge of the pons. The pontine and thalamic structures of these sections are discussed in Chapters 4 and 7, respectively. A salient feature of this section is the massive cerebral peduncles that cradle the midbrain and thalamus.

PRETECTAL NUCLEI (PrTecNu)

The pretectal nuclei (PrTecNu) are positioned between the superior colliculi caudally and the thalamus rostrally (Fig. 6-3). They receive information bilaterally, from the retina, thereby representing the contralateral visual hemisphere. Pretectal axons project di-

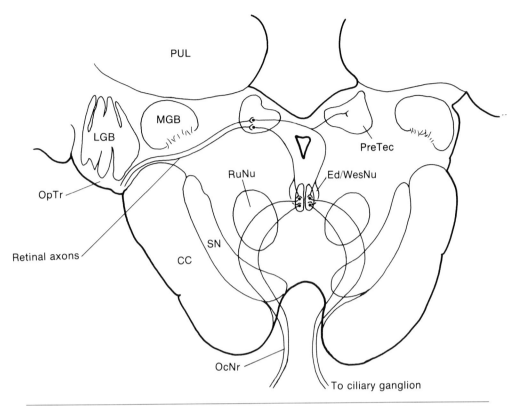

Figure 6-3. This diagram of the pretectal nuclei illustrates their role in the pupillary light reflex.

rectly to the ipsilateral Edinger-Westphal nuclei of the oculomotor complex as well as through the posterior commissure to the contralateral Edinger-Westphal nucleus. From the Edinger-Westphal nucleus parasympathetic fibers travel with the oculomotor nerve to reach the ipsilateral ciliary ganglion in the eye. Short ciliary or postganglionic fibers from the ciliary ganglion innervate the pupillary sphincter muscles of the iris and the ciliary body (see Fig. 6-3). The pretectal system is involved in the pupillary light reflex and the accommodation–constriction response (see discussion in Barr and Kiernan[28]). Light shined in one eye will, acting through the bilateral projections from the pretectum, constrict both pupils.[11]

CLINICAL DEFICIT

Bilateral damage to the pretectal area causes the loss of convergence movements and pupillary light reflex that occur in Parinaud's syndrome or the syndrome of the dorsal midbrain.[29]

Partial damage to the retina or to the retinopretectal fibers in the optic nerve or contralateral optic tract, although not eliminating the light reflex, can weaken that side's ability to maintain pupillary constriction. When light is shined into the eye contralateral to the damage, a consensual response rapidly constricts both pupils. However, when it is quickly moved over to the ipsilateral eye, the pupils dilate because of the weak-

ened constrictor tone from the damaged pretectum. This phenomenon of paradoxical dilation is called the **Marcus Gunn pupil** and is a sign of damage to the pretectal afferent fibers.

ROSTRAL INTERSTITIAL NUCLEUS OF THE MEDIAL LONGITUDINAL FASCICULUS (RINMLF)

The rostral interstitial nucleus of the medial longitudinal fasciculus (RINMLF) is located in the central gray at the rostral end of the medial longitudinal fasciculus. It controls vertical gaze[30] and pursuit movements[31] through a complex set of efferent projections. Fibers influencing downward vertical saccades project caudally along the medial longitudinal fasciculus to reach the ipsilateral oculomotor and trochlear nuclei. Those influencing upward vertical saccades project superiorly to cross the midline in the posterior commissure and then descend in the medial longitudinal fasciculus to reach the contralateral oculomotor and trochlear nuclei.

CLINICAL DEFICITS

Lesions involving the area around the medial longitudinal fasciculus, rostral to the oculomotor or trochlear nuclei, can affect vertical conjugate gaze.[32] Dorsally positioned, small infarctive lesions affecting the rostral interstitial nucleus or its efferent fibers in the posterior commissure can produce Parinaud's syndrome or loss of upward conjugate gaze,[33] whereas more ventrally placed lesions that spare the posterior commissure can compromise downward conjugate gaze.[34] Larger lesions in this region result in complete vertical gaze palsy.[33] Because of the interaction between sides, even unilateral lesions involving the rostral interstitial nucleus can result in a bidirectional (vertical) gaze paresis.[31]

POSTERIOR COMMISSURE (PoCom)

Fibers from the pretectal nuclei and the accessory optic nuclei decussate through the posterior commissure (PoCom) of the thalamus. These include fibers from those portions of the pretectal nuclei involved in the pupillary light reflex that are crossing to innervate the contralateral Edinger-Westphal nucleus.

CLINICAL DEFICIT

Damage to the posterior commissure and its surrounding nuclei can interrupt conjugate vertical gaze, particularly upward gaze.[32]

RADIATIONS OF THE OCULOMOTOR NERVE (OcNr)

Axons of the oculomotor neurons (OcNr) leave the nucleus in a series of fascicles fanning out in an inferolateral direction and passing through the red nucleus forming the radiations of the oculomotor nerve. These fibers coalesce into a unified bundle on the edge of the interpeduncular fossa and leave the brain stem along the medial aspect of the cerebral peduncle. The axons in each fascicle innervate a specific muscle in the orbit. An orderly arrangement of fascicles for each of the extraocular eye muscles[35] has been reported (Fig. 6-2). From medial to lateral the representation is as follows: inferior rectus, medial rectus, superior rectus, and inferior oblique. The fascicle for the levator palpebrae is located in close association with that for the medial rectus, whereas the axons of general visceral efferent neurons form a separate fascicle that courses on the extreme medial border of the oculomotor radiations.

CLINICAL DEFICIT

Complete section of the oculomotor radiations is similar to destruction of the nucleus; the globe is abducted, and slightly depressed, and the pupil is dilated and unreactive to light. Small infarctions in the ventral midbrain can damage a limited number of third-nerve radiations. A specific lesion of the fascicles to the inferior oblique muscle, the lateral-most fascicle, has been reported.[35] Axons for the visceral motor component run separated from, and medial to, the general somatic component. Thus, they can be spared in small lesions of the midbrain tegmentum producing a paresis of the globe in the presence of a reactive pupil. In such cases, the patient presents with a third-nerve palsy but with functioning pupils.[36]

RED NUCLEUS (RuNu)

A large spherical mass of cells in the ventral midbrain forms the red nucleus (RuNu). Afferent fibers to this structure arrive from the cerebral cortex and dentate nucleus of the cerebellum. Two major projections arise from the red nucleus. The rubrospinal tract innervates the ventral and intermediate horns of the contralateral spinal cord. This pathway and the corticospinal tract form the descending output of the lateral motor system. The rubro-olivary tract connects the red nucleus with the inferior olive of the medulla. This tract is part of a feedback circuit passing from the cerebellum, to red nucleus, inferior olive, and back to the cerebellum. The integrity of this circuit, although unnecessary for executing established motor patterns, is necessary for learning new motor patterns.[37]

The red nucleus lies in a nest of fiber tracts entering the thalamus. Laterally, it is closely surrounded by the dentothalamic tract (superior cerebellar peduncle) as it passes from the decussation to the thalamus. Rostrally, the border of the red nucleus is in close juxtaposition with the pallidothalamic tract from the globus pallidus to the thalamus. Lesions in the vicinity of the red nucleus can infringe on these tracts, both of which are related to the function of the motor system.

The influence of the red nucleus on motor behavior in man has long been questioned. Recently, it has been postulated that this nucleus and its tract (rubrospinal) are activated when automated movements are being executed, whereas the corticospinal tract is involved with nonautomated movements.[38]

CLINICAL DEFICIT

The clinical significance of damage of the red nucleus in man is questionable. Most likely, the rubral deficits are masked by the other component of the lateral motor system, the corticospinal tract. Lesions in the area of the red nucleus can present with limb tremor, hypokinesia, and ataxia. However, these clinical signs are most likely due to damage to the surrounding dentothalamic tract and pallidothalamic fibers rather than an expression of the rubral dysfunction (see Chaps. 5 and 10).

DENTOTHALAMIC TRACT OR CEREBELLOTHALAMIC TRCTSs (CThT)

After its decussation, the superior cerebellar peduncle, containing the dentothalamic tract, passes laterally around the red nucleus and ascends into the thalamus. Between the decussation and the thalamus, these axons are also called the cerebellothalamic tract (CThT). Fibers from the dentate nucleus terminate in the contralateral ventrolateral thalamic nucleus. As the tract approaches the thalamus, it joins other fibers to form the thalamic fasciculus (ThFas, Plate 22).

CLINICAL DEFICIT

Section of the superior cerebellar peduncle presents with limb tremor, hypokinesia, and ataxia (see Chap. 5). The clinical signs, resulting from section of the dentothalamic fibers superior to their decussation in the midbrain, present on the contralateral side.

Review Structures From Preceding Plates

Identify the following structures from previous sections:

Brachium of the inferior colliculus (IC, Br)

Substantia nigra (SN)

Ventral tegmental area (VTA)

Central gray (CeGy)

Medial lemniscus (ML)

Anterolateral system (ALS)

Ventral trigeminothalamic tract (VTTr)

Dorsal trigeminothalamic tract (DTTr)

Dorsal longitudinal fasciculus (DLF)

Medial longitudinal fasciculus (MLF)

Central tegmental tract (CTT)

Midbrain reticular formation (MidRetF)

Crus cerebri (CC)

Rostral interstitial nucleus of the medial longitudinal fasciculus (RINMLF)

UNIT B

Case Study 6-2

A 79-year-old man with sensory loss, strabismus, and tremor in the lower extremity

A 79-year-old, right-handed retired business executive was brought to his general practitioner's office by his son after suffering a momentary loss of consciousness, followed by double vision and a tremor in his left arm. He also complained of frequent dizzy periods over the last 5 months.

Past Medical History

He had been married for 40 years; his wife had died 5 years earlier. He had been an executive for a large firm. After retirement he has been active socially and played sports. His past medical history was positive for rheumatic fever at age 6. For the past 5 months he had been experiencing periods of dizziness and fatigue. He had a 30-pack-year history of smoking but quit completely 3 years before. He drank 2 to 3 ounces of alcohol socially per week.

General Physical Examination

He was alert and oriented, well nourished, and of average weight; he appeared his stated age. The patient frequently had to cover his right eye with his hand in order to move about the room. Optic discs were clear with sharp borders. External auditory canals were patent. His neck was supple; there where no bruits over the carotid artery. His larynx and pharynx were nonreddened. His chest was clear to auscultation and percussion; abdomen was soft

127

without rigidity, tenderness, or organomegaly. Heart rate was irregularly irregular. Peripheral pulses were intact; a pulse deficit was present, with the auscultated apical rate exceeding the radial pulse rate. Blood pressure was 135/93, temperature was 37°C, and respirations were 16/min. No cervical, axillary, or inguinal lymphadenopathy was present.

Neurologic Examination

Mental Status. The patient was alert and oriented to time and place with memory and knowledge appropriate for his age. He was articulate in speech and had good comprehension of spoken and written language. He gave a comprehensive history.

Cranial Nerves. On forward gaze, with the lid forcibly elevated, the right eye had an external strabismus; on attempted left lateral gaze, the right eye drifted toward the midline. The right pupil was larger than the left. The right pupil was unresponsive to light shined in either eye; the left pupil was responsive to direct and consensual light. The right eyelid elevated 4 mm, whereas the left elevated 13 mm on forward gaze. With the right eyelid forcibly elevated, its visual field was full to confrontation. The visual field in the left eye was also full. The patient noted diplopia on attempted forward gaze. The diplopia was absent with the right eye covered and exacerbated when the right eyelid was fully elevated. Hearing was normal in both ears. He had a full range of facial expressions. Jaw-jerk and corneal reflexes were normal; the palate was elevated on the midline; gag reflex was normal; and tongue protruded on the midline.

Motor Systems. Strength was slightly diminished in the left limbs; deep tendon reflexes were +2/5 on the right and +3/5 on the left. No Babinski response was present. A tremor of intent was present in the left arm. Finger-to-nose testing was normal on the right but he was slightly off target when using the left upper limb. The left arm and hand displayed an occasional jerky movement that the patient could not suppress.

Sensation. Pinprick and temperature sensation were normal throughout body and face; position sense and vibratory sensation on the left side of his body was diminished. This sensory loss was more noticeable in the upper than in the lower extremity.

QUESTIONS

1. Does the patient exhibit a language or memory deficit or an alteration in consciousness or cognition?

2. Are signs of cranial nerve dysfunction present?

3. Are there any changes in motor functions, such as reflexes, muscle tone, movement, or coordination?

4. Are any changes in sensory functions detectable?

5. At what level in the central neuraxis is this lesion most likely located?

6. Is the pathology focal, multifocal, or diffuse in its distribution within the nervous system?

7. What is the clinical–temporal profile of this pathology: acute or chronic; progressive or stable?

8. Based on your answers to the previous two questions, decide whether the symptoms in this patient are most likely caused by a vascular accident, a tumor, or a degenerative or inflammatory process.

9. If you feel this is the result of a vascular accident, what vessels are most likely involved?

► DISCUSSION
Midbrain Vasculature

The vasculature of the midbrain is relatively complex (Fig. 6-4). The basilar artery and its two terminal branches, the posterior cerebral arteries, contribute many penetrating and circumferential branches. In addition, the midbrain is the only portion of the brain stem distal to the thalamus to receive arteries from the anterior circulation; this is accomplished by the anterior choroidal arteries.

POSTERIOR CIRCULATION

The **basilar artery** divides at its rostral end to form the two posterior cerebral arteries; this occurs in the cisternal space ventral to the midbrain. Short, **anteromedial branches** from the top of the basilar artery and from the proximal segment of the two posterior cerebral arteries supply the median zone to the midbrain. This tuft of vessels, which can arise from a common stem, extends rostrally, giving rise to the thalamic paramedian arteries supplying the medial nuclei of the thalamus, subthalamus, and hypothalamus. If considered all together, the arterial branches at the top of the basilar and proximal posterior cerebral arteries supply a central zone in the midbrain and thalamus (see Plates 19 to 25) and are responsible for the paramedian syndrome of the mesencephalic–thalamic border.[39] Specific midbrain areas serviced by the paramedian branches are the interpeduncular nucleus, the red nucleus, the decussation of the superior cerebellar peduncle, the oculomotor nucleus and its associated structures, and the ventral portion of the central gray.

Two groups of long, circumferential branches from the basilar artery wrap around the brain stem to reach the colliculi (see Fig. 6-4). The caudal group contains the **superior cerebellar arteries (SCA** in

Fig. 6-4), which give off only a few branches to the midbrain until reaching the colliculi. The rostral group contains the **collicular arteries (CA** in Fig. 6-4). Penetrating branches from the collicular arteries service the cerebral peduncles, substantia nigra, medial lemniscus, and dentothalamic tract. The distal twigs of the collicular arteries reach around the lateral and posterior aspect of the brain stem to end in the superior and inferior colliculi.

The **posteromedial choroidal arteries (PMChA** in Fig. 6-4) branch off the proximal segment of the posterior cerebral artery, turn posteriorly, and extend around the cerebral peduncles, running in an arc, parallel but rostral to the collicular arteries. Penetrating branches from posteromedial choroidal arteries perfuse the cerebral peduncles, substantia nigra, medial lemniscus, and dentothalamic tract. The distal twigs of these arteries reach around the posterior aspect of the brain stem to end in the superior and inferior colliculi.

ANTERIOR CIRCULATION

The **anterior choroidal artery (AChA** in Fig. 6-4) branches off the proximal segment of the anterior cerebral artery and passes caudally around the cerebral peduncle, giving off penetrating twigs as it travels. It courses in an arc parallel to the posteromedial choroidal and collicular arteries. Its penetrating branches supply a ventrolateral arc around the brain stem, including cerebral peduncles, substantia nigra, medial lemniscus, and dentothalamic tract.

MIDBRAIN LESION SYNDROMES

Perfusion of the midbrain can be divided into several zones[40]: anterior, lateral, and posterior (see Plates 19 and 20). Each zone consists of numerous penetrating vessels derived from a group of circumferential

129

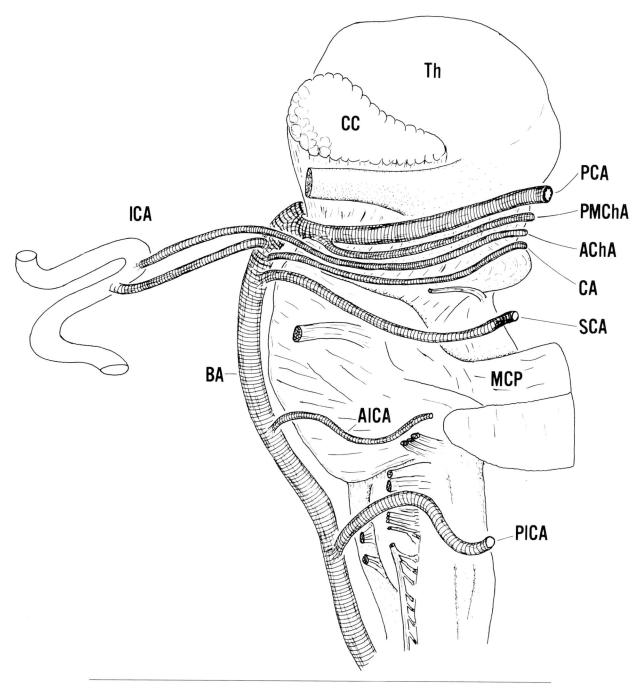

Figure 6-4. Diagram illustrates blood supply to midbrain. (Modified from Mettler FA. Neuroanatomy. 2nd ed. St Louis: CV Mosby, 1942:160)

arteries. The anterior zone is further partitioned into anteromedial (or medial paramedian) and anterolateral (or lateral paramedian) regions.

Several arterial syndromes can be defined in the midbrain. These syndromes represent vascular territory damaged by perfusion failure. A pattern exists in their distribution. The **paramedian syndrome** can occur when the anteromedial penetrating arteries in

the anterior zone are compromised; **Weber's syndrome** can occur when the anterolateral penetrating branches in the anterior zone are damaged; **Benedict's syndrome** can result when arteries in the lateral zone of penetrating branches are damaged; and **Parinaud's syndrome** arises from either the penetrating branches of the posterior zone or tumors of the pineal gland.

130

Paramedian Syndrome

Oculomotor palsy and/or vertical gaze palsy, bilateral limb ataxia, and dysmetria are the presenting signs of the paramedian syndrome. It can occur due to occlusion of the anteromedial branches of the basilar or proximal posterior cerebral arteries. In this syndrome damage is done to the oculomotor nerve, oculomotor nucleus, rostral interstitial nucleus (vertical gaze center), and decussation of the superior cerebellar peduncle (Table 6-1). Extension of the ischemic zone can occur into the midline thalamus, resulting in dementia as well as sleep and memory disturbances. (See Chap. 7.)

Weber's Syndrome

Oculomotor palsy and contralateral spastic paralysis are the cardinal signs of Weber's syndrome.[41] Akinesia and tremor can also be associated, as well as supranuclear palsy of the facial nerve. Conversely, all sensory systems can be intact in this syndrome. Damage is done to the roots of the oculomotor nerve, substantia nigra, and cerebral peduncles (see Table 6-1). Anterolateral branches of the basilar, posterior cerebral, collicular, or anterior choroidal arteries can be involved in the genesis of this syndrome.

Table 6-1.

NEUROLOGIC SIGN	ANATOMIC SOURCE
PARAMEDIAN SYNDROME	
Oculomotor palsy	Oculomotor nerve or nucleus
Vertical gaze paresis	Preoculomotor nuclei
Limb ataxia	Dentothalamic fibers
Memory loss	Median thalamus
Dementia	Median thalamus
Sleep dysfunction	Median thalamus
WEBER'S SYNDROME	
Oculomotor palsy	Oculomotor nerve or nucleus
Spastic paresis	Cerebral peduncle
Akinesia, tremor	Palladiothalamic fibers, substantia nigra, or its tracts
Dystaxia	Dentocerebellar fibers
BENEDICT'S SYNDROME	
Oculomotor palsy	Oculomotor nerve or nucleus
Dyskinesia	Palladiothalamic fibers, substantia nigra, or its tracts

Table 6-2.

NEUROLOGIC SIGN	ANATOMIC SOURCE
PARINAUD'S SYNDROME	
Upgaze palsy	Preoculomotor syndrome
"TOP OF THE BASILAR" SYNDROME	
Oculomotor palsy	Oculomotor nerve or nucleus
Vertical gaze palsy	Preoculomotor nuclei
Visual field defects	Optic radiations or occipital (visual) cortex
Behavior dysfunction	Medial aspect of temporal lobe

Benedict's Syndrome

Ipsilateral oculomotor palsy and contralateral motor dysfunction (hyperkinesia or akinesia) are the cardinal signs of Benedict's syndrome.[41] Damage is done to the root of the oculomotor nerve, red nucleus, dentothalamic fibers, and substantia nigra (see Table 6-1). Distal tips of the lateral paramedian branches of the basilar, posterior cerebral, collicular, posteromedial choroidal, or anterior arteries can also be casual factors.

Parinaud's Syndrome

Upgaze palsy is the characteristic sign of Parinaud's or dorsal midbrain syndrome.[41] Damage is done to the superior colliculus and to the area at the rostral end of the medial longitudinal fasciculus (Table 6-2). The type of eye movement dysfunctions (upgaze palsy) suggests interruption of supranuclear control on the oculomotor nucleus.[42] Causative factors include the following: occlusion of the collicular or posterior choroidal arteries supplying the tectum, expansion of a pineal tumor applying pressure to the tectum and underlying tissue, or giant aneurysm in the posterior cranial fossa.[43]

"Top of the Basilar" Syndrome

The basilar artery is larger in diameter than its two sources, the vertebral arteries. Emboli that survive the trip upward through the vertebrals target the top of the basilar, where they can lodge in and around its bifurcation. Occlusion of the distal (rostral) end of the basilar artery can infarct the midbrain, portions of the thalamus, and medial temporal lobe of the cerebrum.[44] A complex constellation of neurologic signs and symptoms arises, as is illustrated in Table 6-2. The major neurologic presentations resulting from midbrain damage in the "top of the basilar" syndrome are disturbances in alertness, behavior, visual fields, and eye movements, such as oculomotor palsy and vertical gaze palsy, and the presentation of amnesia.[45] The deficits due to thalamic and cerebral damage will be considered in Chapters 7 and 8.

► Bibliography

Adams RD, Victor M. Disorders of ocular movement and pupillary function. In: Principles of neurology. New York: McGraw-Hill, 1989; Chap. 13:206–225.

Adams RD, Victor M. Cerebrovascular diseases. In: Principles of neurology. New York: McGraw-Hill, 1989; Chap. 34:617–693.

Barr ML, Kiernan JA. Brain stem nuclei and tracts. In: The human nervous system: an anatomical viewpoint. Philadelphia: JB Lippincott, 1988; Chap. 7:92–120.

Barr ML, Kiernan JA. Cranial nerves. In: The human nervous system: an anatomical viewpoint. Philadelphia: JB Lippincott, 1988; Chap. 8:121–147.

Barr ML, Kiernan JA. Reticular formation. In: The human nervous system: an anatomical viewpoint. Philadelphia: JB Lippincott, 1988; Chap. 9:148–159.

Brazis PW. The localization of lesion affecting the brainstem. In: Brazis PW, Masdeu JC, Biller J, eds. Localization in clinical neurology. Boston: Little, Brown, 1990; Chap. 14:269–286.

Daube JR, Ragan TJ, Sandok BA, Westmoreland BF. The consciousness system. In: Medical neurosciences. Boston: Little, Brown, 1986; Chap. 8:138–155.

Daube JR, Ragan TJ, Sandok BA, Westmoreland BF. The posterior cranial fossa level. In: Medical neurosciences. Boston: Little, Brown, 1986; Chap. 14:324–373.

Haines DE. Neuroanatomy: an atlas of structures, sections, and systems. Baltimore: Urban & Schwarzenberg, 1987 *(see especially Figs. 5-21 to 5-26)*.

Masdeu JC, Brazis PW. The localization of lesions in the ocular motor system. In: Brazis PW, Masdeu JC, Biller J, eds. Localization in clinical neurology. Boston: Little, Brown, 1990; Chap. 7:127–187.

Nieuwenhuys R, Voogd J, van Huijzen C. The human central nervous system. Berlin: Springer-Verlag, 1988:179–220.

► References

1. Howe JR, Miller CA. Midbrain deafness following head injury. Neurology 1975;25:286–289.

2. Cascino GD, Adams RD. Brainstem auditory hallucinosis. Neurology 1986;36:1042–1047.

3. Jenkins WM, Masterton RB. Sound localization: effects of unilateral lesions in central auditory system. J Neurophysiol 1982; 47:987–1016.

4. Sand JJ, Biller J, Corbett J, Adams HP, Dunn, V. Partial dorsal mesencephalic hemorrhages: report of three cases. Neurology 1986;36(4):529–533.

5. Nieuwenhuys R, Voogd J, van Huijzen C. The human central nervous system. Berlin: Springer-Verlag, 1988.

6. Bender MB. Brain control of conjugate horizontal and vertical eye movements. A survey of the structural and function correlates. Brain 1980;103:23–69.

7. Plum F, Posner JB. The diagnosis of stupor and coma. Philadelphia: FA Davis, 1982:377.

8. Watson RT, Heilman KM, Miller BD, King FA. Neglect after mesencephalic reticular formation lesions. Neurology 1974;24: 294–298.

9. Sparks, DL Translation of sensory signals into commands for control of saccadic eye movements: role of primate superior colliculus. Physiol Rev 1986;66:118–171.

10. Barbur JL, Ruddock KH, Waterfield VA. Human visual responses in the absence of the geniculo-calcarine projection. Brain 1980;103:905–928.

11. Masdeu JC, Brazis PW. The localization of lesions in the ocular motor system. In: Brazis PW, Masdeu JC, Biller J, eds. Localization in clinical neurology. Boston: Little, Brown, 1990:127–187.

12. Ropper AH, Miller DC. Acute traumatic midbrain hemorrhage. Ann Neurol 1985;18(1):80–86.

13. Durward QJ, Barnett HJM, Barr HWK. Presentation and management of mesencephalic hematoma. J Neurosurg 1982;56:123–127.

14. Rush JA, Younge BR. Paralysis of cranial nerves III, IV, and VI: cause and prognosis in 1,000 cases. Arch Ophthalmol 1981;99:76–79.

15. Lavin PM, Troost BT. Traumatic fourth nerve palsy. Arch Neurol 1984;41:679–680.

16. Gonyea EF. Superior oblique palsy due to a midbrain vascular malformation. Neurology 1990;40:554–555.

17. Bernard JF, Peschanski M, Besson JM. Afferents and efferents of the rat cuneiformis nucleus: an anatomical study with reference to pain transmission. Brain Res 1989;490:181–185.

18. Groenewegen HJ, Ahlenius S, Haber SN, Kowall NW, Nauta WJH. Cytoarchitecture, fiber connections, and some histochemical aspects of the interpeduncular nucleus in the rat. J Comp Neurol 1986;249:65–102.

19. Alexander GF, Crutcher MD. Functional architecture of basal ganglia circuits: neural substrates of parallel processing. Trends Neurosci 1990;13:266–271.

20. DeLong MR. Primate models of movement disorders of basal ganglia origin. Trends Neurosci 1990;13:281–285.

21. Moore RY. Catecholamine neuron systems in the brain. Ann Neurol 1982;12:321–327.

22. Bird ED, Spokes EGS, Iverson LL. Increased dopamine concentration in limbic areas of the brain from patients dying with schizophrenia. Brain 1979;102:347–360.

23. Warabi T, Miyasaka K, Inoue K, Nakamura N. Computed tomographic studies of the basis pedunculi in chronic hemiplegic patients: topographic correlation between cerebral lesion and midbrain shrinkage. Neuroradiology 1987;29:409–415.

24. Warabi T, Inoue K, Noda H, Murakami S. Recovery of voluntary movement in hemiplegic patients. Brain 1990;113:177–189.

25. Fisher CM, Curry HB. Pure motor hemiplegia of vascular origin. Arch Neurol 1965;13:30–44.

26. Helweg-Larsen S, Larsson H, Henriksen O, Sorensen PS. Ataxic hemiparesis: three different locations of lesions studied by MRI. Neurology 1988;38:1322–1324.

27. Bucy PC, Keplinger JE. Section of the cerebral peduncles. Arch Neurol 1961;5:132–139.

28. Barr ML, Kiernan JA. The human nervous system: an anatomical viewpoint. Philadelphia: JB Lippincott, 1988, Chap. 8.

29. Waga S Okada M, Ymanoto Y. Reversibility of Parinaud syndrome in thalamic hemorrhage. Neurology 29 1979;3:407–409.

30. Buttner-Ennever JA, Buttner U, Cohen B, Baumgartner G. Vertical gaze paralysis and the rostral interstitial nucleus of the medial longitudinal fasciculus. Brain 1982;105:125–149.

31. Ranalli PJ, Sharpe JA, Fletcher WA. Palsy of upward and downward saccadic, pursuit, and vestibular movements with unilateral midbrain lesion: pathophysiological correlations. Neurology 1988;38:114–122.

32. Christoff N. A clinicopathologic study of vertical eye movements. Arch Neurol 1974;31:1–8.

33. Pierrot-Deseilligny CH, Chain F, Gray F, Serdaru M, Escourolle R, Lhermitte F. Parinaud's syndrome: electro-oculographic and anatomical analysis of six vascular cases with deductions about vertical gaze organization in the premotor structures. Brain 1982;105:667–696.

34. Jacobs L, Anderson PJ, Bender MB. The lesions producing paralysis of downward but not upward gaze. Arch Neurol 1973;28:319–323.

35. Castro O, Johnson LN, Mamourian AC. Isolated inferior oblique paresis from brain-stem infarction. Arch Neurol 1990;47:235–237.

36. Keane JR. Isolated brain-stem third nerve palsy. Arch Neurol 1988;45:813–814.

37. Thach WT, Goodkin HP, Keating JG. The cerebellum and adaptive coordination of movement. Ann Rev Neurosci 1992;15:403–442.

38. Kennedy PR. Corticospinal, rubrospinal, and rubro-olivary pro-jections: a unifying hypothesis. Trends Neurosci 1990;13:474–479.

39. Castaigne P, Lhermitte F, Buge A, Escourolle R, Hauw JJ, Lyon-Caen O. Paramedian thalamic and midbrain infarcts: clinical and neuropathological study. Ann Neurol 1981;10:127–148.

40. Duvernoy HM. Human brainstem vessels. Berlin: Springer-Verlag, 1978.

41. Brazis PW. The localization of lesions affecting the brainstem. In: Brazis PW, Masdeu JC, Biller J, eds. Localization in clinical neurology. Boston: Little, Brown, 1990:269–285.

42. Baloh RW, Furman JM, Yee RD. Dorsal midbrain syndrome: clinical and oculographic findings. Neurology 1985;35:54–60.

43. Coppeto JR, Lessell S. Dorsal midbrain syndrome from giant aneurysm of the posterior fossa: report of two cases. Neurology 1983;33:732–736.

44. Caplan LR. "Top of the basilar" syndrome. Neurology 1980;30:72–79.

45. Caplan LR. Vertebrobasilar system syndromes. Handbook Clin Neurol 1989;53:371–408.

7 *THALAMUS*

► Introduction

The diencephalon is located at the dorsal end of the brain stem surrounded by the internal capsule laterally and the lateral ventricle and corpus callosum superiorly (Fig. 7-1). It is divided into two elongated hemispheres, which are separated by the narrow third ventricle. Each hemisphere is partitioned into dorsal and ventral portions by the hypothalamic sulcus (Fig. 7-2). The dorsal thalamus is composed of the **thalamus proper** (usually called the *thalamus*) and **epithalamus;** the ventral portion is composed of the **hypothalamus** and **subthalamus.** The nuclei of the thalamus proper form reciprocal connections with the ipsilateral cerebral cortex, whereas those of the hypothalamus are involved in regulating endocrine and autonomic nervous systems. The diencephalon receives its blood supply from penetrating arteries derived from the Circle of Willis or its immediate branches.

135

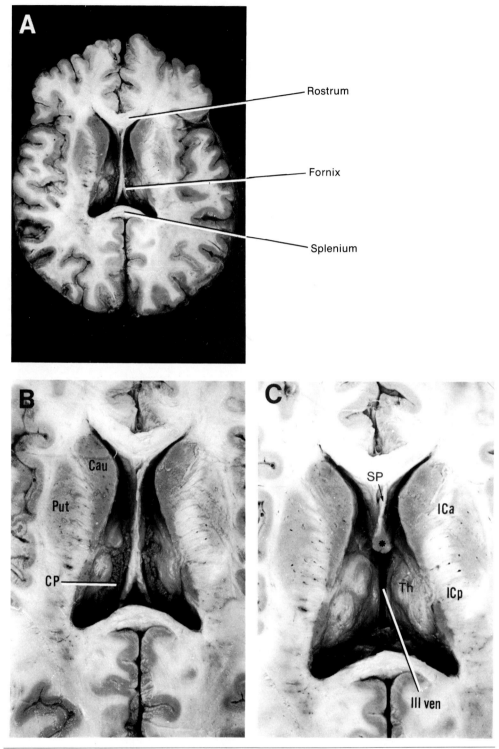

Figure 7-1. A horizontal section revealing a dorsal view of the thalamic hemispheres. **(A)** A horizontal section through the lateral ventricles providing orientation for the magnified views in **B** and **C. (B)** A view of the fornix and septum pellucidum separating the two lateral ventricles. The fornix is the rounded border closely associated with the choroid plexus (CP). **(C)** A view similar to that in **B,** with a portion of the septum pellucidum (SP) and fornix (labeled with an asterisk) removed to reveal the narrow third ventricle separating the two thalamic hemispheres (Th). The septum pellucidum is the thin membrane extending from the fornix to the rostrum of the corpus callosum. (The rostrum and splenium refer to the anterior and posterior portions of the corpus.)

136

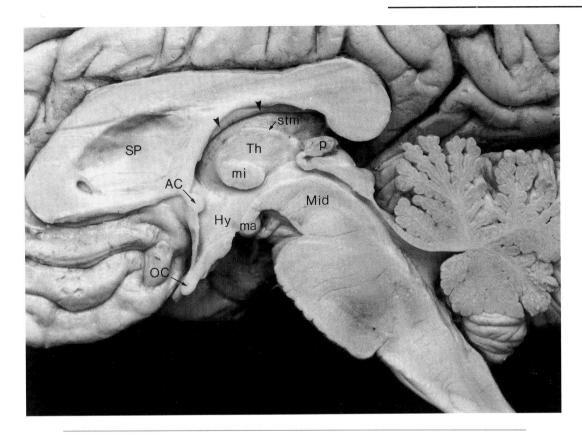

Figure 7-2. A midsagittal section of the brain demonstrating the location of the thalamic hemisphere at the rostral end of the brainstem. The arrowheads indicate the curved arch of the fornix. The hypothalamic sulcus separates the hypothalamus from the thalamus. It is seen as a groove in the lateral wall of the third ventricle passing ventral to the massa intermedia. (AC, anterior commissure; Hy, hypothalamus; ma, mamillary bodies; mi, massa intermedia; Mid, midbrain; OC, optic chiasm; p, pineal; SP, septum pellucidum; stm, stria medullaris.)

GENERAL OBJECTIVES

1. To identify the location of major thalamic nuclei and learn their relationship to the cerebral cortex
2. To identify the major hypothalamic regions and learn their relationships with the endocrine and autonomic nervous systems
3. To learn the presenting signs and symptoms consequent to lesions involving major nuclei and tracts in the thalamus where they are known
4. To apply this knowledge to understanding the clinical manifestations of major thalamic vascular lesions

INSTRUCTIONS

In this chapter you will be presented with one or more clinical case studies. *Each study will be followed by a list of questions that can best be answered by using a knowledge of regional and functional neuroanatomy and by referring to outside reading material.* Following the questions will be a section devoted to structures from a specific region of the central nervous system. Before you attempt to answer the questions, compile a list of the patient's neurologic signs and symptoms; then examine the structures and their functions and study their known clinical deficits. After becoming familiar with the material, reexamine the list of neurologic signs and symptoms and answer the questions. Be aware that some of the questions can have multiple responses or require information beyond the scope of this manual. It may be necessary to obtain material or advice from additional resources, such as specialty texts, a medical dictionary, or clinical personnel.

MATERIALS

1. A human brain sectioned on the midsagittal plane
2. A brain stem model with thalamus
3. A medical dictionary

UNIT A

Case Study 7-1

A 65-year-old man with right-sided hemiparesis, homonymous hemianopsia, dysarthria, and confusion

This 65-year-old, right-handed man was brought to the emergency room early in the morning by his family. They complained that he could not use his right hand, had slurred speech, and was acting confused. He had been that way since shortly after he awoke that morning.

Past Medical History

He was in good health until 7 years before, when he was diagnosed as having hypertension. One year later he was admitted to the community hospital, the day after he experienced a brief episode of quadriparesis, blurred vision, and nausea. At that time Doppler studies of the carotids were normal, as were lumbar puncture, electroencephalogram, and a computed tomographic (CT) scan. Diabetes was detected and he was given a regimen of insulin and discharged. During the next 4 years, no known transient ischemic episodes occurred.

Family History

At the time of admission he was married, retired from military service, and had two children, both of whom are married. His father had had hypertension and died at 55 of coronary artery disease; his mother was still living.

General Physical Examination

He was a well-hydrated, well-nourished man in no acute distress who appeared the stated age. Funduscopic examination revealed arterial–venous nicking without hemorrhage or papilledema. His heartbeat was regular without murmurs or gallops. Blood pressure was 180/100. Respiration and pulse were normal. Lungs were clear to auscultation. Abdomen was soft without masses. Skin was of good texture and temperature. Several small areas of active keratosis on the right posterior scalp were evident.

Neurologic Examination

Mental Status. He was disoriented with respect to time, place, and personal information, relying on his family members to supply much of the history. He had impaired recent memory and fund of knowledge. (He said Kennedy was president.) He confused the left and right sides of his body. A mild sensory neglect, detectable with extinction testing, was apparent on his right side. His speech was poorly articulated and perseverative, and he used word substitutions and mispronounced words frequently; however, he had normal repetition of speech.

Cranial Nerves. He had a full range of eye movements. There was a right homonymous hemianopia. Pupils were symmetric and bilaterally responsive to light both direct and consensual. Hearing was normal in both ears. Corneal, jaw-jerk, and gag reflexes were intact. His face was asymmetric on spontaneous emotional expression (*e.g.,* smiling) but not on voluntary movement (right "emotional" facial paralysis). Discriminative touch was intact across his face, bilaterally. The uvula was elevated on the midline; the tongue protruded on the midline. Shoulder shrug was symmetric.

Motor Systems. Strength in the limbs was +5/5 in the left arm and leg and +3/5 in the right arm and +4/5 in the right leg. Deep tendon reflexes were elevated in the right arm more than the right leg; they were physiologic on the left. A Babinski sign was noted on the right.

Sensation. Pain, light touch, and vibration sense were normal, but discriminative touch and proprioception were impaired in the right hand.

QUESTIONS

1. Does the patient exhibit a language or memory deficit or an alteration in consciousness or cognition?

2. Are signs of cranial nerve dysfunction present?

3. Are there any changes in motor functions, such as reflexes, muscle tone, movement, or coordination?

4. Are any changes in sensory functions detectable?

5. At what level in the central neuraxis is this lesion most likely located?

6. Is the pathology focal, multifocal, or diffuse in its distribution within the nervous system?

7. What is the clinical–temporal profile of this pathology: acute or chronic; progressive or stable?

8. Based on your answers to the previous two questions, decide whether the symptoms in this patient are most likely caused by a vascular accident, a tumor, or a degenerative or inflammatory process.

9. If you feel this is the result of a vascular accident, what vessels are most likely involved?

10. Destruction of what structure could account for the visual dysfunction?

11. Damage to what structure would account for the patient's paralysis?

12. Damage to what thalamic structure(s) would provide an explanation for the impairment of memory?

Case Study 7-2

A 47-year-old man with bitemporal hemianopsia and endocrinopathy

A 47-year-old, left-handed man was admitted to the hospital with a primary complaint of chest pain of 3 weeks' duration. He also complained of a progressive narrowing of his visual fields.

Past Medical History

He had a recent history of angina on exertion, and electrocardiographic analysis documented an acute myocardial infarct. Since childhood he had consumed at least a gallon of water a day and had had thirst, polyuria, and nocturia. Having grown up with these symptoms, he had considered them normal.

Family History

At the time of admission, he was not married, lived alone, and admitted to having very little libido throughout his life. His mother, father, and two siblings were alive and in good health. No one else in his family had exhibited his chief complaints.

General Physical Examination

He appeared to be a well-hydrated, well-nourished man, alert but with an anxious demeanor. He appeared his stated age. He weighed 240 pounds and his height was 66 inches. His head was normocephalic. Funduscopic examination revealed normal cup-to-disc ratio; soft cotton wool patches were noted two disc spaces from the disc in the superior temporal retina bilaterally; no aneurysms, hemorrhages, or papilledema was evident. His heartbeat was regular without gallops or thrills; an SII systolic murmur was noted at the left sternal border. Abdominojugular reflux was noted on application of abdominal pressure. Respiration was labored, breath sounds were decreased; crackles and wheezes were heard at the base of the lungs on auscultation. The abdomen was soft, without masses or tenderness. Temperature was elevated at 37.5°C and oscillated between 37.3°C and 37.9°C over a 24-hour period. Skin was moist with good texture and turgor. Pretibial edema (+2) was present in the lower extremity.

Neurologic Examination

Mental Status. The patient was awake and oriented for time and place; memory and knowledge were appropriate for his education. His speech was articulate and meaningful. Although he was cooperative most of the time, he experienced bouts of rage when he yelled at the attending staff and physician.

Cranial Nerves. He had a full range of eye movements, visual acuity was normal in the center of his fields but diminished rapidly to the sides, vision in the temporal fields was absent altogether. Corneal, jaw-jerk, and gag reflexes were intact. His face was symmetric, with normal expression on emotion. Hearing was diminished in the right ear more than in the left. Uvula and palate were symmetric and elevated on the midline; the tongue protruded on the midline. Shoulder shrug was symmetric.

Motor Systems. Gross motor strength was equal in upper and lower extremities; deep tendon reflexes were 2/4 and equal in upper and lower extremities. Babinski response was physiologic with no muscular atrophy or hypertrophy. No drift or involuntary motion was detected.

Sensation. There was no loss of vibration or proprioceptive sense, and no loss of pain or thermal senses was evident.

Follow-up

During his hospital admission, marked thirst and daily intake of 4000 to 17,000 mL of fluid were noted. Urine outputs of 3500 to 18,000 mL daily were recorded. The specific gravity of his urine was always below 1.005. One month after admission, the patient died of congestive heart failure.

QUESTIONS

1. Does the patient exhibit a language or memory deficit or an alteration in consciousness or cognition?

2. Are signs of cranial nerve dysfunction present?

3. Are there any changes in motor functions, such as reflexes, muscle tone, movement, or coordination?

4. Are any changes in sensory functions detectable?

5. At what level in the central neuraxis is this lesion most likely located?

6. Is the pathology focal, multifocal, or diffuse in its distribution within the nervous system?

7. What is the clinical–temporal profile of this pathology: acute or chronic; progressive or stable?

8. Based on your answers to the previous two questions, decide whether the symptoms in this patient are most likely caused by a vascular accident, a tumor, or a degenerative or inflammatory process.

9. If you feel this is the result of a vascular accident, what vessels are most likely involved?

10. Destruction of what region(s) of the brain could result in obesity, excessive thirst, fluctuant temperature, and sexual dysfunction?

11. How can you explain the visual dysfunction in this patient?

12. Discuss the possible problems in "compliance" that this patient would have experienced had he lived.

► DISCUSSION
Thalamic Structures

The medulla, pons, and midbrain were derived embryologically from the alar and basal plates of the neural tube. This pattern changes in the diencephalon. The dorsal thalamus (or thalamus proper) arises from the alar plate; the basal plate plays a much smaller role, giving rise to portions of the ventral thalamus only. The dorsal thalamus has extensive connections with the overlying mantle of neocortex, whereas the ventral thalamus is related through its connections

141

with the older portions of the cerebral cortex, such as the allocortex, as well as with the brain stem and spinal cord. The alteration in embryogeny along with the changes in connectivity contribute to a substantially different organizational pattern for the diencephalon than that present throughout the more caudal portions of the brain stem.

GROSS ANATOMIC ORGANIZATION

If all telencephalic structures of the forebrain are removed, the diencephalon would appear as two large, egg-shaped masses at the rostral end of the brain stem. A horizontal section passing through the lateral ventricles superior to the diencephalon illustrates its position between the fiber bundles of the internal capsule (see Fig. 7-1). The anterior limb (ICa in Fig. 7-1**C**) of the internal capsule separates caudate from putamen (portions of the basal ganglia; see Chap. 10); the posterior limb (ICp in Fig. 7-1**C**) of the internal capsule separates the putamen laterally from the diencephalon medially. A strand of choroid plexus lies along the dorsal surface of the diencephalon (Fig. 7-1**B**). The narrow third ventricle separates the two diencephalic hemispheres (Th in Fig. 7-1**C**).

The diencephalon is divided into two major regions by the hypothalamic sulcus (Fig. 7-2), each with separate functions. Its dorsal portion is intimately related through reciprocal connections to neocortex, modulating both the information traveling to, and the levels of neuronal activity in, the cerebral cortex. The ventral portion of the thalamus integrates sensory information from external and internal environments and regulates visceral and emotional behaviors through control over the autonomic nervous system via the brain stem and spinal cord, as well as its control over the endocrine system via the pituitary gland.

INTERNAL STRUCTURE

The dorsal thalamus can be divided into two regions: epithalamus and thalamus proper (usually called *thalamus*). The epithalamus contains a nuclear group, the habenular nuclei, and a fiber tract, the stria medullaris (stm in Fig. 7-2), which courses along the medial border of the thalamus. The epithalamic structures have strong connections to the limbic system (see Chap. 9).

The thalamus proper is divided into several groups of nuclei separated by thin bands of fibers and cells called medullary laminae. Four major groups of tha-

lamic nuclei are recognized: anterior, medial, ventral, and lateral-posterior (Fig. 7-3). These groups are separated from each other by the internal medullary lamina. An external medullary lamina surrounds the entire mass, to the outside of which lies the thalamic reticular nucleus (see Plates 21 to 25). Within each of the major groups, several individual nuclei exist, each nucleus being mapped to a specific region of the ipsilateral neocortex (Table 7-1) through reciprocal connections.

The ventral thalamus is also divided into two regions: subthalamus and hypothalamus. The subthalamus forms the border between the diencephalon and midbrain, located very close to the substantia nigra. It is involved in regulating motor activity and is connected to the basal ganglia.

The hypothalamus is separated from the thalamus proper by the hypothalamic sulcus; this appears as a narrow, curved groove passing ventrally around the massa intermedia (mi) on Figure 7-2. The rostral border of the hypothalamus is the lamina terminalis, which stretches between the optic chiasm (OC in Fig. 7-2) and a large fiber bundle called the anterior commissure (AC in Fig. 7-2). The lateral borders of the hypothalamus are formed by the optic tract and cerebral peduncle; caudally, the hypothalamus ends with the mamillary bodies (ma in Fig. 7-2). The ventral surface of the hypothalamus is raised into a ventrally directed dome called the median eminence. At the center of this eminence is the infundibulum, or stalk, of the pituitary.

Within the hypothalamus are several diffuse nuclei whose connections pass through three large fiber bundles: the mamillothalamic fasciculus, the fornix, and the median forebrain bundle. The hypothalamus receives projections from the spinal cord, brain stem, and the older portions of forebrain: the hippocampus and amygdala. Through its projections to the autonomic nuclei of the brain stem and spinal cord and its connections to the pituitary via the median eminence and infundibulum, the hypothalamus exerts control over visceral and emotional behavior.

The nuclei and tracts of the thalamus and hypothalamus are packed closely together. This presents two major problems when studying the deficits consequent to thalamic infarctions. (1) Even small lesions can damage multiple thalamic structures, presenting with a varied mixture of clinical signs and symptoms, many of which are similar to those seen in much larger lesions of the cerebral cortex. (2) In addition, the thalamocortical and corticothalamic fibers pass across the medial to lateral axis of the thalamus going to or from the internal capsule; small lesions in the lateral portions of thalamus can damage lateral nuclei

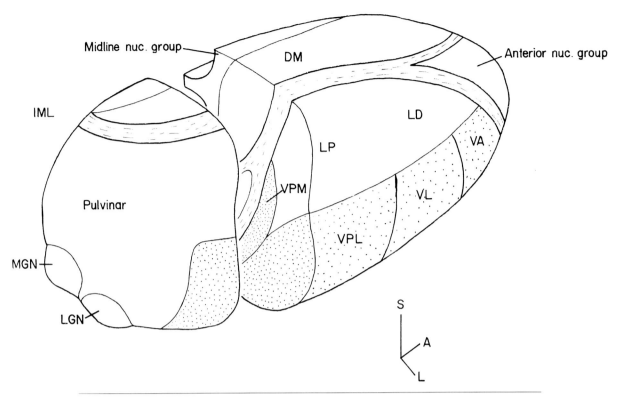

Figure 7-3. View of the thalamus partitioned into its nuclear groups. The internal medullary lamina forms a boundary separating the ventral and posterior groups from the medial, lateral, and anterior groups. (DM, dorsomedial nucleus; IML, intramedullary lamina; LD, lateral dorsal nucleus; LP, lateral posterior nucleus; MGM, medial geniculate nucleus; LGN, lateral geniculate nucleus; VPM, ventroposteromedial nucleu; VPL, ventroposterolateral nucleus; VA, ventroanterior nucleus; VLS, ventrolateral superior; L, lateral; A, anterior.)

as well as the axons of more medially placed nuclei. Again, the resulting clinical presentation can be quite complex. This is further emphasized by studies of cerebral metabolism consequent to thalamic lesions.[1] Even small lesions in specific areas of thalamus were capable of significantly decreasing cortical metabolism, as observed by using positron emission tomography to image the uptake of labeled isotope of glucose. Thus it is difficult to ascertain whether the patient's presenting signs are due to the small thalamic lesion or to a more global shutdown of cerebral cortex.

Bearing these caveats in mind as well as the warnings concerning the use of the lesion method in human neuroanatomy,[2] it is possible to glean information on thalamic structure and function from the clinical literature on intracerebral infarctions. Recent studies employing magnetic resonance imaging (MRI) and CT scanning have attempted to identify complexes of neurologic signs and symptoms that occur with damage to specific vessels supplying the diencephalon.[3–7] Although there are signs and symptoms that can be associated with specific vascular territories (see pp. 157–159), only a few can be associated with specific thalamic nuclei or fiber tracts. Where they are known, an attempt will be made to include relevant comments on deficits of each thalamic nucleus or

Table 7-1.
Thalamo-Cortical Relationships

THALAMIC NUCLEI	CORTICAL TARGET
Anterior nuclei	Cingulate
Medial nuclei	Prefrontal
Ventral nuclei	Parietal, frontal
Lateral nuclei	Parietal, occipital, temporal
Lateral geniculate	Occipital
Medial geniculate	Temporal

structure. A summary of vascular territories and the neurologic sequelae associated with damage in these territories will be included with the section on blood supply.

▷ **Atlas Plate 20**

The dorsal portion of this section passes through the caudal thalamus; the ventral portion passes through the midbrain and an extreme rostral edge of the pons. The pontine and midbrain structures were discussed in Chapters 4 and 6, respectively. Characteristic of sections through the caudal thalamus is the large, pillowlike profile of the dorsally positioned pulvinar, a thalamic nucleus.

PINEAL

The pineal gland lies in a matrix of arachnoid tissue, straddling the caudal end of the third ventricle between the two masses of the pulvinar. It is also directly anteroinferior to the great vein of Galen. Rostrally, it is attached to the habenular nucleus of the thalamus by two peduncles, or stalks; caudally, the body of the pineal overlies the superior colliculus. The gland is composed of pinealocytes supported by a meshwork of neuroglia and is involved in the production of melatonin.

Although the pineal gland is not directly connected to the central nervous system by fiber tracts, it does receive a sympathetic autonomic innervation from the hypothalamus via thoracic spinal cord and superior cervical ganglion. The portion of the hypothalamus involved in this circuit receives projections from the retina. The pineal nerves, which hitchhike on the internal carotid and its branches, are called the *nervi conarii*,[8] in reference to the original name for the pineal, *konareion* ("cone-shaped"). Through this innervation the pineal receives a signal indicating the presence or absence of light. Sympathetic output is stimulated by darkness and increases the production and release of melatonin from the gland. This mechanism allows the pineal, through its periodic release of melatonin, to act as a circadian clock.[8]

Melatonin has been demonstrated to have an antigonadotrophic effect. In humans, circulating levels of melatonin fall with puberty. This hormone is also suspected of influencing the activity of the thyroid and adrenal glands, but the mechanism appears quite complex.[8] A link between pineal dysfunction, abnormal secretion of corticotrophin, and major depressive disorders has also been proposed.[9]

CLINICAL DEFICIT

Removal of the pineal gland is compatible with human life; however, its removal in prepubescent males can result in precocious puberty. The major neurologic significance of the pineal arises when tumors cause expansion of the gland and compression of the tectal plate and underlying midbrain tegmentum. This presents as loss of conjugate vision and vertical gaze paresis (Parinaud's syndrome; see Chap. 6). Low levels of melatonin, measured nocturnally, were found in patients suffering from Cushing's disease and from major depressive disorders. Higher than normal levels of melatonin have been reported in manic-depressive patients who were supersensitive to light.[9] These observations point to a relationship between melatonin and the release of corticotrophin-releasing factor that can significantly influence endocrinologic and neuropsychological activity.

PULVINAR NUCLEUS (PulNu)

The pulvinar nucleus (PulNu) is the largest of the thalamic nuclei. It is associated with the lateral posterior nucleus in the caudal portion of the thalamus and has reciprocal connections with areas of cerebral cortex located around the parieto-occipito-temporal junction, called posterior parietal association cortex. It also has well-developed connections with portions of the occipital cortex.

The pulvinar contains representations of the contralateral visual hemispheres; thus, the nucleus is considered part of the extrageniculate visual system in the thalamus, even though it does not receive direct projections from the retina.[10] It has been suggested that the pulvinar is involved in providing the appropriate amount of cortical attention for language-related tasks on the dominant side and for mechanicospatial tasks on the nondominant side of the brain.[11]

CLINICAL DEFICIT

Deficits expressed following lesions in the vicinity of the lateroposterior/pulvinar complex show a strong preference for laterality. Small hemorrhagic lesions on the nondominant side present with disturbances of topographic memory, constructional apraxia,[4,11] and visual neglect.[11] Lesions on the dominant side present with a speech deficit called thalamic aphasia; it is similar in composition to a mixed transcortical aphasia.[4,11]

LATERAL GENICULATE NUCLEUS (LGNu)

The thalamic relay for the visual system is the lateral geniculate nucleus (LGNu). It consists of multiple layers of cells and fibers wrapped in a dense capsule of efferent axons called the optic radiations. The major afferent projections to the lateral geniculate arise from retinal ganglion cells via the optic nerve and tract. In addition, the nucleus receives projections from the occipital (visual) cortex via the internal capsule. Since the lateral geniculate is distal to the optic chiasm in the ascending visual pathway, it contains a representation of contralateral visual space (see Barr and Kiernan[12]). The superior portion of the retina is represented in the superomedial part of the geniculate; the inferior portion of the retina is represented in the inferolateral part of the nucleus.

CLINICAL DEFICIT

Destruction of the lateral geniculate, optic tract, or optic radiations results in the loss of the contralateral visual hemisphere, called **hemianopsia.** Complete destruction of the nucleus results in dense hemianopsia without the macular sparing that is seen even in large lesions of visual cortex (for a diagram see Barr and Kiernan[12]).

The anterior choroidal artery supplies portions of the lateral geniculate nucleus. Occlusion of this artery can result in contralateral loss of the superior and inferior visual fields with sparing of a narrow, horizontal, central stripe.[13] The reduction of the visual field into a horizontal visual stripe is pathognomonic for lesions of the lateral geniculate.

OPTIC RADIATIONS (OpRad)

The thalamocortical axons from the lateral geniculate form a dense capsule of fibers as they leave the nucleus. Once in the posterior limb of the internal capsule they pass first superiorly and then posteriorly around the inferior horn of the lateral ventricle in route to occipital (visual) cortex.

The curved pathway of the optic radiations (OpRad) is referred to as Meyer's loop. The fibers representing the superior visual fields pass into the temporal lobe, whereas those representing the inferior visual fields pass deep to the parietal lobe.

CLINICAL DEFICIT

After leaving the area of the nucleus, the optic radiations fan out to sweep around the border of the temporal and parietal lobes. Here it is possible to achieve partial lesions of the tract. Such lesions present as **quadrantanopsia,** or "visual field cuts," in the contralateral visual hemisphere (for a diagram see Barr and Kiernan[12]). Loss in the superior visual field suggests damage to the temporal lobe or inferior lip of calcarine cortex; loss in the inferior visual field sug-

gests damage in the parietal lobe.[13] Complete section of the optic radiations should be similar to a lesion of the lateral geniculate, loss of vision from the contralateral hemisphere, or **hemianopsia.**

MEDIAL GENICULATE NUCLEUS (MGNu)

The medial geniculate nucleus (MGNu) is a complex cluster of cells on the caudal border of the thalamus, positioned medial to the lateral geniculate.[14] The ascending auditory pathways from the inferior colliculus relay through the medial geniculate nucleus en route to ipsilateral cerebral cortex. This nucleus is located in a fiber capsule on the caudal end of the thalamus, lateral to the superior colliculus and ventral to the pulvinar. The fiber capsule is composed of ascending afferent fibers from the brachium of the inferior colliculus and efferent fibers forming the auditory radiations to temporal (auditory) cortex.

The auditory cortex is not an exclusive target of the medial geniculate nucleus; it also has projections to limbic system structures such as the amygdala. These limbic connections of the thalamic auditory nuclei have been implicated in the reflex pathways relating acoustic stimuli to specific autonomic functions such as heart rate.[15]

CLINICAL DEFICIT

Very little is written concerning lesions of the medial geniculate nucleus in humans. Since the auditory system has bilateral representation above the trapezoid body, the loss in hearing after unilateral lesions will not be as profound as that of visual losses following thalamic lesions. Bilateral lesions of the human thalamus, which did not appear to involve the cortex, resulted in an auditory agnosia for nonverbal sounds.[16] However, this defect may result more from cortical hypofunction resulting from loss of thalamic input than from thalamic damage. Lesions of the medial geniculate nucleus or of its afferent or efferent fiber systems in cats result in diminished hearing functions in the contralateral auditory hemisphere.[17]

▷ **Atlas Plate 21**

The dorsal portion of this section passes through the caudal thalamus, above the level of the hypothalamus; the ventral portion of the section passes through the rostral midbrain. The midbrain structures on this section have been presented in Chapter 6. A characteristic feature of this section is the encapsulated lateral geniculate nucleus.

STRIA MEDULLARIS (StMed)

The stria medullaris (StMed) courses from septal nuclei to habenular nuclei, forming a prominent landmark positioned along the dorsomedial border of the thalamus (see Plates 21 to 25). It is part of the pathway for limbic system information moving from the septal area to the brain stem and spinal cord (see Chap. 9).

HABENULAR NUCLEUS (Hab)

The habenular nucleus (Hab) is located on the dorsomedial boundary of the caudal thalamus. It receives afferent projections from the septal nuclei via the stria medullaris and projects to the interpeduncular nuclei over the fasciculus retroflexus. Thus, the habenula forms a relay station in the flow of limbic system information from the septal area to the brain stem and spinal cord (see Chap. 9).

HABENULOPEDUNCULAR TRACT (HPTr)

Projections from the habenular nucleus reach the interpeduncular nucleus of the midbrain by passing over the habenulopeduncular tract (HPTr). This tract is also known as the fasciculus retroflexus. The pathway involving the stria medullaris, habenular nuclei, habenulo-interpeduncular tract, and interpeduncular nuclei represents a route over which olfactory information from the forebrain can gain access to the nuclei of the brain stem.

VENTROPOSTERIOR NUCLEI (VPL and VPM)

The ventroposterior nuclei (VPL and VPM) are the major somatic sensory nuclei in the thalamus. They represent an elongated structure, which is tipped onto a diagonal line coursing from superolateral to inferomedial, and is divided into lateral and medial nuclei (Fig. 7-3). The lateral nucleus of this complex receives fibers from the medial lemniscus (contralateral body representation; Fig. 7-4), whereas the medial portion receives fibers from the trigeminothalamic tracts (contralateral head representation). The edges of the nuclei receive fibers from the anterolateral system.

The ventroposterior nuclei project to the ipsilateral somatic sensory cortex of the postcentral gyrus in a topographic manner. The ventroposterior lateral nucleus (body representation) projects medially; the ventroposterior medial (face representation) projects laterally, thus establishing the homunculus in somatic sensory cortex. These two nuclei form an important link in the transfer of somatic sensory information from spinal cord and brain stem to the cerebral cortex.

CLINICAL DEFICIT

Small lesions, restricted to the ventroposterior nuclear group, can present with a pure somatic sensory loss from portions of the contralateral face and body.[18,19] Larger lesions can present with a feeling of numbness across the contralateral extremities and down the torso, maintaining a sharp demarcation at the midline.[11] This vertical border of sensory loss along the midline is a characteristic of lesions in the somatic sensory portion of thalamus.

Lesions in the area of the ventroposterior nuclei and pulvinar complex can also present as dysesthesia.[5] Numbness and tingling are perceptions commonly encountered with lesions of the area of the ventroposterior nuclei.[3,19] In cases where large lesions destroy the ventroanterior and ventrolateral nuclei as well, the dysesthesia can take the form of severe, burning pain, the Dejerine-Roussy syndrome of thalamic pain.[19] The medial and lateral nuclei of the ventroposterior complex have different blood supplies. The medial nucleus (face representation) lies in the midline vascular territory, while the lateral nucleus (body representation) lies in the posterolateral territory. Consequently, infarctions restricted to a specific vascular territory can result in sensory dissociation between the face and body.

MEDIAL LEMNISCUS (ML)

The medial lemniscus (ML) arises in the contralateral dorsal column nuclei (see Chap. 3). Its fibers represent the sensory modalities of discriminative touch, vibratory sense, and proprioception. Axons from the medial lemniscus terminate in the ventroposterior lateral nucleus (Fig. 7-4). As it enters the nucleus, the homunculus (fiber topography) is arranged with its feet positioned laterally and its arms positioned medially.

CLINICAL DEFICIT

Damage to the medial lemniscus will produce hemisensory loss on the contralateral side of the body. The modalities lost are proprioception, two-point discriminative touch, and vibratory sense.

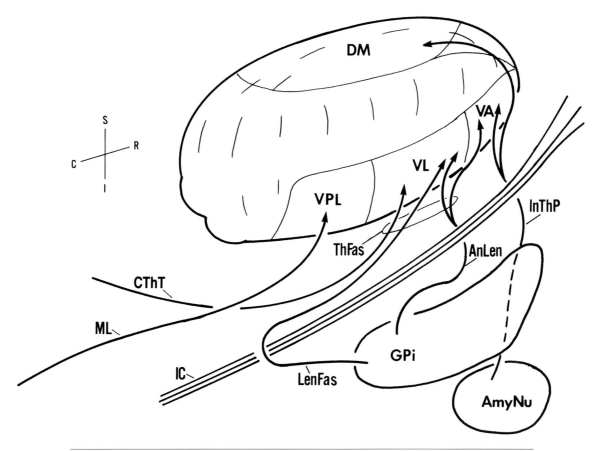

Figure 7-4. Diagram illustrates the major inputs to the ventral group of thalamic nuclei. The thalamic mass is depicted in the same profile as that seen in Figure 7-3. The major input pathways are illustrated with lines and arrows. (AmyNu, amygdaloid nucleus; AnLen, ansa lenticularis; C, caudal; CThT, cerebellothalamic tract; DM, dorsomedial nucleus; GPi, internal segment of globus pallidus; I, inferior; IC, internal capsule; InThP, inferior thalamic peduncle; LenFas, lenticular fasciculus; ML, medial lemniscus; R, rostral; S, superior; ThFas, thalamic fasciculus; VA, ventroanterior nucleus; VL, ventrolateral nucleus; VPL, ventroposterolateral nucleus.)

CENTROMEDIAN NUCLEUS (CM)

The centromedian nucleus (CM)—a large, spherical mass—is located in the posterior portion of the thalamus and is surrounded by a capsule of fibers, the internal medullary lamina (Fig. 7-3). The centromedian nucleus receives connections from the forebrain, globus pallidus, ventrolateral thalamic nucleus, and mesencephalic reticular formation. Its axons project to prefrontal cortex, ventrolateral nucleus, putamen, and caudate. Most of these connections suggest a role for the centromedian nucleus in the motor system. The input from the midbrain is part of the reticular activating system and plays a role in preparing the aroused individual for making a motor response to a specific sensory stimulus.[20]

The exact role played by the centromedian nucleus in thalamic processing is not at all clear, and studies in humans using the lesion method of analysis are confounded by its adjacent structures. The internal medullary lamina, which surrounds the centromedian nucleus, receives projections from the anterolateral system and from the midbrain reticular activating system. Lesions in this area of the thalamus can result in analgesia and a neglect syndrome. However, it is possible that neither of these two syndromes arises from the centromedian nucleus but is related instead to its surrounding fiber systems.

CLINICAL DEFICIT

Unilateral lesions of the centromedian nucleus and adjacent internal medullary lamina can cause contralateral thalamic neglect. The patient does not attend to all objects on the contralateral side of the body and is hypokinetic in both limbs in response to stimuli from the affected side. However, the limbs are not paralyzed, since they respond to stimuli from the ipsilateral side of the body. Bilateral lesions of the centromedian complex–internal medullary lamina result in bilateral neglect, considered a form of akinetic mutism.[20]

Lesions of the area including the centromedian nucleus, posterior internal medullary laminae, and rostral end of the midbrain have produced unarousable sleep.[21] This may be due to damage to the fibers of the ascending reticular activating system that reach the internal medullary lamina.

Stereotaxic lesions in the area of the centromedian nucleus have been used to counter intractable thalamic pain; however, it is unclear that this nucleus actually plays a role in pain processing. These lesions may be affecting the anterolateral tract fibers that pass close to the nucleus, or they may be producing a form of neglect.[10]

DORSOMEDIAL NUCLEUS (DMNu)

The dorsomedial nucleus (DMNu) is a large mass of cells lying along the dorsal and medial border of the thalamus (Fig 7-3). It is bounded laterally by the internal medullary lamina and medially by the third ventricle. This nucleus is divided into several components, one of which has extensive reciprocal connections with the prefrontal cortex. The other portions of the nucleus are connected to the amygdala and olfactory cortex through the inferior thalamic peduncle as well as to the substantia nigra. Based on its connections, it has been suggested that the dorsomedial nucleus integrates somatic and visceral information and is involved in maintaining consciousness. When an analysis of lesion data is considered, it appears that the dorsomedial nucleus is also involved in the thalamic pathways related to memory processing and the maintenance of cognitive functions.[11]

CLINICAL DEFICIT

Destruction of the dorsomedial nucleus or the surrounding area results in various neuropsychological dysfunctions.[3,22] This may take the form of dysfunctions in verbal memory[23] and topographic memory.[4] Familial degeneration of the dorsomedial nucleus and anterior thalamic nuclei produced insomnia and dysautonomia in a patient.[24] Lesions of dorsomedial nucleus or its connections to the prefrontal cortex can

present with components of the frontal lobe syndrome.[21]

LATEROPOSTERIOR NUCLEUS (LP)

The lateroposterior nucleus is a member of the lateral nuclear group, which consists of the pulvinar, lateroposterior, and laterodorsal nuclei. The pulvinar is the most posterior of the three; rostrally, it is replaced by the lateroposterior nucleus (LP) and finally by the laterodorsal nucleus (see Fig. 7-3). Although its connections in humans are not well known, the lateroposterior nucleus in cats receives afferent fibers from visual cortex and superior colliculus, thus creating multiple representations of the visual hemisphere. Its efferent connections go to posterior parietal (association) cortex, and it has been suggested that the structure is involved in visuomotor activity.[25]

CLINICAL DEFICIT

Exact clinical deficits associated with lesions in the lateral posterior nucleus are unknown. Lesions in the lateral posterior–pulvinar complex result in disturbances of topographic memory and in constructional apraxia.[4]

INTERNAL MEDULLARY LAMINA (IML)

The internal medullary lamina (IML) is a thin velum of cells and fibers that divides the ventral nuclear groups from the medial nuclear groups (dorsomedial nucleus) in the thalamus. Caudally, it surrounds the centromedian nucleus; rostrally, it encapsulates the anterior nuclei. Ascending fibers from the anterolateral system and the mesencephalic reticular formation terminate on cells in the internal medullary lamina. Cells in the internal medullary lamina provide a diffuse innervation of most regions of the ipsilateral cerebral cortex. Since these efferent fibers do not target discrete cortical areas, they are often referred to as nonspecific projections. The internal medullary lamina is involved in the transmission of pain and, through the reticular activating system, in maintenance of the arousal state in cerebral cortex.

CLINICAL DEFICIT

Sleep dysfunctions and altered levels of consciousness are reported features of lesions in the internal medullary lamina or closely related nuclei.[6,21] Stereotaxic lesions have been placed in the vicinity of the centromedian nucleus,[10] a structure surrounded by the internal medullary lamina, to control intractable thalamic pain (see pp. 147–148).

EXTERNAL MEDULLARY LAMINA (EML)

A band of fibers, the external medullary lamina (EML), makes up the lateral border of the thalamus, separating the major thalamic nuclei from the thin reticular thalamic nucleus (see Plates 21 to 25). This lamina is composed of the thalamocortical and corticothalamic fibers passing in and out of the internal capsule.

THALAMIC RETICULAR NUCLEUS (ThRetNu)

The external medullary lamina forms a thin velum of fibers around the main body of the thalamus. The thalamic reticular nucleus (ThRetNu) is a thin sheet of cells lying between the external medullary lamina and the internal capsule (see Plates 21 to 25). Although little is known of its organization in humans, in the cat this nucleus receives collateral axons from the corticothalamic and thalamocortical fibers. In turn, it projects to most thalamic nuclei.[26] Thus, the thalamic reticular nucleus could be acting as a gate, sampling the activity occurring between thalamus and cortex and modulating the output of individual thalamic nuclei. It has also been proposed that the thalamic reticular nucleus plays a role in directing attention to novel stimuli and inhibiting attention to repetitive stimuli.[20]

SUBTHALAMIC NUCLEUS (SThNu)

The subthalamic nucleus (SThNu) is located along the medial side of the internal capsule at approximately the midbrain–thalamic junction. It receives fibers from the external segment of the ipsilateral globus pallidus and projects back to the internal segment of this structure. Consequently, the subthalamic nucleus represents a station in the "indirect output pathway" for the basal ganglia (see Chap. 10). Its role in the motor system involves modulation of the activity of the internal segment of the globus pallidus. This latter structure directly inhibits the ventrolateral and portions of the ventroanterior thalamic nuclei.[27]

CLINICAL DEFICIT
Lesions of the subthalamic can result in a loss of excitation to the internal segment of the globus pallidus, which then fails to repress the ventral lateral and ventral anterior nuclei of the thalamus. The elevated output from these two thalamic nuclei to the premotor cerebral cortex results in increased output of motor patterns from the neocortex.[28] The patient experiences violent, uncontrollable, ballistic movements in the proximal muscles of the contralateral extremities.

CEREBELLOTHALAMIC TRACT (CThT)

The thalamic fasciculus (ThFas, see Plate 22) is composed of axons from the dentate nucleus (cerebellothalamic fibers [CThT]) and from the globus pallidus (pallidothalamic fibers). The cerebellothalamic fibers are visible in Plate 21 and in Figure 7-4. These axons originate in the dentate and interpositus nuclei of the contralateral cerebellum. They cross the midline in the decussation of the superior cerebellar peduncle, pass around the red nucleus, and terminate in the ventrolateral nucleus of the thalamus. On Plate 21, the cerebellothalamic fibers are seen as they encapsulate the red nucleus. The pallidothalamic fibers are present on Plates 22 to 25 (ansa lenticularis and lenticular fasciculus).

CLINICAL DEFICIT
Lesion of the cerebellothalamic fibers is similar to section of the superior cerebellar peduncle and can present with ataxia and dysmetria in the contralateral limb.[19] If the lesion is superior to the decussation of the dentothalamic fibers in the midbrain, the presentation is on the contralateral side of the body.

BODY OF THE FORNIX

The fornix is a major efferent pathway of the hippocampus. Arising from the dorsal surface of the hippocampus, its body passes over the caudal thalamus, and its columns descend through the rostral thalamus to terminate in the hypothalamus and septal area. The body of the fornix is present in Plate 21. It will be discussed further in Chapter 9.

CLINICAL DEFICIT
Lesions of the fornix, interrupting the hippocampal–hypothalamic connections, have been associated with amnesia (reviewed by Grafman et al[29]).

Review Structures From Preceding Plates
Identify the following structures from previous sections:

Lateral geniculate nucleus (LGNu)

Optic radiations (OpRad)

Optic tract (OpTr)

Pulvinar nucleus (PulNu)

149

▷ **Atlas Plate 22**

The dorsal portion of this section passes through the center of the thalamus; the ventral portion lies on the caudal border of the hypothalamus. A salient feature of Plate 22 is the mamillothalamic tract wrapped around the medial border of the mamillary nuclei.

VENTROLATERAL NUCLEUS (VL)

The ventral group of nuclei extend along the entire posterior to anterior axis of the thalamus (see Fig. 7-3). This group contains the ventroposterior, ventrolateral, and ventroanterior nuclei. The ventrolateral nucleus (VL) lies anterior to the ventroposterior nuclei. It receives afferent fibers from the contralateral dentate nucleus in the cerebellum (see Fig. 7-4) and from the ipsilateral globus pallidus of the basal ganglia. These two projections end in separate regions of the ventrolateral nucleus; those from the cerebellum are more posterior than those from the basal ganglia.[30] A somatotopic representation of the body is present in the ventrolateral nucleus[30] and is in register with that found in the adjacent ventroposterior nucleus. The ventrolateral nucleus projects to the ipsilateral primary motor cortex, its output is excitatory, and at least that from the portion of the nucleus receiving the pallidothalamic fibers most likely sets the level of neural activity in motor cortex, thus influencing the tonic activity of muscles through the output of motor cortex.[10]

CLINICAL DEFICIT

Large lesions in the vicinity of the ventrolateral nucleus can produce hemiplegia; this most likely reflects the involvement of the corticospinal fibers in the internal capsule. Pure lesions of the ventrolateral nucleus can result in hypotonia, diminished emotional expression, and a neglect that is transitory.[11]

Loss of cerebellar input (dentothalamic tract) to the ventrolateral nucleus can present as contralateral limb hemiataxia. Lesions in the inhibitory input from the basal ganglia (pallidothalamic tract) that spare the internal capsule can induce unwanted motion (*i.e.,* the choreiform or athetotic movements). Conversely, stereotaxic lesions of the nucleus have been used to block uncontrolled movements and tremor.[31]

Language dysfunctions, usually transient, have also been associated with lesions in the ventrolateral thalamus.[11,21] These are characterized by reduced spontaneous speech, paraphasic errors, perseveration, and reduced comprehension in the face of preserved repetition. A small lesion in the ventrolateral nucleus along its border with the lateral–posterior nuclear group presented with astasia.[32]

THALAMIC FASCICULUS (ThFas)

In this section, the ascending cerebellothalamic fibers are joined by axons from the ipsilateral globus pallidus (pallidothalamic fibers) traveling in the lenticular fasciculus; the combined fiber bundle is called the thalamic fasciculus (ThFas). The cerebellothalamic fibers terminate in the caudal portion the ventrolateral nucleus; the pallidothalamic fibers terminate in the rostral portions of the nucleus as well as in the ventroanterior nucleus (see Fig. 7-4).

CLINICAL DEFICIT

Lesions of the thalamic fasciculus can result in cerebellar ataxia and dysmetria of the contralateral extremities due to damage to the cerebellothalamic fibers, and sudden, unexpected, chorealike or dystonic movements of the contralateral limbs caused by loss of the pallidothalamic fibers.[19]

ZONA INCERTA (Zi)

The zona incerta (Zi) is a narrow strip of cells wedged between the thalamic fasciculus dorsally and the lenticular fasciculus ventrally. It receives fibers from ipsilateral motor cortex and projects to the red nucleus and superior colliculus. Its function and clinical neurology are poorly understood.

LENTICULAR FASCICULUS (LenFas)

Fibers from the globus pallidus (pallidothalamic fibers) traveling to the rostral portion of the ventrolateral nucleus pass through the internal capsule to enter the thalamus as the lenticular fasciculus (LenFas). Once in the thalamus, this fasciculus joins with the ascending cerebellothalamic fibers to form the thalamic fasciculus (see Fig. 7-4).

CLINICAL DEFICIT

Lesions of the lenticular fasciculus can result in sudden, unexpected, chorealike, or dystonic movements of the contralateral limbs.[19] This expression of unwanted motion most likely comes from the loss of the inhibition pallidothalamic fibers have on the ventrolateral nucleus (see Chap. 10).

MAMILLARY BODY (MB)

The posterior end of the hypothalamus contains a prominent external structure, the mamillary body (MB). Each body is partitioned into several nuclei.

This structure is integrated into the limbic circuit, receiving projections from the hippocampus and septal area via the fornix and sending efferent projections to the anterior thalamic nuclei (which then project to cingulate cortex). This circuitry is involved in processing memory and in learning.

CLINICAL DEFICIT

Neurodegenerative changes in the mamillary nuclei are prominent in chronic alcoholism. This observation has led to the theory that destruction of the mamillary nuclei is involved in the diencephalic amnesia associated with chronic alcoholics. However, the dorsomedial nuclei also exhibit necrosis with prolonged alcohol abuse,[33] and recent evidence has suggested that lesions of the dorsomedial thalamic nuclei alone can produce a severe memory impairment.[23] Controlled lesions of the mamillary nuclei in primates resulted in a form of spatial memory impairment, not the global diencephalic amnesia of alcoholics.[34] Thus, it appears that necrosis of the mamillary nuclei, while contributing to the overall amnesic syndrome in alcoholics, is not responsible for its entirety.

MAMILLOTHALAMIC TRACT (MTTr)

The projection from the mamillary nuclei to the thalamus is the mamillothalamic fasciculus (MTTr). This prominent fiber bundle can be seen passing rostrally and dorsally from the mamillary nuclei to the base of the fiber capsule surrounding the anterior thalamic nucleus (see Plate 25).

CLINICAL DEFICIT

Lesions of this tract or its surrounding territory can present with amnesia.[35,36]

POSTERIOR HYPOTHALAMUS (PHyTh)

Surrounding the mamillary bodies are the nuclei of the posterior hypothalamus (PHyTh). This diffuse mass of neurons has descending projections onto the autonomic nuclei of the brain stem and spinal cord and is involved in controlling activity of the sympathetic nervous system.

CLINICAL DEFICIT

Lesions in the posterior hypothalamus can disrupt autonomic regulation. Symptoms that have been reported are hypothermia or poikilothermy, and Horner's syndrome. Apathy and hypersomnia or coma have also been noted in lesions of this area.[37]

Review Structures From Preceding Plates

Identify the following structures from previous sections:

Stria medullaris (StMed)

Lateroposterior nucleus (LPNu)

Dorsomedial nucleus (DM)

Internal medullary lamina (IML)

External medullary lamina (EML)

Subthalamic nucleus (SThNu)

Fornix (Fx)

Thalamic reticular nucleus (ThRetNu)

▷ Atlas Plate 23

This section passes through thalamus and hypothalamus. It is characterized by the mamillothalamic tract in the thalamus, the fornix in the hypothalamus, and the prominent optic tracts bordering the hypothalamus and cerebral peduncles.

LATERAL DORSAL NUCLEUS (LD)

The lateral nuclear group is composed of three nuclei: lateral dorsal, lateral posterior, and pulvinar (see Fig. 7-3). The lateral dorsal nucleus (LD) is housed in a separate, myelinated fiber capsule along the dorsal surface of the thalamus. Projections to this nucleus arise in the hippocampus, pretectum, and lateral geniculate. In turn, the nucleus sends projections to the cingulate and parahippocampal cortex. It has been suggested that the lateral dorsal nucleus is a gateway for visual sensory information reaching the limbic system.[38] Specific clinical deficits have not been associated with the lateral dorsal nucleus.

MASSA INTERMEDIA (MI)

In approximately 80% of brains examined, the midline nuclear group is continuous with the opposite thalamus (see Fig. 7-2). This continuity, composed of neurons and fibers, represents a bridge of gray matter; it is not a fiber tract.

ANSA LENTICULARIS (AnLen)

The ansa lenticularis (AnLen) is a fiber tract that passes out of the globus pallidus, ventral to the internal capsule, and curves dorsally to join the thalamic fasciculus, eventually terminating in the rostral portion of the ventrolateral nucleus and the ventroanterior nucleus of the thalamus (Fig. 7-4). These pallidothalamic fibers are inhibitory in their actions on the thalamic neurons. The clinical deficits associated with interruption of the pallidothalamic fibers have been presented with the lenticular fasciculus (p. 150).

LATERAL HYPOTHALAMIC AREA (LHyTh)

The lateral hypothalamic area (LHyTh) extends from the midbrain tegmentum to the preoptic area, situated lateral to the fornix. Distinct nuclear boundaries are difficult to locate in this zone of the hypothalamus. Stimulation of the lateral hypothalamic area can result in the desire to eat.

CLINICAL DEFICIT

Lesions of the lateral hypothalamus can present with loss of appetite, emaciation, adipsia, and apathy.[37]

MEDIAL HYPOTHALAMUS (MHyTh)

The region medial to the fornix is the medial hypothalamus (MHyTh). Like the lateral hypothalamic area, it lacks distinct nuclear boundaries. The medial hypothalamic area contains a satiety center that if lesioned can result in obesity. Several of its nuclei also produce regulatory factors that function in controlling the pituitary gland.

CLINICAL DEFICIT

Destruction of the medial hypothalamus can result in diabetes insipidus and hyperdipsia. Hyperphagia to the point of obesity can occur as well as the syndrome of inappropriate antidiuretic hormone release and dwarfism. Behavioral dysfunctions, such as rage or amnesia, can also occur with these lesions.[37]

OPTIC TRACT (OpTr)

The anterior boundary of the hypothalamus is the optic tract (OpTr). This tract contains the axons of the retinal ganglion cells.

CLINICAL DEFICIT

Pressure on the optic tract, resulting from a mass expanding lesions in the hypothalamus, can result in visual field defects such as **hemianopsia.**

Review Structures From Preceding Plates

Identify the following structures from previous sections:

Stria Medullaris (StMed)

Thalamic reticular nucleus (ThRetNu)

External medullary lamina (EML)

Internal medullary lamina (IML)

Ventrolateral nucleus (VL)

Dorsomedial thalamus (DM)

Zona incerta (Zi)

Mamillothalamic tract (MTTr)

Thalamic fasciculus (ThFas)

Lenticular fasciculus (LenFas)

Fornix (Fx)

▷ Atlas Plate 24

The dorsal portion of this section passes through the thalamus; the ventral portion traverses the rostral border of the hypothalamus and preoptic area. The inferior thalamic peduncle and ansa lenticularis are seen entering the ventral aspect of the thalamus.

ANTERIOR HYPOTHALAMUS (AHyTh)

The anterior hypothalamus (AHyTh) is located rostrally in the hypothalamus. At the level of the optic chiasm it merges into the preoptic area. Cells in the anterior hypothalamic nucleus contain receptors for sex hormones and produce regulating factors for the anterior pituitary gland. Neural circuits that determine set points for the control of temperature in the body are also located in the anterior hypothalamus. This area is involved in control of the pituitary gland and the parasympathetic nervous system.

CLINICAL DEFICIT

Lesions of the anterior hypothalamus can result in hyperthermia. This alteration in temperature can be cyclic and accompanied by fever, shivering, and chills. Diabetes insipidus and insomnia can also present with lesions in this area.[37]

152

INFERIOR THALAMIC PEDUNCLE (InThP)

The inferior thalamic peduncle (InThP) enters the thalamus from the ventral surface and carries fibers from the orbitofrontal cortex, medial temporal cortex, and amygdala to the dorsomedial nucleus of the thalamus.

Review Structures From Preceding Plates

Identify the following structures from previous sections:

Stria medullaris (StMed)

Dorsomedial thalamic nucleus (DM)

Internal medullary lamina (IML)

Ventrolateral thalamic nucleus (VL)

Lateral dorsal thalamic nucleus (LD)

Ansa lenticularis (AnLen)

Fornix (Fx)

Lateral hypothalamic area (LHyTh)

External medullary lamina (EML)

Hypothalamus (HyTh)

▷ **Atlas Plate 25**

The superior portion of this section passes through the rostral pole of the thalamus; the inferior portion passes through the central portion of the hypothalamus. Its salient feature is the encapsulated anterior thalamic nucleus.

ANTERIOR THALAMIC NUCLEUS (AN)

The mamillothalamic tract rises out of the hypothalamus (see Plates 22 to 24) into the anterior portion of the thalamus, where it meets the internal medullary lamina. These two structures form a fibrous capsule surrounding the anterior thalamic nucleus (AntNu) (see Plate 25). The major afferent connections of this nucleus are the mamillothalamic tract and the cingulate gyrus of cortex; its efferent projections go to the cingulate gyrus. These projections are part of a major limbic circuit that extends from hippocampus to mamillary bodies via fornix, and from mamillary bodies through the anterior nucleus to the cingulate cortex (see Chap. 9). Given its involvement in this

circuit, the anterior thalamic nucleus joins with the dorsomedial nucleus to form the limbic thalamus.[39]

The functions of the anterior nucleus are not well known. It is associated with a limbic circuit thought to play a role in memory.[39]

CLINICAL DEFICIT

Surgical lesions of the anterior thalamic nuclei have been used to ameliorate agitation and anxiety; they induce some confusion in the patient, especially with relation to time, date, and place. Degeneration of the mamillary bodies, mamillothalamic tract, and, to a lesser extent, the anterior thalamic nucleus is seen in chronic alcoholism. This is accompanied by Korsakoff's psychosis, featuring profound memory loss. It is not clear just how much of a role the thalamic nuclei play in this syndrome, since surgical lesions directed at the anterior thalamic nucleus did not replicate the amnesia.[39]

VENTROANTERIOR THALAMIC NUCLEUS (VA)

The ventroanterior nucleus (VA) is the rostral pole of the ventral group of thalamic nuclei (Fig. 7-3) that includes ventroposterior (see Plate 21) and ventrolateral (see Plates 22 to 24) nuclei. Medially, the ventroanterior nucleus is bounded by the mamillothalamic tract and the anterior thalamic nucleus. The afferent projections to the ventroanterior nucleus arise in the internal segment of the globus pallidus (see Plates 22 to 24) and enter the thalamus through the lenticular fasciculus (see Plates 22 and 23) and the ansa lenticularis (see Plates 23 to 25). The ventroanterior nucleus projects axons to the premotor and supplementary motor portions of frontal cerebral cortex (see Chap. 8). Stimulation of the ventroanterior nucleus produces motor behavior that resembles the movements obtained from stimulation of the supplementary motor cortex.[10]

The ventroanterior nucleus participates in a looped circuit involving cerebral cortex, corpus striatum, globus pallidus, ventroanterior nucleus, and cerebral cortex. The circuit functions to set the scale of intensity in motor system[27] as well as other systems (see Chap. 10). Unfortunately, little is known concerning lesions restricted to the ventroanterior nucleus.[10]

Review Structures From Preceding Plates

Identify the following structures from previous sections:

Stria medullaris (StMed)

Internal medullary lamina (IML)

153

Fornix (Fx)

Ansa lenticularis (AnLen)

Thalamic reticular nucleus (ThRetNu)

Hypothalamus (HyTh)

External medullary lamina (EML)

Optic tract (OpTr)

Mamillothalamic tract (MTTr)

Stria terminalis (StTer)

Lenticular fasciculus (LenFas)

UNIT B

Case Study 7-3

A 55-year-old man with sudden-onset left-sided sensory loss and athetotic movements in his left hand

This 55-year-old man experienced a sudden onset of numbness in his left upper limb while eating supper. When it persisted, he consulted his family physician.

Past Medical History

At the time of examination he was unmarried and worked in a factory performing quality-control inspections. Both of his parents were alive, and he had lived with them all his life. He was diagnosed with myotonic dystrophy at 33 years of age; its course had been a slow, progressive increase in proximal muscle weakness since that time.

General Physical Examination

The patient was an awake, alert, oriented man with significant muscle wasting, especially in the proximal limb muscles. His movements were punctuated by occasional tonic muscle contractions of considerable force. He appeared older than his stated age. The center of the lens in each eye was significantly, grayed obscuring observation of the optic discs. His blood pressure, respiration, and temperature were all within normal ranges. His chest was clear to auscultation; the abdomen was soft, with no tenderness. A reducible mass was present in the inguinal region on the right. The cataracts, myotonia, and proximal muscle weakness are of long duration.

Neurologic Examination

Mental Status.   He was awake and oriented for time and place. Normal mental status was found on all tests except for a short-term visual memory deficit discovered during a neuro-psychological examination at a latter date; there was no significant amnesia or aphasia.

Cranial Nerves.   Visual fields were full to confrontation (however, visual acuity was poor), a full range of eye movements was possible, and no nystagmus was present. Facial expression was full, and smiling was symmetric. His hearing was normal in both ears. Jaw-jerk and corneal reflexes were physiologic. The palate was elevated midline, and tongue protruded midline. Shoulder shrug was bilaterally symmetric. Swallowing and voice were normal.

Motor Systems.   Extended periods of tonic muscle contractions followed some of his movements; these lessened with repetitive motion. Muscle strength was diminished, with considerable wasting present in the proximal muscles of the shoulders and pelvis. His tendon reflexes were diminished but symmetric in all extremities, and plantar reflexes were flexor. His left hand exhibited athetoid movements but only when he closed his eyes.

Sensation. He had loss of sensation on the left side of his torso and face and left extremities for pinprick, light touch, proprioception, vibration, two-point discrimination, graphesthesia, and stereognosis. There was an abrupt vertical boundary to the sensory loss along the midline of the torso. No hyperesthesia or dysesthesia was noted.

QUESTIONS

1. Does the patient exhibit a language or memory deficit or an alteration in consciousness or cognition?

2. Are signs of cranial nerve dysfunction present?

3. Are there any changes in motor functions, such as reflexes, muscle tone, movement, or coordination?

4. Are any changes in sensory functions detectable?

5. At what level in the central neuraxis is this lesion most likely located?

6. Is the pathology focal, multifocal, or diffuse in its distribution within the nervous system?

7. What is the clinical–temporal profile of this pathology: acute or chronic; progressive or stable?

8. Based on your answers to the previous two questions, decide whether the symptoms in this patient are most likely caused by a vascular accident, a tumor, or a degenerative or inflammatory process?

9. If you feel this is the result of a vascular accident, what vessels are most likely involved?

Case Study 7-4

A 78-year-old woman with confusion, memory dysfunction, and sleep disturbances

This 78-year-old woman was brought to the emergency room from a local nursing home after she became very agitated and disoriented, alarming the other residents.

Past Medical History

At the time of admission she had been retired for 13 years from her position as an elementary school teacher. She had been married, and her husband was deceased. She had no children. Five years previously she had moved from her house to a nursing home. Two years previously she had experienced a period of right facial weakness with language dysfunction; this had resolved over a 2-week period. Until the day of admittance she had been a pleasant person, sociable with other residents of the nursing home, and with good memory.

General Physical Examination

She was in an agitated state and uncooperative, making a detailed examination difficult. She was well nourished and well hydrated and appeared her stated age. She had increased pulse, respiration, and blood pressure (190/100 mmHg). She appeared flushed, and her skin was moist.

Neurologic Examination

Mental Status. She was disoriented with respect to time and place. She insisted she was going shopping and that the driver had let her out at the hospital by mistake. She was aggravated and abusive with the attending personnel. She was a poor historian. At the time of admission she could not be tested for memory, since she refused to answer most questions.

Cranial Nerves. Visual fields appeared full to confrontation, a full range of eye movements was possible, and no nystagmus present was. Facial expression was full and hearing was normal. Jaw-jerk reflex was normal, and corneal reflex was present. Palate was elevated midline, and tongue protruded midline. Shoulder shrug was bilaterally symmetric. Swallowing and voice were normal.

Motor Systems. Movements were normal; strength and deep tendon reflexes were physiologic throughout the patient's body.

Sensation. Response to pinprick was normal; no detectable loss of proprioception was found. Testing was complicated by her uncooperative nature.

Follow-up

The patient was insomnic for 3 days while under observation in the hospital. On discharge she was calm but had marked memory dysfunction and continued to confabulate explanations covering the memory loss. One month after returning to the nursing home she developed hypersomnia and was difficult to arouse. She returned to the hospital, where she died 1 week later.

QUESTION

1. Does the patient exhibit a language or memory deficit or an alteration in consciousness or cognition?

2. Are signs of cranial nerve dysfunction present?

3. Are there any changes in motor functions, such as reflexes, muscle tone, movement, or coordination?

4. Are any changes in sensory functions detectable?

5. At what level in the central neuraxis is this lesion most likely located?

6. Is the pathology focal, multifocal, or diffuse in its distribution within the nervous system?

7. What is the clinical–temporal profile of this pathology: acute or chronic; progressive or stable?

8. Based on your answers to the previous two questions, decide whether the symptoms in this patient are most likely caused by a vascular accident, a tumor, or a degenerative or inflammatory process.

9. If you feel this is the result of a vascular accident, what vessels are most likely involved?

10. Is this patient exhibiting Alzheimer's syndrome? Why or why not?

► DISCUSSION
Thalamic Vascular Supply

The blood supply to the thalamus is complex and highly variable. It comes from numerous penetrating vessels that branch from the circle of Willis, closely related portions of the basilar artery, posterior cerebral artery, and middle cerebral artery. Rather than consider the distribution of each artery, it is more instructive to describe groups of arteries that supply a reasonably constant thalamic territory. Infarction within a vascular territory can be related to a reasonably specific constellation of neurologic signs and symptoms.

Although terminology varies, most clinical authors recognize three major thalamic territories that can be described by their related blood supply: midline (paramedian), anterolateral, and posterolateral (see Plates 20 to 25). Some authors describe an additional lateral thalamic–internal capsule territory.[5]

The *paramedian group* is supplied by a tuft of small arteries that branch off of the top of the basilar and proximal cerebral arteries (PMbr in Fig. 7-5**A**). They supply the midline of the diencephalon, being more prevalent posteriorly and diminishing in number anteriorly. In some cases many of the bilateral branches arise from a common stem at the top of the basilar artery. In such situations, a stem infarction can present with bilateral signs.

The *anterolateral* group consists of the posterior communicating artery and its tuberothalamic branches (PComA and TuTh in Fig. 7-5**B**). Small penetrating arteries from the posterior communicating artery supply a band of tissue along the lateral and anterior borders of the thalamus.

The *posterolateral group* consist of several long, circumferential arteries, such as the posteromedial choroidal, that arise from the posterior cerebral artery (PMChA and PCA in Fig. 7-5**C**). These circumferential arteries wrap around the cerebral peduncle, curve dorsally to arch over the posterior end of the thalamus, and finally course rostrally along the superior aspect of the thalamus, diminishing in prevalence from caudal to rostral. These vessels course in close association with the stria terminalis and stria medullaris; their penetrating branches enter the thalamic tissue from its superior surface.

The *lateral group* consists of the anterior choroidal artery and its penetrating branches. The anterior choroidal arises from the internal carotid and passes posteriorly around the cerebral peduncle (AChA Fig. 7-5). Penetrating branches from this artery perfuse a zone along the lateral border of the thalamus involving the posterior limb of the internal capsule and globus pallidus. The anterior choroidal terminates as small branches wrapping around the caudal border of the thalamus and perfusing portions of the lateral geniculate nucleus.

There is variation and considerable overlap in the distribution of cerebral arteries within the thalamus; thus, it is difficult to assign specific arteries to individual thalamic nuclei. However, general zones of the thalamus can be related to the vascular territory of specific groups of cerebral arteries. Constellations of neurologic signs and symptoms are associated with perfusion failure within these vascular territories.[4,5,40]

The following is a compilation of vascular territories, their distribution within the thalamus, and the known neurologic sequelae caused by perfusion compromise.

Midline Territory[5,19]

Arteries. The paramedian branches arise from the apex of the basilar artery or proximal portion of the posterior cerebral artery (other names for these branches include *interpeduncular profundus a., thalamoperforating a.,* and *thalamic–subthalamic a.*

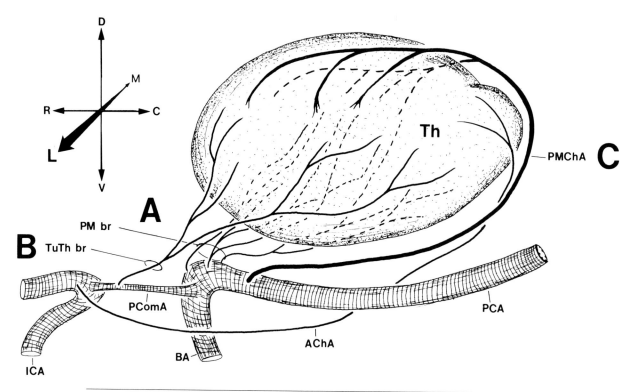

Figure 7-5. The arterial supply of the left thalamus. (AChA, anterior choroidal artery; BA, basilar artery; PCA, posterior cerebral artery; PComA, posterior communicating artery; PM br, paramedian branches; PMChA, posteromedial choroidal artery; Th, thalamic hemisphere; TuTh br; tuberothalamic branches.)

Distribution. The midline territory is widest caudally and narrows to a point rostrally. It contains the midline nuclei, centromedian nucleus, dorsomedial nucleus, posterior portion of the internal medullary lamina, and rostral portion of ventrolateral nucleus, as well as subthalamic nucleus and rostral interstitial nucleus of the median longitudinal fasciculus.

Deficit. Coma or drowsiness, confusion, amnesia, confabulation, disorientation, hypersomnolence (bilateral lesions), cognitive impairment, gaze palsies, constructional apraxias and sometimes ataxia, and delayed movements.

Anterolateral Territory[3–5,19,41,42]

Arteries. Tuberothalamic arteries branch from the posterior communicating artery (other names for these branches include *polar artery, anterior optic artery, centralis anterolaterales artery,* or *premamillary pedicle*).

Distribution. The anterolateral territory is a ventral wedge coursing from a lateral position in the caudal thalamus to a medial position in the rostral thalamus. Structures serviced by these vessels are the paraventricular nuclei; massa intermedia; ventrolateral and ventroanterior nuclei; portions of the thalamic reticular, dorsomedial, and posterior nuclear groups; mamillothalamic tract; and posterior limb of the internal capsule.

Deficit. Neuropsychological deficits in language, temporal orientation, intellect, memory (amnesias), and visual perception, as well as constructional apraxias, dysphasia (lesion on dominant side), neglect, abulia (including facial paresis for emotion, and transient hemiparesis). Speech is characterized by reduced volume and quantity, paraphasic errors, and verbal perseveration.

Posterolateral Territory[3–5,32,43]

Arteries. Thalamogeniculate and posterior choroidal arteries that branch off the posterior cerebral artery (other names for these branches include thalamoperforating, posterior thalamic, or posteroinferior arteries).

Distribution. The posterolateral territory is a dorsal wedge extending from a lateral position caudally to a medial position rostrally. These vessels service the ventroposterior and portions of the ventrolateral nuclei, pulvinar and portions of the lateroposterior nuclear group, and make contributions to the centromedian nucleus.

Deficit. Hemibody sensory loss and paresthesia; hemianopsia, hemiparesis, and choreiform or athetotic movements; astasia; visual memory and visual perceptual dysfunction.

Lateral Thalamic/Internal Capsule Zone[5,43]
Arteries. Anterior choroidal arteries that branch off the internal carotid or middle cerebral artery.

Distribution. This territory forms a cusp along the lateral border of the thalamus. It contains the posterior limb of internal capsule, lateral portion of ventrolateral nucleus, and both segments of globus pallidus.

Deficit. Hemiparesis, diminished pinprick, and light touch sensation.

► Bibliography

Adams RD, Victor M. The hypothalamus and neuroendocrine disorders. In: Principles of neurology. New York: McGraw-Hill, 1989; Chap. 27:445–454.

Masdeu JC. The localization of lesions of the hypothalamus and pituitary gland. In: Brazis PW, Masdeu JC, Biller J. Localization in clinical neurology. Boston: Little, Brown, 1990; Chap. 16:299–318.

Masdeu JC, Brazis PW. The localization of lesions in the thalamus. In: Brazis PW, Masdeu JC, Biller J, eds. Localization in clinical neurology. Boston: Little, Brown, 1990; Chap. 17:319–343.

Daube JR, Ragan TJ, Sandok BA, Westmoreland BF. The consciousness system. In: Medical neurosciences. Boston: Little, Brown, 1986; Chap. 8:138–155.

Daube JR, Ragan TJ, Sandok BA, Westmoreland BF. The supratentorial level. In: Medical neurosciences. Boston: Little, Brown, 1986; Chap. 15:374–417.

Haines DE. Neuroanatomy: an atlas of structures, sections, and systems. Baltimore: Urban & Schwarzenberg, 1987 *(see especially Figs. 5-29 to 5-37).*

Nieuwenhuys R, Voogd J, van Huijzen C. The human central nervous system. Berlin: Springer-Verlag, 1988:237–246.

► References

1. Szelies B, Herholz K, Pawlik G, Karbe H, Hebold I, Heiss W-D. Widespread functional effects of discrete thalamic infarction Arch Neurol 1991;48:178.
2. Damasio H, Damasio AR. Lesion analysis in neuropsychology. New York: Oxford University Press, 1989.
3. Bogousslavsky J, Regli F, Uske A. Thalamic infarcts: clinical syndromes, etiology, and prognosis. Neurology 1988;38:837.
4. Kawahara N, Sato K, Muraki M, Tanaka K, Kaniko M, Uemura K. CT classification of small thalamic hemorrhages and their clinical implications. Neurology 1986;36(2):165.
5. Graff-Radford NR, Damasio H, Yamada T, Eslinger PJ, Damasio AR. Nonhaemorrhagic thalamic infarction. Brain 1985;108:485.
6. Castaigne P, Lhermitte F, Buge A, Escourolle R, Hauw JJ, Lyon-Caen O. Paramedian thalamic and midbrain infarcts: clinical and neuropathological study. Ann Neurol 1981;10:127.
7. Walshe TM, Davis DR, Fisher CM. Thalamic hemorrhage: a CT clinical correlation. Neurology 1977;27(3):217.
8. Erlich SS, Apuzzo MLJ. The pineal gland: anatomy, physiology, and clinical significance. J Neurosurg 1985;63:321.
9. Wetterberg L. The relationship between the pineal gland and the pituitary adrenal axis in health, endocrine and psychiatric conditions. Psychoneuroendocrinology 1983;8:75.
10. Ohye C. Thalamus. In: Paxinos G, ed. The human nervous system. San Diego: Academic Press, 1990:439–468.
11. Masdeu JC, Brazis PW. The localization of lesions in the thalamus. In: Brazis PW, Masdeu JC, Biller J, eds. Localization in clinical neurology. Boston: Little, Brown, 1990:319–343.
12. Barr ML, Kiernan JA. The human nervous system: an anatomical viewpoint. Philadelphia: JB Lippincott, 1988, Chap. 20.
13. Masdeu JC. The localization of lesions affecting the visual pathways. In: Brazis PW, Masdeu JC, Biller J, eds. Localization in clinical neurology. Boston: Little, Brown, 1990:127–187.
14. Winer JA. The human medial geniculate body. Hear Res 1984;15:225.
15. Jarrell TW, Gentile CG, McCabe PM, Schneiderman N. The role of the medial geniculate region in differential Pavlovian conditioning of bradycardia in rabbits. Brain Res 1986;374:126.
16. Motomura N, Yamadori A, Mori E, Tamaru F. Auditory agnosia. Brain 1986;109:379.
17. Jenkins WM, Masterton RB. Sound localization: effects of unilateral lesions in central auditory system. J Neurophysiol 1982;47:987.
18. Fisher CM. Thalamic pure sensory stroke: a pathologic study. Neurology 1978;28(11):1141.
19. Caplan LR. Posterior cerebral artery syndromes. Hdbk Clin Neurol 1988;53(9):409.
20. Watson RT, Valenstein E, Heilman KM. Thalamic neglect: possible role of the medial thalamus and nucleus reticularis in behavior. Arch Neurol 1981;38:501.
21. Graff-Radford N, Eslinger PJ, Damasio AR, Yamada T. Nonhemorrhagic infarction of the thalamus: behavioral, anatomic, and physiologic correlates. Neurology 1984;34:14.
22. Choi D, Sudarsky L, Schachter S, Biber M, Burke P. Medial thalamic hemorrhage with amnesia. Arch Neurol 1983;40:611.
23. Squire L, Moore RY. Dorsal thalamic lesion in a noted case of human memory dysfunction. Ann Neurol 1979;6:503.
24. Lugaresi E, Medori R, Montagna P, et al. Fatal familial insomnia and dysautonomia with selective degeneration of thalamic nuclei. N Engl J Med 1986;315:997.
25. Chalupa LM, Abramson BP. Receptive-field properties in the tecto- and striate-recipient zones of the cat's lateral posterior nucleus. Prog Brain Res 1988;75:85.
26. Steriade M, Parent A, Hada J. Thalamic projections of nucleus reticularis thalami of cat: a study using retrograde transport of horseradish peroxidase and fluorescent tracers. J Comp Neurol 1984;229:531.
27. Alexander GF, Crutcher MD. Functional architecture of basal ganglia circuits: neural substrates of parallel processing. Trends Neurosci 1990;13:266.
28. DeLong MR. Primate models of movement disorders of basal ganglia origin. Trends Neurosci 1990;13:281.
29. Grafman J, Salazar AM, Weingartner H, Vance SC, Ludlow C.

Isolated impairment of memory following a penetrating lesion of the fornix cerebri. Arch Neurol 1985;42:1162.

30. Thach WT, Goodkin HP, Keating JG. The cerebellum and adaptive coordination of movement. Ann Rev Neurosci 1992;15:403.

31. Bullard DE, Nashold BS. Stereotaxic thalamotomy for treatment of posttraumatic movement disorders. J Neurosurg 1984;61:316.

32. Masdeu JC, Gorelick PB. Thalamic astasia: inability to stand after unilateral thalamic lesions. Ann Neurol 1988;23:596.

33. Mair WG, Warrington EK, Weiskrantz L. Memory disorder in Korsakoff's psychosis. A neuropathological and neuropsychological investigation of two cases. Brain 1979;102:749.

34. Aggleton JP, Mishkin M. Mammillary-body lesions and visual recognition in monkeys. Exp Brain Res 1985;58:190.

35. von Cramon DY, Heibel N, Schuri U. A contribution to the anatomical basis of thalamic amnesia. Brain 1985;108:993.

36. Graff-Radford NR, Tranel D, Van Hoesen GW, Brandt JP. Diencephalic amnesia. Brain 1990;113:1.

37. Masdeu JC. The localization of lesions of the hypothalamus and pituitary gland. In: Brazis PW, Masdeu JC, Biller J, eds. Localization in clinical neurology. Boston: Little, Brown, 1990.

38. Thompson SM, Robertson RT. Organization of subcortical pathways for sensory projections to the limbic cortex II. Afferent projections to the thalamic lateral dorsal nucleus in the rat. J Comp Neurol 1987;265:189.

39. Armstrong E. Limbic thalamus: anterior and mediodorsal nuclei. In: Paxinos G, ed. The human nervous system. San Diego: Academic Press, 1990:469–481.

40. Percheron G. The anatomy of the arterial supply of the human thalamus and its use for the interpretation of thalamic vascular pathology. Z Neurol 1973;205:1.

41. Gorelick PB, Hier DB, Benevento L, Levitt S, Tan W. Aphasia after left thalamic infarction. Arch Neurol 1984;41(12):1296.

42. Mori E, Yamadori A, Mitani Y. Left thalamic infarction and disturbance of verbal memory: a clinicoanatomical study with a new method of computed tomographic stereotaxic lesion localization. Ann Neurol 1986;20:671.

43. Caplan LR, DeWitt D, Pessin MS, Gorelich PB, Adelman LS. Lateral thalamic infarcts. Arch Neurol 1988;45:959.

8 CEREBRAL HEMISPHERES: NEOCORTEX

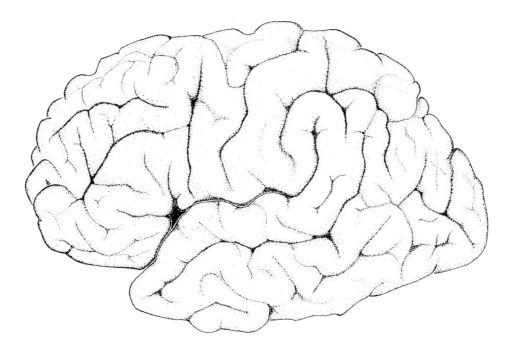

► Introduction

The cerebral hemispheres are the most prominent structures of the brain. Starting as small, lateral protrusions off the diencephalon, they expand rapidly during development to eventually envelop the rostral end of the brain stem as well as portions of the cerebellum. When mature, each hemisphere is composed of a thin, folded cortical mantle of neurons overlying a massive accumulation of white matter. The axons of the white matter form an elaborate network of intracerebral communication, both within a hemisphere and between hemispheres. In addition, some of these axons represent the efferent projections of the cerebral cortex, which descend through the white matter, enter the internal capsule, and eventually reach the brain stem and spinal cord.

The cortical mantle can be divided into two general regions: *neocortex* and *allocortex*. Neocortical areas form the prominent convoluted mantle on the surface of the hemisphere. They establish reciprocal connections with thalamic nuclei and also project axons to the brain stem and spinal cord.

The allocortex lies along the medial edge or limbus of the cortical mantle. This region represents the oldest portions of the cerebral cortex. Information from the neocortex is passed to allocortical structures via pathways referred to collectively as the limbic system. Through these circuits, sensory input from neocortical areas is processed and complex behavioral responses involving somatomotor and secretomotor, as well as intellectual activities, are generated (see Chap. 9).

Buried deep inside the white matter of the cerebral hemisphere, and in close association with the thalamus, are the *subcortical nuclei* or basal ganglia (the corpus striatum, globus pallidus, and amygdala). The neocortex has extensive projections onto these subcortical nuclei that in turn feed back to the neocortex through the thalamus. This network is involved in modulating or scaling the amount of neural activity in specific portions of neocortex (see Chap. 10).

The organization of the neocortical mantle of the cerebral hemisphere and its connections will be examined in this chapter. Using data derived from the lesion method of analysis,[1] the clinical effects of neocortical damage will be described and several related clinicopathologic cases will be presented.

GENERAL OBJECTIVES

1. To learn the locations and functions of the major sensory, motor, and association areas of neocortex
2. To learn the clinically detectable deficits associated with destruction of specific neocortical areas

3. To use the preceding information to localize the extent of cerebral damage based on a patient's clinical signs and symptoms

INSTRUCTIONS

In this chapter you will be presented with one or more clinical case studies. *Each study will be followed by a list of questions that can best be answered by using a knowledge of regional and functional neuroanatomy and by referring to outside reading material.* Following the questions will be a section devoted to structures from a specific region of the central nervous system. Before attempting to answer the questions, compile a list of the patient's neurologic signs and symptoms, then examine the structures and their functions and study their known clinical deficits. After becoming familiar with the material, reexamine the list of neurologic signs and symptoms and answer the questions. Be aware that some of the questions can have multiple responses or require information beyond the scope of this manual. It may be necessary to obtain material or advice from additional resources, such as specialty texts, a medical dictionary, or clinical personnel.

MATERIALS

1. A whole brain
2. A sagittal brain
3. Brain sections
4. A medical dictionary

UNIT A

Case Study 8-1

A 73-year-old right-handed male with rapid onset of right-sided weakness and aphasia

This 73-year-old, right-handed male was in excellent health until 7 o'clock on the evening of his admission, when he suddenly dropped his pipe out of his right hand while sitting on back porch of his daughter's house. Although he did not experience a syncopal episode, his family reported that he was obtunded for a few minutes. Since this episode, he has been unable to speak. He was brought directly to the emergency room.

Past Medical History

At the time of admission, the patient had been retired for 4 years from his position as an executive with a large firm in the southern portion of the country. He had been active in recreation for the past 10 years. He was in Maine visiting his daughter's family as part of an extended vacation touring the country in a recreation vehicle. His past medical history was unremarkable. There was no history of peptic ulcer disease or of any previous myocardial infarction or rheumatic fever.

General Physical Examination

The patient was an elderly male who appeared younger than his stated age. He was sitting with the head of the bed at less than 30 degrees. He was alert, cooperative, and followed two- and three-step commands. His neck was supple with bilateral high-pitched carotid bruits. No hemorrhages were present in the conjunctiva. No nailbed hemorrhages were present. Heart was regular with no murmurs, rub, or gallops. No easy bruising, bleeding, hematochezia, hemoptysis, or hematuria were noticeable. He denied any stomach pain. Skull and spine were atraumatic. No cranial or orbital bruits were heard. Also, no history of migraine or other neurologic illnesses was given.

Neurologic Examination

Mental Status.   The patient was awake and oriented to place and time. He had a markedly decreased output of speech and answered only in monosyllables of *yes* or *no*. If asked for names, he pointed to the object or person, rather than responding with the word. By using yes or no responses and by following commands, he could demonstrate that he comprehended spoken and written language. He was incapable of writing his name or the days of the week, but could point to the correct day from a list. He quickly recognized family members and attending hospital staff as they entered the room. He could follow two- and three-step commands accurately with his left arm and hand.

Cranial Nerves.   The optic disks were flat; visual fields were intact. No hemorrhages or other embolic phenomenon were present. He had a full range of extraocular motion. His pupils had a range of motion of 2.5 mm to 1.5 mm to both direct and consensual light reflexes. Both eyes could close tightly. Wrinkle lines were symmetric across the forehead, and eyebrows elevated symmetrically. The lower right quadrant of his face showed some paresis when he was asked to grimace or smile. Corneal, jaw-jerk, and gag reflexes were intact. His uvula elevated symmetrically, his tongue protruded along the midline, and his shoulder shrug was symmetric.

Motor Systems.   Motor examination reveals a right upper limb monoparesis with a right pronator drift. Motor power was approximately $4^+/5$ in the right upper extremity. Motor power in the right leg was 5/5. There was right hyperreflexia in the upper extremity, and the right toe was up-going.

Sensation

Sensation to touch, vibration, proprioception, and pain were decreased on the right arm and thigh but was intact on the left side of his body. This portion of the examination was somewhat equivocal because of the the patient's poor communication skills.

QUESTIONS

1. Does the patient exhibit a language or memory deficit or an alteration in consciousness or cognition?

163

2. Are signs of cranial nerve dysfunction present?

3. Are there any changes in motor functions, such as reflexes, muscle tone, movement, or coordination?

4. Are any changes in sensory functions detectable?

5. At what level in the central neuraxis is this lesion most likely located?

6. Is the pathology focal, multifocal, or diffuse in its distribution within the nervous system?

7. What is the clinical–temporal profile of this pathology: acute or chronic; progressive or stable?

8. Based on your answers to the previous two questions, decide whether the symptoms in this patient are most likely caused by a vascular accident, a tumor, or a degenerative or inflammatory process.

9. If you feel this is the result of a vascular accident, what vessels are most likely involved?

10. Is the sparseness of spontaneous speech consistent with the retention of comprehension?

11. Explain the increased paresis in the upper extremity over that of the lower extremity.

► DISCUSSION
Cerebral Structures

The cerebral cortex can be divided into two general regions based on anatomic, phylogenetic, and embryologic studies. These are the following: **neocortex** (six-layered cortex) and **allocortex** (three-layered cortex). The allocortex is divided further into olfactory cortex (paleocortex) and hippocampus (archicortex). The allocortical structures will be discussed in Chapter 9.

The neocortex is the youngest and largest portion of the cerebrum. Its outermost velum, or cortical ribbon, is distinguishable by its six layers of cells and fibers. Its surface is divided into six lobes, four of which can be seen in a lateral view: frontal, parietal, occipital, and temporal (Fig. 8-1). The fifth, the limbic lobe, can be seen in a sagittal view (Fig. 8-2); the sixth, the insula lobe, is tucked deep into the lateral fissure and requires dissection for exposure (Fig. 8-3). (Some of the borders between lobes of the cerebrum are not well defined and different partitioning schemes are employed by various texts.) Each cerebral lobe encompasses several specific gyri (folded ridges) and sulci (valleys between the gyri).

The cerebral lobes are further divided into specific cortical areas, each of which is characterized by its cytology, afferent projections, and efferent targets. These areas, of which there are approximately 50, were described initially by Brodmann and given numeric designations. Although this work was done around the turn of the century, these areas have proven useful in recent physiologic studies and have become a standard for describing territory in the human cerebral cortex. Only the most prominent of the Brodmann areas will be presented in this text. (For details on cortical cytology and a map of the Brodmann areas see Barr and Kiernan.[2])

The Brodmann areas of cerebral cortex can be arranged in a hierarchy of functional groupings (summarized by Changeux[3]). The subcortical sensory systems relay information to the **primary sensory cortex,** the first level in the cortical hierarchy. Well-organized, topographic maps of the external environment exist in these areas. Surrounding the primary sensory areas are regions of the **secondary sensory cortex,** representing the second level in the hierarchy. The secondary areas are involved in feature extraction from the sensory data represented in primary sensory cortex. Examples of such features are motion

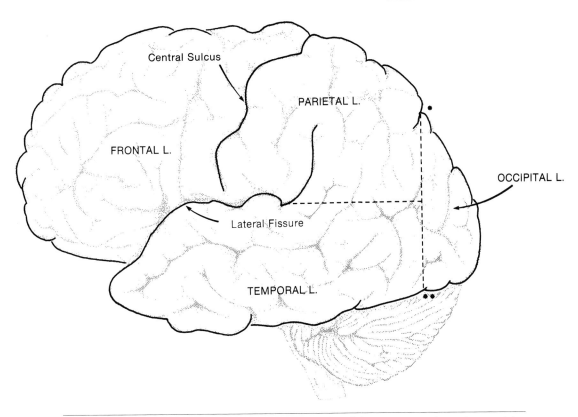

Figure 8-1. This schematic outline illustrates the four lobes seen on a lateral view of the cerebral cortex. The junction separating parietal, occipital, and temporal cortex is defined by dashed lines connecting the parieto-occipital sulcus (∗) to the preoccipital notch (∗∗) and the distal one-third of the lateral fissure.

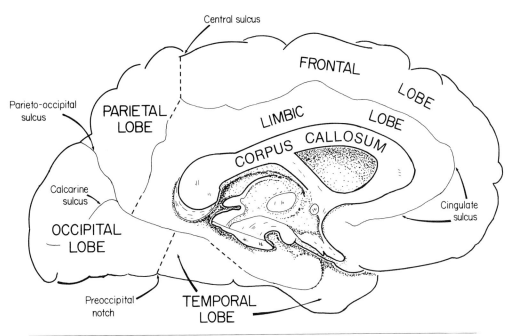

Figure 8-2. This schematic outline illustrates the lobes of the seen on a medial view of the cerebral cortex. Where there are no outward landmarks, the dashed lines have been used to approximate the borders of lobes.

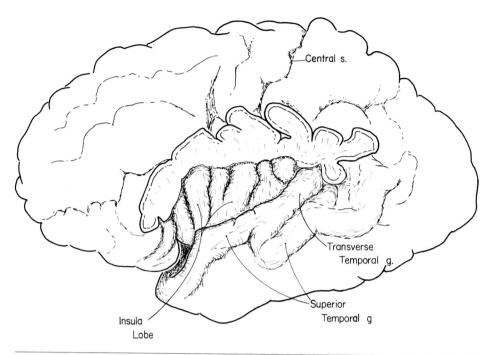

Central s.

Transverse
Temporal g.

Superior
Temporal g

Insula
Lobe

Figure 8-3.   This drawing illustrates the insular cortex after walls of lateral fissure have been removed.

and color and texture of the stimulus. Finally, surrounding the primary and secondary areas are large regions called the **association cortex,** the tertiary level in the hierarchy. Here polymodal sensory convergence from the cortical sensory areas takes place; it is speculated that the image of the environmental event is formed and behavioral patterns are initiated in the association cortex.

Although information flows into the cortex in a hierarchic fashion, processing of this information for attention, memory, language, and cognition cannot be thought of as being derived strictly from the hierarchy array. Numerous interconnections exist between primary, secondary, and tertiary regions of the cerebral cortex, forming vast neural networks. Simultaneous processing of information occurs in these networks in a parallel fashion rather than in a serial order.[4] This mechanism of **parallel distributed processing** affords the brain a far more powerful strategy for extracting features from information than a serial method of processing.

FRONTAL LOBE

The frontal lobe extends rostrally from the central sulcus to the frontal pole (see Figs. 8-1 and 8-2). It is divided into three regions: prefrontal, premotor, and

motor cortex. Each region is composed of multiple gyri and sulci (Fig. 8-4). The motor cortex contains the primary motor representation; the premotor cortex is a secondary level; and the prefrontal cortex is a tertiary or associational level.

Prefrontal Cortex

The rostral portions of three longitudinal gyri (*superior, middle,* and *inferior frontal*) form the prefrontal cortex (see Fig. 8-4). The three gyri are separated by two sulci. The superior and middle gyri are separated by the superior frontal sulcus; the middle and inferior gyri are separated by the inferior frontal sulcus. The inferior frontal gyrus has three named parts (from caudal to rostral): the pars *opercularis, triangularis,* and *orbitalis* (see Fig. 8-4).

In fulfilling its role as an associational level in the cortical hierarchy, the prefrontal cortex has established extensive connections with the rest of the brain. It receives a major fiber projection from the dorsomedial nucleus of the thalamus as well as from other regions of the cerebral cortex, particularly the secondary sensory areas of the parietal, temporal, and occipital cortex, as well as the posterior parietal and inferotemporal association cortex. Thus, neurons in the prefrontal association cortex are heteromodal in their response to sensory stimuli. The efferent fibers from

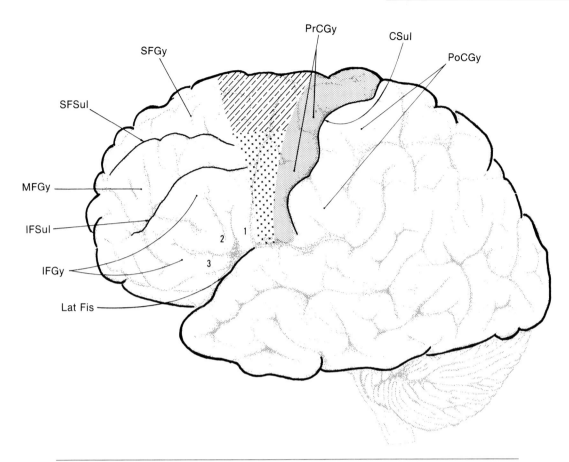

Figure 8-4. Schematic diagram of the gyri and sulci of the frontal cortex. Primary motor cortex is indicated by the gray shading; supplementary motor cortex, by the diagonal lines; and premotor cortex, by the small crosses. The three horizontal gyri (superior middle, and inferior frontal gyri) are collectively called prefrontal cortex. CSul, central sulcus; IFGy, inferior frontal gyrus; 1, pars opercularis; 2, pars triangularis; 3, pars orbitalis; IFSul, inferior frontal sulcus; LatFis, lateral fissure; MFGy, middle frontal gyrus; PoCGy, postcentral gyrus; PrCGy, precentral gyrus; SFGy, superior frontal gyrus; SFSul, superior front sulcus.

the prefrontal cortex radiate out to association areas of the parietal, occipital, temporal, and cingulate cortex as well as to allocortical areas (parahippocampal gyrus). Its descending efferent fibers provide considerable innervation to the corpus striatum (corticostriate fibers), cerebellum (frontopontocerebellar fibers), and many brain stem nuclei (frontonuclear fibers) as well.

In summary, the prefrontal association cortex can be depicted as receiving input from multiple secondary cortical sensory and motor areas and, after processing, passing this sensory information on to the limbic lobe through the cingulate and parahippocampal gyri. In this sense, the prefrontal cortex represents a gateway from the neocortex into the limbic system. Through these extensive connections, the prefrontal cortex plays a major role in controlling the complex patterns of motor and social behavior elicited by external stimuli.

CLINICAL DEFICIT

The signs and symptoms of prefrontal lobe damage are controversial and have presented considerable confusion in the literature.[5] Given the laterality of function in the cerebrum, any analysis of prefrontal cortex damage is best considered in terms of unilateral and bilateral lesions.[6]

Unilateral lesions can result in an elevation of mood, with increased talkativeness, recitation of silly jokes and inappropriate comments, and a lack of tact characterized by loss of social inhibition. Inability to adapt to changing circumstances and a loss of initiative can also be seen. Bilateral prefrontal cortex lesions

167

can result in a general depression of activity, an idleness of thought and speech, an inability to sustain attention, a rigidity or concreteness in thinking, bland affect, and labile mood. The general reduction in activity takes the form of diminished movement, spoken words, and thoughts per unit of time. In mild cases, this is referred to as *abulia;* profound cases result in *akinetic mutism.*[6]

Characteristic of some prefrontal lobe lesions is a perseveration of behavior. The patient fixes on a particular step (usually an early step) in a sequence and repeats that step even though it means that the overall task is not completed correctly.[5] This perseveration of task can occur even though the patient acknowledges that it is not the correct sequence. The underlying deficit may be the patient's inability to adjust to changing circumstances in the external environment.[7]

Memory loss also occurs in some prefrontal lobe lesions. Loss of memory resulting from anterolaterally positioned lesions tends to be a failure to assimilate new material; whereas lesions in the ventral portion of prefrontal cortex result in memory loss resembling the Korsakoff's amnesic syndrome.[6]

Recently, a common theme of behavioral disturbance has been proposed for frontal lobe damage.[7] It is characterized by a loss of attention, shallowness and impulsiveness of thought (increased distractibility), and a disintegration of those behaviors that lack a pronounced external guidance. Typifying this *environmental dependency syndrome* stemming from frontal lobe damage are the "imitation behaviors" and "utilization behaviors" described by Lhermitte and colleagues.[8]

Premotor and Supplementary Motor Cortex

The caudal portions of the superior and middle frontal gyri, as well as the rostral border of the precentral gyrus, are involved in motor functions controlling the axial and proximal limb musculature and constitute the premotor and supplementary motor cortex (see Fig. 8-4). These two regions are considered part of the *medial motor system* of Kuypers (as described in Nieuwenhuys et al[9]).

Premotor and supplementary motor cortex are located in area 6 and part of area 8. Afferent projections to these portions of cortex are received from the ipsilateral ventroanterior and ventrolateral thalamic nucleus and from the ipsilateral posterior parietal cortex. The premotor and supplementary motor cortices have many targets for their efferent projections. Corticocortical fibers interconnect these portions of frontal cortex with primary motor cortex bilaterally. Descending corticonuclear fibers terminate in the reticular formation of the brain stem, and corticospinal fibers terminate in the contralateral medial portions of the ventral horn of the spinal cord.

A distinction between premotor and supplementary motor cortex is seen in the subtleties of their afferent connections and their proposed function (reviewed in Kandel et al.[10]) The premotor cortex receives afferent fibers from the ventrolateral thalamic nucleus (the portion of the thalamus receiving the dentothalamic fibers) and is reported to function by guiding limb trajectory based on sensory information derived from the cerebellum. The supplementary motor cortex receives thalamic afferent axons from the ventroanterior nucleus (the recipient of pallidothalamic fibers) and is reported to function in programming motor sequences derived from the basal ganglia.

Precentral Cortex

The posterior portion of the frontal cortex is the *precentral gyrus* (area 4), which contains the primary motor cortex. This region is involved in controlling distal limb musculature and is considered part of the *lateral motor system* of Kuypers (as described in Nieuwenhuys et al[9]).

The motor cortex contains the large pyramidal neurons of Betz; it receives afferent fibers from the ventrolateral nucleus of thalamus, the primary somatic sensory cortex, and the premotor and supplementary motor cortex. It gives rise to corticospinal fibers that terminate in the lateral portions of the ventral horn.

Cells in the motor cortex are arranged in a body map; the head is represented lateral and inferior along the precentral gyrus, and the arm is found medial and superior. The representation of the leg is found on the medial aspect of the precentral gyrus as it rolls over the edge of the longitudinal fissure to become the anterior paracentral lobule.

The cells of the primary motor cortex exert control over the reflex circuits in the spinal cord and directly control activity of alpha motoneurons, especially over those innervating the distal musculature of the limbs. Stimulation of the primary motor cortex with weak currents produces twitches in one or several related muscles in the extremity (reviewed by Henneman[11]).

Apparently, one role of the primary motor cortex is to encode the force of contraction of the muscle groups about a joint and to prepare these ventral horn neurons to act by adjusting the spinal reflex circuits. However, prior to sending instructions from motor cortex to spinal cord, they are tempered with data concerning the programming of muscle groups around surrounding joints, and the guidance of trajectory derived from the supplementary motor and premotor cortices. These modified instructions are delivered to the spinal neurons producing smooth, coordinated, and balanced movements of the extremities (reviewed in Kandel et al[10]).

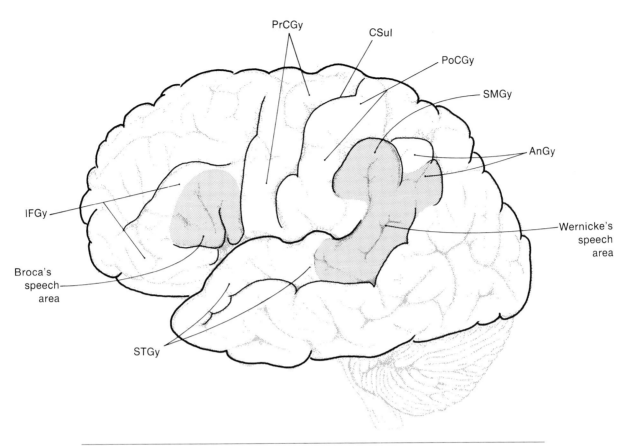

Figure 8-5. A diagram of sensorimotor structures at the parietofrontal junction and the major language areas of cerebral cortex. AnGy, angular gyrus; CSul, central sulcus; IFGy, inferior frontal gyrus; PoCGy, postcentral gyrus; PrCGy, precentral gyrus, SMGy, supramarginal gyrus; STGy, superior temporal gyrus.

Two specialized areas of motor cortex extend rostrally into the premotor cortex. These regions are concerned with eye movements and speech. The frontal eye fields (inferior portion of area 8 plus part of areas 6 and 9) are found on the caudal border of the middle frontal gyrus; they direct the movement of the eyes into the opposite visual hemisphere.

On the inferior border of the precentral gyrus and spreading onto the pars opercularis of the inferior frontal gyrus is Broca's speech area (areas 44 and 45; Fig. 8-5). Broca's area contains the motor patterns for speech. Right-handed persons have Broca's area only in the left or dominant cortex. Superior to Broca's area is a related region of cortex controlling the hand and containing the motor patterns for writing.

CLINICAL DEFICIT

Damage to the precentral gyrus (motor cortex) results in spasticity and hemiplegia on the contralateral side of the body. If the lesion is confined to the lateral portion of the precentral gyrus, supplied by the middle cerebral artery, the paresis affects movements of the arm (monoparesis) as well as producing a paresis of the muscles in the lower quadrant of the face. If the lesion involves the medial portion of the gyrus, supplied by the anterior cerebral artery, the resulting paresis involves the lower extremity. In primates, experimental lesions in motor cortex (area 4) resulted in spasticity and paresis of the affected limb. Recovery from the paresis followed; however, the animal never regained dexterity in the digits or exploratory behavior with the affected extremity (reviewed in Henneman[11]).

Lesions of the premotor cortex in man can result in weakness of the proximal limb muscles.[12] However, the weakness was characterized, on EMG study, by significant delays in the preactivation of proximal limb muscles, an event that interfered with the normal sequencing of contractions between the proximal and distal musculature of the limb.

A notable result of damage to the supplemental motor cortex seems to be the expression of the grasp response (reviewed in Henneman[11]). Slight contact with the hands leads to instinctive grasping of the object. Unilateral lesions involving the left supplemen-

169

tary motor cortex in right-dominant individuals produced a form of apraxia bilaterally in the upper extremities as well as the grasp reflex in the right hand.[13]

Damage to Broca's area can result in nonfluent speech called motor, or anterior, aphasia. The patient's vocabulary is reduced to a few monosyllabic words or sounds, such as *yes* or *no*. Speech is agrammatic, effortful, and slow. However, comprehension may be intact, as may the ability to write. Larger lesions can infringe on the premotor areas of hand representation dorsal to Broca's and interfere with writing. Although the patient may have only a mild paresis of the dominant extremity, when attempting to write he may produce scribbling or illegible characters (dysgraphia) or be unable to move the instrument at all (agraphia). The signs and syndromes of Broca's aphasia are reviewed by Damasio[14] and by Levine and Sweet.[15]

If the damage involves premotor cortex representation of the hand, apraxias can be present unilaterally or bilaterally.[16] Although the patient can hear and understand a command, he is unable to access the hand representation in motor cortex volitionally and thus cannot initiate the requested movement. Yet the hand is not paralyzed and can be moved in other tasks.

Damage to the medial frontal lobe can result in transcortical motor aphasia as well as hemiplegia of the lower portion of the lower limb. In transcortical motor aphasia the patient has nonfluent aphasia but maintains good repetition of words or phrases and some comprehension of language.[17]

PARIETAL LOBE

The parietal lobe extends from the central sulcus to the parieto-occipital sulcus (see Fig. 8-1). Inferiorly, it blends with the temporal and occipital cortex at the base of the supramarginal and angular gyri. Superiorly, it wraps over the medial edge of the longitudinal fissure and descends along the medial wall to reach the limbic lobe (see Fig. 8-2).

The parietal lobe contains several subdivisions (Fig. 8-6); these are the *postcentral gyrus, posterior parietal lobule,* and *medial parietal lobule.* The posterior parietal lobule is separated from the postcentral gyrus by the postcentral sulcus and is divided into superior and inferior portions by the intraparietal sulcus. The inferior portion contains two important gyri: supramarginal, surrounding the distal terminus of the lateral fissure, and angular, surrounding the distal terminus of the superior temporal sulcus. The medial parietal lobule is located on the wall of the longitudinal fissure and is divided into two areas: the posterior paracentral cortex, located rostrally, and the precuneate cortex, located caudally.

Postcentral Gyrus

The postcentral gyrus is immediately posterior to the central sulcus. Contained in this gyrus is the primary somatic sensory cortex, composed of Brodmann's areas 3, 1, and 2. These areas are arranged as three bands parallel to the long axis of the postcentral gyrus. Medially, the postcentral gyrus extends over the edge of the longitudinal fissure and onto the medial parietal lobule.

The primary somatic sensory cortex receives afferent fibers from the ventroposterior medial and lateral nuclei of thalamus. Its cells are arranged in a topographic body map in register with the motor map present in the precentral gyrus directly across the central sulcus. The head representation is located on the edge of the lateral fissure; the leg representation is positioned in the longitudinal fissure. Projections from postcentral gyrus travel to the superior and inferior parietal lobule (collectively called posterior parietal cortex) and to primary motor cortex.

Secondary somatic sensory areas are also present in the cerebral cortex. One such area is found on the upper bank of the lateral fissure at the lateral end of the postcentral gyrus. It has a separate body representation. Another area is the supplementary somatic sensory cortex on the medial wall of the longitudinal fissure, opposite the supplementary motor cortical area. The function of these secondary areas is unclear; however, it is known that they receive information from the primary somatic sensory cortex and that they project to the posterior parietal association cortex and the limbic system through the cingulate cortex (see Chap. 9 and review by Kaas[18]).

CLINICAL DEFICIT

Damage to the "body map" in the postcentral gyrus results in a dysfunction of somatic sensation from the contralateral portion of the body. This is characterized by loss of position sense and two-point discrimination, as well as astereognosis, which is an inability to identify objects by tactile sense of size and shape alone.[18] Damage to only a small portion of the cortical map results in dysfunction of sensory input from the corresponding portion of the body. However, the losses tend to be most profound when they involve the contralateral distal extremities, since they receive the greatest amount of cortical representation.

Paresthesias, such as a tingling sensation, are common features of lesions in the postcentral gyrus.[19] In addition, poorly localized pain and thermal sensation can remain intact in the presence of discriminative sensory loss.

It is also possible to dissociate localization of touch from discrimination of the object. Patients with cortical lesions have been observed who are capable of

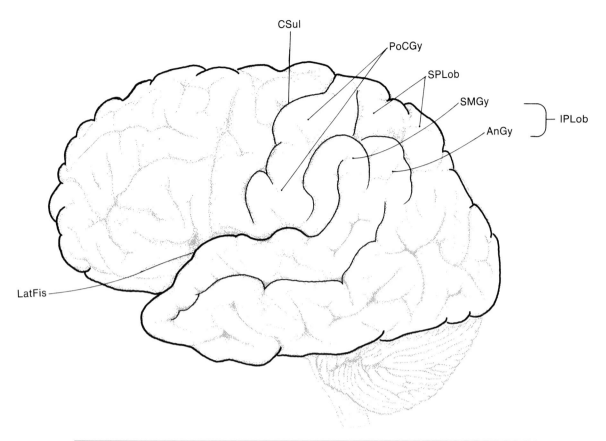

Figure 8-6. Diagram of general organization of parietal cortex. The parietal lobe is bounded by the dashed line posteriorly and by the central sulcus anteriorly. The inferior parietal lobule is composed of the angular gyrus (ANGy) and supramarginal gyrus (SMGy). CSul, central sulcus; IPLob, inferior parietal lobe; LatFis, lateral fissure; PoCGy, postcentral gyrus; SPLOb, superior parietal lobe.

identifying the approximate location of the touch on their affected limb while being unable to recognize the object with which they were touched.[20]

Medial Parietal Lobule

The parietal cortex wraps over the medial wall of the longitudinal fissure (see Fig. 8-2). This portion of cortex is the medial parietal lobule and is composed of posterior paracentral cortex and precuneate cortex. The posterior paracentral cortex is a direct continuation of the postcentral gyrus. It contains the body representation for the lower part of the leg and foot. Also present is a second body map, analogous to that of the supplementary motor cortex.[18] The major source of afferent fibers to the medial parietal lobule is the ventroposterior lateral nucleus of thalamus. The precuneate extends caudally to the occipital cortex. Its major source of afferent fibers is the pulvinar nucleus of thalamus.

CLINICAL DEFICIT

Lesions of the posterior paracentral cortex affect the sensory representation of the distal lower extremity, resulting in loss of two-point discrimination and position sense. Since this region is supplied by branches of the anterior cerebral artery, it is possible to disassociate it from the head, torso, and upper-extremity representation located laterally in the postcentral gyrus. This latter region is supplied by branches of the middle cerebral artery.

Posterior Parietal Lobule

The posterior parietal lobule is divided into two parts, superior and inferior, by the intraparietal sulcus (see Fig. 8-6). Both portions receive thalamic afferent fibers from the lateral posterior nucleus and pulvinar nucleus. The posterior parietal lobule is considered association cortex; it receives polysensory input from somatic, visual, and auditory cortical areas. Its major

171

efferent projections extend to premotor cortex, prefrontal association cortex, and inferior temporal association cortex as well as to lateral posterior thalamic nuclei.

The inferior portion of posterior parietal cortex is composed of the *supramarginal* and *angular gyri* (see Fig. 8-6). These association levels of cortex receive projections from the somatic, auditory, and visual sensory areas. In the dominant hemisphere, this region, along with portions of the superior temporal gyrus, contains Wernicke's area (see Fig. 8-5) and represents a location involved in language comprehension.[21] In the nondominant hemisphere the analogous region is thought to function in the comprehension of mechanicospatial relationships.

The superior portion of the posterior parietal cortex (reviewed in Kaas[18]) includes areas 5 and 7 of Brodmann. This portion of the neocortex receives projections from the primary somatic sensory cortex and the superior temporal cortex (visual information) and from several thalamic nuclei, such as the ventroposterior nucleus, pulvinar, and lateral posterior nucleus. The superior portion of posterior parietal cortex projects axons to the other portions of the parietal cortex bilaterally, and to the prefrontal cortex, premotor cortex, limbic cortex, and the superior temporal gyrus ipsilaterally. Its subcortical projections reach the basal ganglia, thalamus, and pons ipsilaterally and the spinal cord contralaterally. A particularly strong connection exists between the neocortex along the walls of the intraparietal sulcus and the frontal eye fields; these are involved in guiding the eyes toward an object to which we want to attend. The region around the junction of the superior posterior parietal cortex with the supramarginal gyrus on the dominant side is involved with the spatial representation of writing and directs the learned motor patterns in the extremities for forming letters.[22]

It is clear from its pattern of connections that the posterior parietal lobule, a tertiary level in the cortical hierarchy, serves to integrate polymodal sensory stimuli and communicate with other areas of association cortex. It has been hypothesized that, through this process, our awareness of the extrapersonal world is transformed into a sensory map that attaches relevance to the specific sensory experience.[23]

CLINICAL DEFICIT

Damage to Wernicke's area (dominant hemispheres) can result in a form of *fluent or posterior aphasia;* such patients can produce an effortless volume of words rapidly, but they are not related meaningfully to each other.[14,24] This is sometimes called a "word salad," for obvious reasons, and it affects both the volitional and repetitive forms of speech. Damage to a broad belt around Wernicke's area, including the medial parietal cortex, can result in *transcortical sensory aphasia.*[17] The patient demonstrates fluent aphasia on attempted volitional speech, however, unlike pure fluent aphasia, the patient can repeat words as well as complex phrases accurately after the examiner. Right homonymous hemianopsia frequently accompanies lesions to the inferior parietal lobule, since the optic radiations pass close to this portion of cortex on their way to the occipital lobe.

A hemorrhagic lesion in the superior portion of the posterior parietal cortex on the dominant side, verified by computed tomography, resulted in an apraxia for the geometric aspects of writing called **apraxic agraphia.**[22] The patient initially expressed paresis in the right extremity, which resolved with time. Although the patient had fluent speech with only mild word-finding difficulties and could spell orally as well as type correctly, she was unable to write with either hand despite having a knowledge of the letters and words. Over several weeks a limited writing capability returned; however, at best, her writing was described as laborious and time consuming and letters had poor geometric order.

The nondominant inferior parietal lobule seems to be involved in mechanicospatial perception. Along with left homonymous hemianopsia, patients with damage to the nondominant inferior parietal lobule displayed constructional apraxia,[25] an inability to construct models of common objects with blocks or cards due to a lack of spatial order.

Large lesions in the nondominant posterior parietal lobule result in a *neglect syndrome* (asomatognosis) and loss of topographic memory.[19] Varying degrees of the neglect syndrome exist, ranging from only mild extinction of bilateral sensory information on the affected side to extreme neglect of the entire affected hemisphere of personal and extrapersonal space.[18,23] In the extreme form, the hapless patient refuses to acknowledge that the contralateral side of his or her body belongs to him or her and fails to recognize contralateral extrapersonal space as well!

TEMPORAL LOBE

There are four longitudinally oriented gyri in the temporal lobe: the *superior temporal gyrus* (with its extension, the *superficial transverse temporal gyrus,* on which auditory functions are located [see Fig. 8-3]), the *middle temporal gyrus,* the *inferior temporal gyrus,* and the *occipitotemporal gyrus.* The first three are located on the lateral and inferolateral surfaces of the temporal lobe (Fig. 8-7). The latter is located on the inferior surface of the temporal lobe, and its medial border with the parahippocampal gyrus is determined by the collateral sulcus (Fig. 8-8).

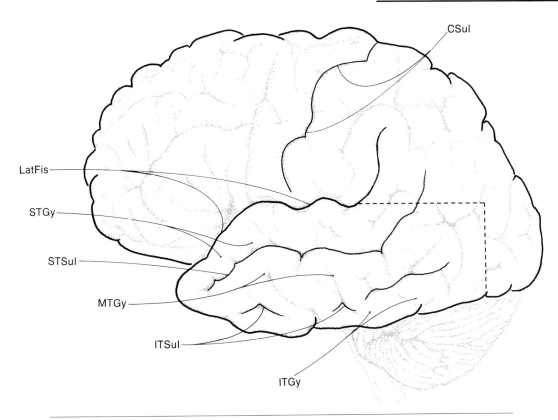

Figure 8-7. Diagram of general organization of temporal cortex. CSul, central sulcus; ITGy, inferior temporal gyrus; ITSul, inferior temporal sulcus; LatFis, lateral fissure; MTGy, middle temporal gyrus; STGy, superior temporal gyrus; STSul, superior temporal sulcus.

The superficial transverse temporal gyrus and adjacent portions of the superior temporal gyrus receive thalamic afferent fibers from the medial geniculate nuclei and represent the primary auditory cortex (Brodmann's area 41 and part of 42). The neural components of this cortex are arranged in a topographic map of frequency representation on the basilar membrane. This organization is referred to as tonotopy.[26,27] Its efferent projections are to the adjacent temporal cortex, Wernicke's area, and the posterior parietal cortex. The auditory cortex is necessary for discerning the temporal component of language.

The primary auditory area, like that of the somatic sensory cortex, is surrounded by secondary areas. Several secondary auditory areas, each with tonotopic representations, are present in the temporal cortex. The specific functions of these areas are unknown at this time.

The remaining temporal gyri (collectively called the inferior temporal association cortex) are influenced by the pulvinar nuclei and the visual cortex. Superiorly, this region blends with the posterior parietal association cortex; posteriorly, it blends with the occipital association cortex. They are involved in visual and acoustic cognition, visual discrimination, and pattern perception. The general function of this large expanse of the association cortex was discussed on pp. 171–172.

CLINICAL DEFICIT

Damage to the primary auditory cortex is not readily detectable unless it is bilateral. Damage on both sides results in loss of the ability to hear speech, called *cortical deafness,* although in at least one reported case, sounds could be detected.[27] Apparently, the auditory cortex is necessary for us to understand the temporal pattern (acuity) of sounds involved in speech. *Verbal auditory agnosia* can result from either bilateral or unilateral lesions of the region in or around the auditory cortex. Affected individuals are capable of identifying environmental sounds but cannot recognize speech patterns. However, the opposite can also occur; in rare cases temporal lesions can result in a patient who cannot recognize nonverbal (environmental) sounds but can understand speech, called *nonverbal auditory agnosia.*

Lesions that affect the superolateral portion of the superior temporal gyrus can result in auditory illu-

173

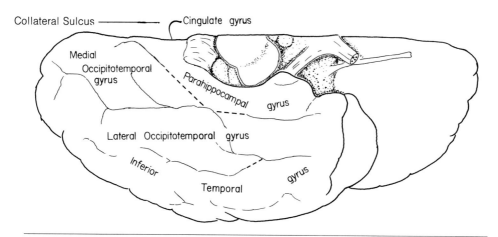

Collateral Sulcus — Cingulate gyrus

Medial Occipitotemporal gyrus

Parahippocampal gyrus

Lateral Occipitotemporal gyrus

Inferior Temporal gyrus

Figure 8-8. This is a ventral view of the brain illustrating the occipitotemporal gyri. The medial occipitotemporal gyrus is also called lingual gyrus; Some authors call the lateral occipitotemporal gyrus the fusiform gyrus.

sions and hallucinations. Damage to any of the rest of the temporal lobe can present with various forms of visual agnosia (loss of the ability to identify common objects when seen), as disturbances of visual perception and visual learning, and as disturbances of time scale, such as diminished capacity to reckon personal events in terms of a time scale.[6]

OCCIPITAL LOBE

The occipital lobe is the caudalmost portion of the cerebrum and is represented on its lateral (see Fig. 8-1), medial (see Fig. 8-2), and inferior (see Fig. 8-8) surfaces. The borders between occipital, parietal, and temporal lobes are not well defined. On the lateral aspect of the cerebrum, these borders have been depicted by a vertical line connecting the parieto-occipital sulcus with the preoccipital notch and a horizontal line at the beginning of the distal one third of the lateral fissure (see Fig. 8-1). On the medial aspect of the cerebrum (Fig. 8-2), the borders of the occipital lobe are formed by the parieto-occipital sulcus, the medial portion of the calcarine sulcus, and a line drawn from the splenium of the corpus callosum to the preoccipital notch.

The medial aspect of the occipital lobe contains a prominent, curvilinear groove on its surface—the *calcarine sulcus* (Fig. 8-9). *Primary visual cortex* (Brodmann's area 17) is located on both sides of this groove, posterior to its junction with the parieto-occipital sulcus. This area is often called striate cortex in recognition of the prominent bands of fibers in the cortical cytoarchitecture. Primary visual cortex is surrounded by bands of secondary visual or extrastriate cortex (Brodmann's areas 18 and 19).

Primary visual cortex is arranged as a visuotopic map of space, superimposed on the calcarine sulcus. The map is generated by thalamic afferent fibers from the lateral geniculate nuclei and is inverted in its representation of space. The superior visual field is represented on the inferior lip of the calcarine sulcus, while the inferior visual field is located on the superior lip (see discussion in Barr and Kiernan[2]).

Several secondary visual cortical areas surrounds area 17. They receive cortical projections from area 17 and thalamic projections from portions of the pulvinar nuclei. Secondary visual cortical areas function in the feature extraction from the sensory information represented in primary visual cortex. Differential activity has been reported for secondary visual cortex. Those regions inferior to area 17 are involved in perception of object shape and color; while the superior regions are involved in spatial relationships.[1] Efferent projections from secondary visual cortex travel to posterior parietal cortex, premotor cortex (frontal eye fields), and inferior temporal cortex.

The remainder of occipital cortex (outside of areas 18 and 19) and portions of the inferior temporal cortex form the association areas. These regions blend with posterior parietal association cortex. Some of the functions of association cortex have been discussed on pages 171 to 172.

CLINICAL DEFICIT

Damage to the area around the calcarine sulcus results in blindness in the affected portion of the visual hemisphere. If total destruction occurs, such as in a large bleeding accident or large tumor, it can lead to complete blindness in the contralateral visual hemisphere. Although such individuals cannot "see" or identify objects within their visual fields, they still have extra-

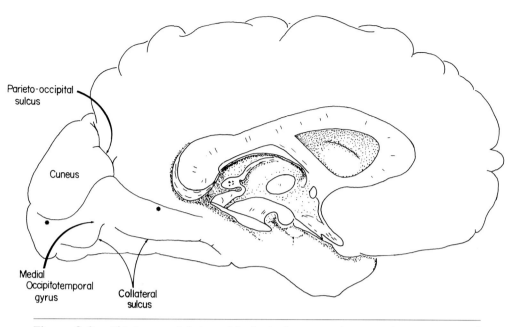

Figure 8-9. This is a medial view of the brain illustrating the general organizations of occipital cortex.

cortical visual pathways and can respond to the presence or absence of light. Their pupillary reflex is present and they have a full range of eye movements. This syndrome is referred to as *cortical blindness* (reviewed by Aldrich et al[28]). Lesions that extend into the visual association cortex can result in Anton's syndrome. The individual is cortically blind but refuses to admit visual loss.[19]

Simultanagnosia (an ability to see the parts of an image but an inability to synthesize the whole) can result from damage to the secondary cortex superior to the primary visual cortex. Cortical blindness is not necessarily present in patients with simultanagnosia. The involvement of the medial aspect of the inferior temporo-occipital cortex can result in color agnosia; if bilateral damage occurs in this area, *prosopagnosia* (loss of recognition of familiar faces) can result.[6]

INSULA LOBE

If the walls of the lateral fissure are separated or cut away (see Fig. 8-3), an island of cortex, the insula, is seen within. Numerous branches of the middle cerebral artery course over the surface of the insula lobe. Afferent fibers to the insular cortex arise in the medial geniculate nuclei (auditory and vestibular input), ventroposterior medial nucleus (gustatory and visceral sensory input), parabrachial nucleus of the pons, solitary nucleus of the medulla, and olfactory bulb. Projections from the insular cortex reach the

brain stem nuclei with autonomic functions, especially those controlling blood pressure and heart rate. This arrangement favors a role for the insular cortex in the convergence of taste, smell, and visceral feelings to control autonomic functions, such as the cardiovascular system.[29,30]

CLINICAL DEFICIT

Isolated, destructive lesions of the insula in humans are rare. However, irritative lesions have been reported to cause seizures. The precursor for insular lobe seizures can involve gustatory hallucinations, such as a perceived bitter taste.[31]

CORPUS CALLOSUM

The two cerebral hemispheres are separated by the longitudinal fissure. A massive fiber bridge, the corpus callosum, spans the longitudinal fissure, interconnecting the hemispheres (see Fig. 8-2). Reciprocal mapping occurs between homologous areas of cortex through these commissural connections. Frontal commissural fibers cross in the rostrum of the corpus callosum, parietal commissural fibers cross in the body, and occipital commissural fibers cross in the splenium. The temporal lobes communicate via the anterior commissure passing through the rostral forebrain (see Plates 23 to 25).

The two hemispheres do not function identically, each being capable of some independent thought processes. The localization of specific functions into a re-stricted hemisphere is called *lateralization*. The corpus callosum normally helps to unite the activity of the two hemispheres. Sectioning callosal fibers can dissociate the two hemispheres and, literally, produce an individual with two rather distinct brains.[32-37]

CLINICAL DEFICIT

Section of the corpus callosum is done to disconnect the hemispheres in intractable epilepsy. Numerous

reviews have summarized the results of these "split-brain" operations.[37,38]

Some split-brain studies can occur naturally; developmental abnormalities leading to partial or complete agenesis of the corpus callosum have been detected in the population using magnetic resonance imaging (reviewed in Kolodny[39]). Agenesis occurs in from one to three of every 1000 births and is more predominant in children with additional cerebral malformations[40] or metabolic diseases.[41] Agenesis or partial genesis of the corpus callosum can appear silent in the patient.[42]

UNIT B

Case Study 8-2

A 52-year-old man with paresis of the distal lower extremity, confusion, and aphasia

This 52-year-old, right-handed male was brought to the emergency room by ambulance after losing consciousness in a restaurant on a Sunday afternoon. Although he maintained vital signs, he remained unconscious for 2 days, after which he began responding to external stimuli. Over a 2-week period he gradually regained consciousness. At this point he was re-examined for evaluation of future course.

Past Medical History

At the time of admission he was a post office employee, married, with three children, all in high school and living at home. His family stated that he did not smoke but admitted that he drank three or four glasses of beer per week. He had been in good health up until the apoplectic episode. His father had died of cerebrovascular disease 10 years before, at the age of 64; his mother was living and in good health.

General Physical Examination

The patient was a well-nourished, well-hydrated male with male-pattern baldness and appeared his stated age. He was awake and fully cooperative but was disoriented for time and place. He had difficulty recognizing family members and hospital staff. He was overweight and appeared anxious. His optic discs were clear and sharp, and visual acuity was good. The neck was supple, with no bruits or lymphadenopathy. The chest was clear to percussion; the abdomen was soft, with no masses or tenderness. Peripheral pulses were intact at the wrist and ankle. Skin was moist and warm.

Neurologic Examination

Mental Status. The patient was an awake, fully cooperative, but disoriented male. His volitional speech was extremely nonfluent, consisting of several short phrases, such as, "No . . . no . . . no . . . no . . . no" or "Tat . . . tat . . . tat." He repeated these phrases many times when attempting to answer questions. He could, however, repeat complicated phrases following the examiner's lead, such as "no ifs, ands, or buts." Yet he could not recite the days of the week or months of the year when asked. Although he could understand simple commands (*e.g.*, "Point to the door"), his comprehension of language was extremely poor. He never understood two- or three-step commands. He could read aloud but could not comprehend what he had read; he could not write or draw even simple figures.

Cranial Nerves. He had a full range of eye movements but tended to keep his eyes positioned to the left when resting. Visual acuity was difficult to test, but he was capable of reading 8-point type. Both pupils were reactive to light, direct, and consensual. Hearing could not be tested accurately. Corneal, jaw-jerk, and gag reflexes were intact. There was a mild weakness in the right lower quadrant of his face. The uvula was elevated on the midline, and the tongue protruded on the midline. Snout, grasp, and suck reflexes were not present.

Motor Systems. Strength was diminished on the right, more so in the leg than in the arm. Deep tendon reflexes were elevated on the right compared to the left. A Babinski sign was present on the right. He was incontinent for urine and feces and was visibly upset when this occurred.

Sensation

The sensorium was difficult to examine because of the patient's poor mental status. Pinprick, temperature, vibratory, and proprioceptive senses appeared intact throughout the body and face, with the exception of some loss in the lower extremity on the right.

QUESTIONS

1. Does the patient exhibit a language or memory deficit or an alteration in consciousness or cognition?

2. Are signs of cranial nerve dysfunction present?

3. Are there any changes in motor functions, such as reflexes, muscle tone, movement, or coordination?

4. Are any changes in sensory functions detectable?

5. At what level in the central neuraxis is this lesion most likely located?

6. Is the pathology focal, multifocal, or diffuse in its distribution within the nervous system?

7. What is the clinical–temporal profile of this pathology: acute or chronic; progressive or stable?

8. Based on your answers to the previous two questions, decide whether the symptoms in this patient are most likely caused by a vascular accident, a tumor, or a degenerative or inflammatory process.

9. If you feel this is the result of a vascular accident, what vessels are most likely involved?

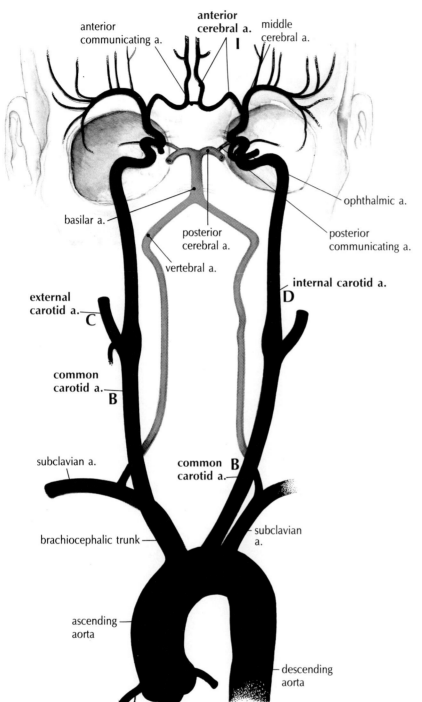

anterior
communicating a.

**anterior
cerebral a.**

middle
cerebral a.

ophthalmic a.

basilar a.

posterior
cerebral a.

posterior
communicating a.

vertebral a.

internal carotid a.

D

**external
carotid a.**

C

**common
carotid a.**

B

subclavian a.

**common B
carotid a.**

subclavian
a.

brachiocephalic trunk

ascending
aorta

descending
aorta

© MELLONI

Figure 8-10.
Source of cerebral vasculature: the carotid and vertebral arterial system. (Reproduced with permission from Melloni BJ, et al, Melloni's illustrated review of human anatomy. Philadelphia: JB Lippincott, 1988:7)

► DISCUSSION
Cerebral Vasculature

ORIGIN OF THE CEREBRAL VASCULATURE

Arterial branches from the arch of the aorta and the subclavian artery are the major source of vessels supplying cerebral circulation (Fig. 8-10). Anteriorly, the carotid system ascends through the neck to the base of the skull; posteriorly, the vertebral system winds through the transverse processes of the vertebrae to reach the foramen magnum. After entering the cranial vault, the internal carotids bifurcate to form the anterior and middle cerebral arteries, and the vertebrals fuse to form the basilar artery. This latter vessel traverses the long axis of the brain stem and subsequently bifurcates in the interpeduncular fossa to form the posterior cerebral arteries. As a result, three

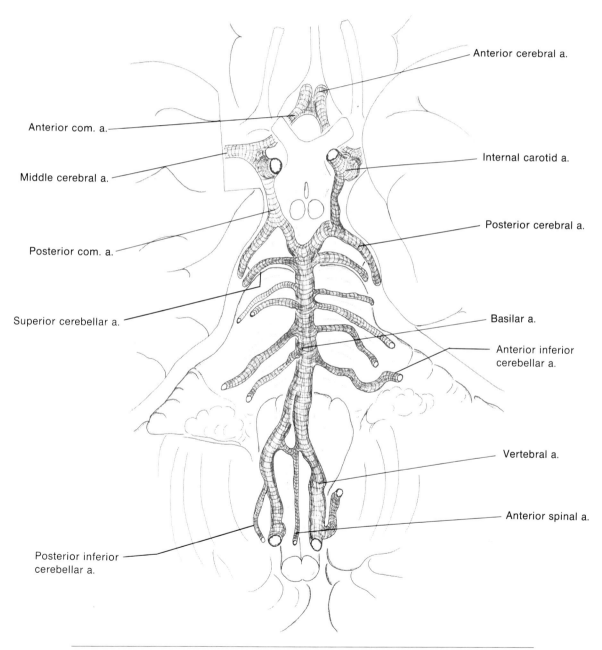

Anterior cerebral a.

Anterior com. a.

Internal carotid a.

Middle cerebral a.

Posterior cerebral a.

Posterior com. a.

Superior cerebellar a.

Basilar a.

Anterior inferior cerebellar a.

Vertebral a.

Anterior spinal a.

Posterior inferior cerebellar a.

Figure 8-11. A diagram of the circle of Willis as seen from the ventral surface of the brain.

paired arterial systems come to lie in close juxtaposition at the base of the brain, surrounding the pituitary stalk (Fig. 8-11).

At the base of the brain, the three paired cerebral arteries are joined into an anastomotic circle by small communicating branches (see Fig. 8-11). The two anterior cerebral arteries are united by the anterior communicating branch; the middle and posterior cerebral arteries are joined by the posterior communicating branch. Finally, the middle and anterior cerebral arteries are united by a common origin from the internal carotid artery. The arterial ring so created is called the circle of Willis; if it is of sufficient size, it can serve to bypass perfusion deficits in any one of the major ascending vessels of the neck.

ANTERIOR CEREBRAL ARTERY (ACA)

The anterior cerebral artery (ACA) arises from the internal carotid artery near the optic chiasm (see Figs. 8-10 and 8-11). (The anatomy and radiology of this arterial system is extensively reviewed by Lin and Kricheff[43] and by Moscow.[44]) This artery turns medially, passing inferior to the medial olfactory stria and superior to the optic tract and giving off the medial striate arteries to the anterior hypothalamus and anterior inferior portion of the striatum. As it approaches the midline, the anterior cerebral arteries are interconnected through the anterior communicating artery, completing the rostral aspect of the circle of Willis. Each anterior cerebral artery enters the longitudinal fissure and arches superiorly and caudally over the rostrum of the corpus callosum.

Once above the corpus callosum, the anterior cerebral artery divides into pericallosal and callosomarginal trunks, which course inferior and superior to the cingulate gyrus, respectively. Each of these trunks gives off cortical branches to supply the walls of the cerebral cortex within the longitudinal fissure, including the anterior cingulate cortex, the medial aspect of frontal and parietal lobes, the anterior corpus callosum, the anterior limb of the internal capsule, and the head of the caudate nucleus (Fig. 8-12). Notable among the cortical areas serviced by this artery are the paracentral lobules, which contain motor and sensory representation of the leg and foot, and the supplementary motor cortex, which is involved in the initiation and regulation of voluntary movement and speech.

CLINICAL DEFICIT

Damage to the anterior cingulate and paracentral distribution of the anterior cerebral artery can present clinically as contralateral paralysis, and/or sensory loss

in the foot and leg, a Babinski sign, urinary incontinence, gait apraxia, akinetic mutism, transcortical aphasia, and cognitive impairment. If damage occurs to deeper tissue around the internal capsule, undercutting the precentral gyrus, paresis of the upper extremity and facial musculature can result.[45] Large lesions of the anterior cerebral artery can affect the frontal eye fields, and the patient may lose volitional control of conjugate eye movement to the contralateral side. In milder cases, the eyes simply drift to the ipsilateral side while resting. Damage to the corpus callosum and/or supplementary motor cortex can produce ideomotor apraxia, alien hand syndrome, and left-handed apraxia and agraphia (reviewed in Hung and Ryu[46]).

The incontinence seen in anterior cerebral artery occlusion results from damage to the superior frontal and anterior cingulate cortex. As the position of the lesion is shifted anteriorly along the cingulate gyrus, the patients become less concerned with their incontinence.[6]

A language deficit can result from damage to the anterior cerebral artery. If it involves damage to the medial frontal lobe alone, it is characterized by a loss of spontaneous speech (nonfluent aphasia) in the face of preserved repetition and comprehension and is called **transcortical motor aphasia.**[17] Damage to the medial parietal lobe results in **transcortical sensory aphasia**, characterized by fluent but paraphasic spontaneous speech, poor comprehension, and preserved repetition. If both medial frontal and parietal lobes are involved in the lesion, **transcortical mixed aphasia** can result. Such individuals present with nonfluent speech, poor comprehension, but good repetition.[47]

MIDDLE CEREBRAL ARTERY (MCA)

The internal carotid ends by bifurcating to form the anterior cerebral and middle cerebral arteries (MCA) (see Figs. 8-10 and 8-11). The larger of the two branches, the middle cerebral is, in reality, a direct continuation of the internal carotid. It passes upward along the medial aspect of the temporal lobe, winds across the insula, and emerges from the lateral fissure onto the cortical surface. (The normal anatomy and radiology of the middle cerebral artery are presented by Ring.[48]) The branches of the middle cerebral artery spread out to supply the lateral portions of frontal, parietal, and temporal cortex, as well as the extreme anterior border of occipital cortex (Fig. 8-13). Anastomoses are established with posterior and anterior cerebral arteries.

The middle cerebral artery can be divided into three regions: a **stem** or horizontal portion and its penetrating branches, an **upper division** (ascending

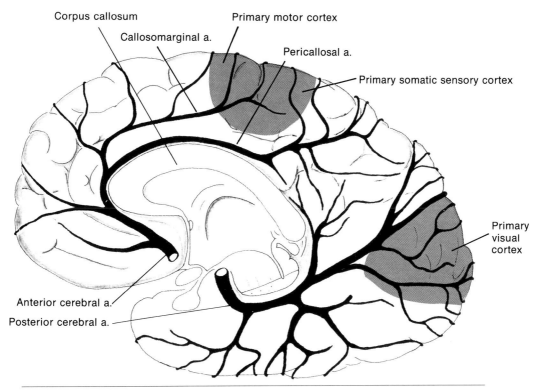

Figure 8-12. A diagram of a midsagittal view of the brain illustrates the distribution of the anterior and posterior cerebral arteries. (Modified from Melloni BJ, et al. Melloni's illustrated review of human anatomy. Philadephia: JB Lippincott, 1988)

frontal branches), and a **lower division.** The stem passes from the carotid trunk into the insular region; its penetrating branches, the lateral striate arteries, supply caudate, putamen, anterior limb of the internal capsule, and globus pallidus (see Plates 22 to 25). The stem ends by bifurcating into upper and lower divisions. The upper division supplies the middle and inferior frontal gyri as well as the pre- and postcentral gyri. The lower division supplies the superior and inferior parietal lobules as well as the superior and inferior temporal gyri.

CLINICAL DEFICIT

Defects in the perfusion of the middle cerebral artery are reviewed by Kase.[49] Complete occlusion of the middle cerebral arterial stem results in massive damage to the cerebral hemisphere. The patient can present with contralateral hemiplegia of the face, arm, and leg. (The whole leg is involved, since damage to the internal capsule undercuts the entire central sulcus.) The paralytic side also experiences hemihyperesthesia, homonymous hemianopsia, and conjugate deviation of the eyes into the opposite hemisphere. (They look toward the lesioned side because the

frontal eye fields are damaged.) If the occlusion is on the dominant side, global aphasia with no ability to repeat phrases can be present; if it is on the nondominant side, hemi-inattention (neglect) can be present.

Occlusion of the upper division can result in hemiparesis of the upper limbs and face. (The lower limb can be spared because of its supply from the anterior cerebral artery.) A somatic sensory defect accompanies the paralysis as well as nonfluent aphasia and agraphia (dominant side lesion) or inattention and neglect (nondominant side lesion). Volitional gaze into the contralateral hemisphere can be impaired due to involvement of the frontal eye fields. Occlusion of the lower division is characterized by a visual field defect and fluent aphasia, alexia and agraphia (dominant side lesion) or hemi-neglect syndromes (nondominant side lesion).

POSTERIOR CEREBRAL ARTERY (PCA)

The posterior cerebral artery (PCA) arises as the termination of the basilar artery near the interpeduncular fossa (see Figs. 8-10 and 8-11). (The normal anat-

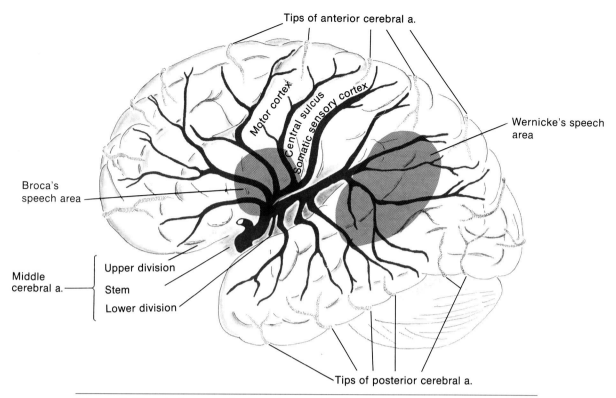

Figure 8-13. A diagram of a lateral view of the brain illustrates the distribution of the middle cerebral artery. (Modified from Melloni BJ, et al. Melloni's illustrated review of human anatomy. Philadelphia: JB Lippincott, 1988)

omy and radiology are presented in Margolis et al.[50]) In the ambient cistern, it passes laterally around the cerebral peduncles to course in a posterior direction along the medial border of temporal and occipital cortex. Branches of the posterior cerebral artery distribute to the midbrain and caudal thalamus (see Plates 20 and 21) and across the inferior surface of the temporal and occipital lobes (Fig. 8-12). The territory supplied by the posterior cerebral artery includes the inferior temporal gyrus, parahippocampal gyrus, hippocampus, medial aspect of superior parietal gyrus, and portions of the occipital lobe. Anastomoses are established with the anterior and middle cerebral arteries.

CLINICAL DEFICIT

A cardinal sign of damage to the posterior cerebral artery is homonymous hemianopsia (cortical blindness). If the damage is restricted to the calcarine area, patients can be aware of their visual field defects; however, if the damage involves the occipitotemporal or occipitoparietal association areas, visual neglect can occur although the patients deny loss of sight. Damage to the area around the visual cortex can also result in

visual hallucinations, such as perseverations and distortions of color vision.

If the pericallosal branch of the posterior cerebral artery on the dominant side is occluded, the splenium of the corpus callosum as well as part of the deep occipital cortex is affected. As a result, the input of visual information to the supramarginal and angular gyri is diminished. The patient can present with alexia without agraphia (*i.e.,* can write but cannot read what has been written).

Infarctions of the posterior cerebral artery in the dominant hemisphere can also result in memory defects, transcortical sensory aphasia, or anomic aphasia. Infarction of posterior cerebral artery in the nondominant hemisphere can result in visual neglect and constructional apraxia (reviewed in Caplan[51]).

► Bibliography

Adams RD, Victor M. Cerebrovascular disease. In: Principles of neurology. New York: McGraw-Hill, 1989: Chap. 34.

Biller J. Vascular syndromes of the cerebrum. In: Brazis PW, Masdeu JC, Biller J, eds. Localization in clinical neurology. Boston: Little, Brown, 1990: Chap. 20.

Daube JR, Ragan TJ, Sandok BA, Westmoreland BF. The supratentorial level. In: Medical neurosciences. Boston: Little, Brown, 1986: Chap. 15;374–417.

Haines DE. Neuroanatomy: an atlas of structures, sections, and systems. Baltimore: Urban & Schwarzenberg, 1987 *(see especially Figs. 2-5 to 2-23, and 3-2 to 3-6).*

Masdeu JC. The localization of lesions of the hypothalamus and pituitary gland. In: Brazis PW, Masdeu JC, Biller J, eds. Localization in clinical neurology. Boston: Little, Brown, 1990: Chap. 19.

► References

1. Damasio H, Damasio AR. Lesion analysis in neuropsychology New York: Oxford University Press, 1989.
2. Barr ML, Kiernan JA. The human nervous system: an anatomical viewpoint. Philadelphia: JB Lippincott, 1988;216–243.
3. Changeux J. Neuronal man. New York: Oxford University Press, 1986.
4. Mesulam M-Marsel. Large scale neurocognitive networks and distributed processing for attention, language, and memory. Ann Neurol 1990;28:597.
5. Nauta WJH. The problem of the frontal lobe: reinterpretation. J Psychiatr Res 1971;8:167.
6. Adams RD, Victor M. Principles of neurology. New York: McGraw-Hill Information Services, 1989.
7. Mesulam M-M. Frontal cortex and behavior. Ann Neurol 1986;19:320.
8. Lhermitte F, Pillon B, Serdaru M. Human autonomy and the frontal lobes. Part I: Imitation and utilization behavior: a neuropsychological study of 75 patients. Ann Neurol 1986;19:326.
9. Nieuwenhuys R, Voogd J, van Huijzen C. The human central nervous system. Berlin: Springer-Verlag, 1988.
10. Kandel E, Schwartz JH, Jessell TM. Principles of neural sciences. New York: Elsevier, 1991.
11. Henneman E. Motor functions of the cerebral cortex. In: Mountcastle VB, eds. Medical physiology. St Louis: CV Mosby, 1980: 859–889.
12. Freund H-J, Hummelsheim H. Lesions of the premotor cortex in man. Brain 1985;108:697.
13. Watson RT, Fleet WS, Gonzalez-Rothi L, Heilman KM. Apraxia and the supplementary motor area. Arch Neurol 1986;43:787.
14. Damasio A. The nature of aphasia: signs and syndromes. In: Sarno MT, eds. Acquired aphasia. New York: Academic Press, 1981:51–65.
15. Levine DN, Sweet E. Localization of lesions in Broca's aphasia. In: Kertesz A , eds. Localization in neuropsychology. New York: Academic Press, 1983:185–208.
16. Geschwind N. The apraxias: neural mechanisms of disorders of learned movement. Am Sci 1975;63:188.
17. Rubens AB, Kertesz A. The localization of lesions in transcortical aphasias. In: Kertesz A, eds. Localization in neuropsychology. New York: Academic Press, 1983:245–268.
18. Kaas JH. Somatosensory system. In: Paxinos G, eds. The human nervous system. San Diego: Academic Press, 1990:813–844.
19. Masdeu JC. The localization of affecting the cerebral hemispheres. In: Brazis PW, Masdeu JC, Biller J, eds. Localization in clinical neurology. Boston: Little, Brown, 1990.
20. Paillard J, Michel F, Stelmach G. Localization without content: a tactile analogue of "blind sight." Arch Neurol 1983;40:548.
21. Williams PL, Warwick R, Dyson M, Bannister LH. Grays's anatomy. Edinburgh: Churchill Livingstone, 1989.
22. Alexander MP, Fischer RS, Friedman R. Lesion localization in apractic agraphia. Arch Neurol 1992;49:246–251.
23. Mesulam M-M. A cortical network for directed attention and unilateral neglect. Ann Neurol 1981;10:309.
24. Kertesz A. The localization of lesions in Wernicke's aphasias. In: Kertesz A, ed. Localization in neuropsychology. New York: Academic Press, 1983:209–230.
25. Caplan LR, Kelly M, Kase CS, Hier DB, White JL, Tatemichi T, Mohr J, Price T, Wolf P. Infarcts of the inferior division of the right middle cerebral artery: mirror image of Wernicke's aphasia. Neurology 1986;36:1015.
26. Clopton BM, Winfield JA, Flammino FJ. Tonotopic organization: review and analysis. Brain Res 1974;76:1.
27. Webster WR, Garey LJ. Auditory system. In: G Paxinos, eds. The human nervous system. San Diego: Academic Press, 1990.
28. Aldrich MS, Alessi AG, Beck RW, Gilman S. Cortical blindness: etiology, diagnosis, and prognosis. Ann Neurol 1987;21:149.
29. Shipley MT, Geinisman Y. Anatomical evidence for convergence of olfactory, gustatory, and visceral afferent pathways in mouse cerebral cortex. Brain Res Bull 1984;12:221.
30. Ruggiero DA, Mraovitch S, Granata AR, Anwar M, Reis DJ. A role of insular cortex in cardiovascular function. J Comp Neurol 1987;257:189.
31. Crosby EC, Schnitzlein HN. Comparative correlative neuroanatomy of the vertebrate telencephalon. New York: Macmillan, 1982:820.
32. Geschwind N, Galaburada AM. Cerebral localization. Biological mechanisms, associations, and pathology: I. A hypothesis and a program for research. Arch Neurol 1985;42:428.
33. Geschwind N, Galaburada AM. Cerebral localization. Biological mechanisms, associations, and pathology: II. A hypothesis and a program for research. Arch Neurol 1985;42:521.
34. Geschwind N, Galaburada AM. Cerebral localization. Biological mechanisms, associations, and pathology: III. A hypothesis and a program for research. Arch Neurol 1985;42:634.
35. Geschwind N. Specializations of the human brain. Sci Am 1979;241:180.
36. Sergent J. A new look at the human split brain. Brain 1987;110:1375.
37. Sperry RW. Lateral specialization in the surgically separated hemispheres. In: Schmitt FO, Worden FG, eds. The neurosciences: third study program. Cambridge: MIT Press, 1974:5–19.
38. Sperry RW. Mental unity following surgical disconnection of the cerebral hemispheres. Harvey Lect 1968;62:293.
39. Kolodny EH. Agenesis of the corpus callosum: a marker for inherited metabolic disease? Neurology 1989;39:847.
40. Atlas S, Zimmermanm RA, Bilaniuk LT, Rorke L, Hackney DB, Goldberg HI, and Grossman RI. Corpus callosum and limbic system: neuroanatomic MR evaluation of developmental anomalies. Radiology 1986;160:355.
41. Dobyns WB. Agenesis of the corpus callosum and gyral malformations are frequent manifestation of nonketotic hyperglycinemia. Neurology 1989;39:817.
42. Davidson HD, Abraham R, Steiner RE. Agenesis of the corpus callosum: magnetic resonance imaging. Radiology 1985;155:371.
43. Lin JP, Kricheff II. Normal anterior cerebral artery complex. In: Newton TH, Potts DG, eds. Radiology of the skull and brain: angiography. St Louis: CV Mosby, 1974:1391–1410.
44. Moscow NP, Michotey P, Salamon G. Anatomy of the cortical branches of the anterior cerebral artery. In: Newton TH, Potts DG, eds. Radiology of the skull and brain: angiography. St Louis: CV Mosby, 1974:1411–1420.
45. Bogousslavsky J, Regli F. Anterior cerebral artery territory in-

183

farction in the Lausanne stroke registry. Arch Neurol 1990;
47:144.

46. Hung T-P, Ryu S-J. Anterior cerebral artery syndromes. Hdbk
Clin Neurol 1988;53(9):339.

47. Ross ED. Left medial parietal lobe and receptive language functions: mixed transcortical aphasia and left anterior cerebral artery infarction. Neurology 1980;30:144.

48. Ring AB. Normal middle cerebral artery. In: Newton TH, Potts
DG, eds. Radiology of the skull and brain: angiography. St Louis:
CV Mosby, 1974;1442–1470.

49. Kase CS. Middle cerebral arterial syndromes. Hdbk Clin Neurol
1988;53(9):353.

50. Margolis MT, Newton TH, Hoyt WF. The posterior cerebral ar-
tery: gross and roentgenographic anatomy. In: Newton TH,
Potts DG, eds. Radiology of the skull and brain: angiography. St
Louis: CV Mosby, 1974:1551–1579.

51. Caplan LR. Posterior cerebral artery syndromes. Hdbk Clin
Neurol 1988;53(9):409.

9 CEREBRAL HEMISPHERES: LIMBIC LOBE

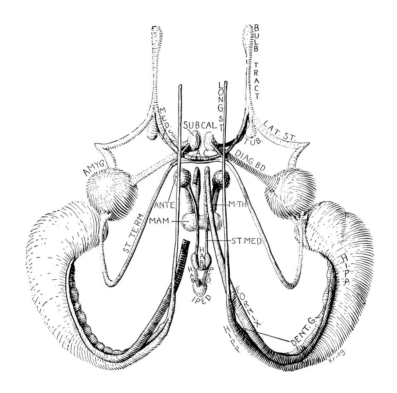

► Introduction

The limbic lobe of the cerebrum consists of the cingulate and parahippocampal gyri: two structures that are wrapped around the rostral portion of the brain stem and that form the medial border of the cerebral cortex. Deep to the parahippocampal gyrus are the *hippocampus* and *amygdala*. The hippocampus represents the oldest portion of the cerebral cortex (archicortex), and the amygdala is a rostral extension of the tail of the caudate nucleus.

The limbic lobe structures can be considered a neural interface between external and internal environments, receiving converging sensory information at the cerebral cortical level from the five sensory systems representing the extrapersonal world as well as that from the visceral sensory system, which represents the intrapersonal world. This information is fun-

185

neled through the hippocampus and amygdala and projected on to the hypothalamus, where it can regulate our behavioral responses. Although they are not well understood, these circuitous neural routes through the limbic system modulate the activity of the autonomic nervous system and the endocrine system, and through these two, influence the activity of the immune system. The limbic structures also play an important role in various aspects of learning, memory, and emotions.

In this chapter the structure and connections of four components of the limbic lobe—cingulate gyrus, parahippocampal gyrus, hippocampus, and amygdala—will be studied, and their functions will be examined. The vasculature of the limbic lobe will be reviewed and several clinicopathologic cases presented.

GENERAL OBJECITVES

1. To learn the location, connections, and function of the limbic lobe structures
2. To learn the major neurologic deficits occurring consequent to damage in specific limbic lobe structure

INSTRUCTIONS

In this chapter you will be presented with one or more clinical case studies. *Each study will be followed by a list of questions that can best be answered by using a knowledge of regional and functional neuroanatomy and by referring to outside reading material.* Following the questions will be a section devoted to structures from a specific region of the central nervous system. Before attempting to answer the questions, compile a list of the patient's neurologic signs and symptoms; then examine the structures and their functions and study their known clinical deficits. After becoming familiar with the material, reexamine the list of neurologic signs and symptoms and formulate answers to the questions. Be aware that some of the questions can have multiple responses or require information beyond the scope of this manual. It may be necessary to obtain material or advice from additional resources, such as specialty texts, a medical dictionary, or clinical personnel.

MATERIALS

1. Horizontal and coronal sections of the human brain
2. A human brain cut in the midsagittal plane

UNIT A

Case Study 9-1

A 38-year-old trauma victim with complex partial seizures

A 38-year-old, right-handed, male received a blow to the right side of his skull with the butt of a rifle 6 years ago. At the time of the accident he suffered no syncope or seizures. A subdural hematoma was removed from the right side of the patient. Nine months subsequent to the trauma, he developed seizures. Recently, because of the increased severity of the seizures, his wife had had to bring him to the emergency room at the hospital for examination. They were now seeking consultation for surgery.

Past Medical History

At the time of examination he was a private with 10 years of service in the army. He had experienced head trauma to the head while on practice maneuvers in the Middle East. He had had several other accidents involving automobiles and at least one involving a motorcycle. He had no history of syncope or seizures prior to the traumatic event with the rifle.

Subsequent to being struck on the head with a rifle butt, he developed seizures characterized by onset of dizziness and followed by an olfactory sensation of foul odor, such as that of vomitus. He then would assume a blank stare and often demonstrate several automatisms, including lip-smacking and rubbing his hands on his shirt. During these periods, he would not respond to questions or statements. He has experienced periods characterized by a sense of light-headedness and mingled thoughts. He occasionally has heard voices that gave him commands, and he has had periods of automatisms during which he lacked conscious awareness of his acts.

General Physical Examination

At the time of examination, he was an alert, well-hydrated, well-nourished male, oriented for time and place, and appeared his stated age. His body had numerous scars, presumably from previous traumatic injuries. Optic discs were sharp, with no hemorrhagic spots. Visual fields were full to confrontation. Chest was clear to auscultation and percussion. Abdomen was soft, with no masses or tenderness. Blood pressure, pulse, temperature, and respirations were normal.

Neurologic Examination

Mental Status. The patient was alert and oriented to time and place. Knowledge and memory seemed appropriate for his age and occupation. Speech, writing, and reading were intact. He complained of periods when he could not recall events; these times coincided with the seizure events as described by his wife.

Cranial Nerves. His visual fields were full to confrontation, and a full range of eye movements was present. His hearing was normal in both ears. His face had a full range of expression; corneal and jaw-jerk reflexes were intact. His palate and uvula elevated midline; the tongue protruded. His shoulders shrugged bilaterally.

Motor Systems. His limb muscles were normotonic with bilaterally symmetric reflexes in all extremities. No weakness, tremor, or dysmetria were present. He exhibited no past pointing or pronator drift.

Sensation. Pinprick, temperature, vibratory, and proprioceptive senses were intact throughout body and face.

Tests

Interictal EEG studies were normal. Those taken during a seizure revealed a predominant right temporal focal involvement.

QUESTIONS

1. Does the patient exhibit a language or memory deficit or an alteration in consciousness or cognition?

2. Are signs of cranial nerve dysfunction present?

3. Are there any changes in motor functions, such as reflexes, muscle tone, movement, or coordination?

4. Are any changes in sensory functions detectable?

5. At what level in the central neuraxis is this lesion most likely located?

6. Is the pathology focal, multifocal, or diffuse in its distribution within the nervous system?

7. What is the clinical–temporal profile of this pathology: acute or chronic; progressive or stable?

8. Based on your answers to the previous two questions, decide whether the symptoms in this patient are most likely caused by a vascular accident, a tumor, or a degenerative or inflammatory process.

9. If you feel this is the result of a vascular accident, what vessels are most likely involved?

10. What was the source of the patient's olfactory hallucinations?

11. What is an aura? What is an automatism?

12. What is meant by consciousness? When is a patient considered unconscious?

13. Develop a short classification scheme for seizures.

CASE STUDY 9-2

A 55-year-old man with profound anterograde amnesia

This is a 55-year-old, male government worker retired because of medical disability. During coronary surgery he suffered several extended periods of anoxia and has experienced severe neurologic consequences. He is presenting for a checkup, *4 years postsurgery*.

Past Medical History

Five years ago, this patient was diagnosed with coronary artery occlusion, and bypass surgery was performed. During recovery, an atrial tear resulted in a significant loss of blood. The patient experienced a 15-minute period of hypoxia. The tear was repaired; however, during this second trip to the operating room, the patient's EEG was flat and his pupils were fixed. The following day, a third trip to the operating room was required by further bleeding; again his pupils were fixed and the EEG was diminished in amplitude.

Over the next 2 days the patient gradually regained consciousness. He had reduced strength and paresthesia in the left arm. He also demonstrated severe memory loss and confusion with respect to time and place. Prior to the surgical event, he had had no history of neurologic signs or symptoms.

General Physical Examination

This was a well-nourished, well-hydrated, obese male who was alert and cooperative and in no acute distress. Carotid auscultation revealed a soft bruit without radiation on the right. Heartbeat was regular; a grade III harsh systolic murmur, auscultated best at the second intercostal space on the right, with an S_4 gallop was present. Peripheral pulses were intact. Lungs were clear to auscultation and percussion. The abdomen was soft, without masses, tenderness, rigidity, or rebound. A +2 peripheral, dependent edema was noted in the lower extremities bilaterally. Skin was sallow in appearance, with poor texture and turgor. A well-healed cicatrix of the anterior chest wall extended from the second intercostal space to the diaphragmatic area; a healed 2-cm cicatrix was noted in the left antecubital fossa; and a healed 1-cm cicatrix was located in the left subclavicular area.

Neurologic Examination

Mental Status. The patient was disoriented with respect to time and place and could not describe the reason for his past hospital confinement or recall the history of his illness. However, his speech, naming, reading aloud, and comprehension were all normal for his age. He rapidly forgot information recently expressed to him; he could not recognize any words presented to him 5 minutes previously. He could not recall the names of staff and physicians in either the office or the hospital. Prior to his illness, he had had a strong interest in American history and politics. During the examination he could recall most of the president's names and supply some details concerning their era, but he could not identify the current president or describe any recent historical events. He frequently relied on his family members to provide any recent descriptions of his life. He did not recall why he was ill or any of the events occurring around the time of his cardiac surgery. No other significant personality changes or cognitive deficits were detectable in the patient.

Cranial Nerves. His visual fields were full to confrontation; funduscopic examination revealed AV nicking and silver wire changes without exudates, hemorrhages, or papilledema. His hearing was slightly diminished in both ears. A full range of facial expression was present, and the jaw-jerk reflex was normal. Palate and uvula elevated symmetrically, and tongue protruded on the midline.

Motor Systems. Although the patient had motion in all extremities, strength was diminished on the left side, with slightly elevated deep tendon reflexes and a Babinski sign. Strength in the left upper extremity was $+3 \neq 5$ and $+4 \neq 5$ in the left lower extremity.

Sensation. Vibratory sense, proprioception, and discriminative touch were diminished but not absent in the left and normal in the right extremities. Paresthesias (tingling sensations) were found involving the patient's left hand and forearm.

QUESTIONS

1. Does the patient exhibit a language or memory deficit or an alteration in consciousness or cognition?

2. Are signs of cranial nerve dysfunction present?

3. Are there any changes in motor functions, such as reflexes, muscle tone, movement, or coordination?

4. Are any changes in sensory functions detectable?

5. At what level in the central neuraxis is this lesion most likely located?

6. Is the pathology focal, multifocal, or diffuse in its distribution within the nervous system?

7. What is the clinical–temporal profile of this pathology: acute or chronic; progressive or stable?

8. Based on your answers to the previous two questions, decide whether the symptoms in this patient are most likely caused by a vascular accident, a tumor, or a degenerative or inflammatory process.

189

9. If you feel this is the result of a vascular accident, what vessels are most likely involved?

10. What are the major regions of the central nervous system involved in memory?

11. What criteria will assist in distinguishing between retrograde and anterograde amnesia?

► DISCUSSION
Limbic Lobe Structures

CINGULATE CORTEX

The cingulate gyrus (areas 23 and 24 of Brodmann) is best seen on a midsagittal section of a whole brain. This structure stretches along the medial wall of cortex (Fig. 9-1) at the base of the longitudinal fissure, in close relationship to the superior surface of the corpus callosum. Rostrally, the cingulate gyrus is continuous, with the inferior frontal cortex, and caudally, with the parahippocampal gyrus through a narrowing called the isthmus. The cingulate and parahippocampal gyri represent the limbic lobe of the cortex and form an annulus (limbus or rim) around the rostral end of the brain stem.[1]

The connections of the primate cingulate cortex are extensive.[2] Cortical fibers to cingulate arise in the association areas, such as prefrontal and posterior parietal. The thalamic fibers to the cingulate cortex arise in the anterior, ventroanterior, and dorsomedial nuclei. Projections from the cingulate cortex return to the prefrontal and posterior parietal cortex as well as targeting the parahippocampal cortex. Axons from the parahippocampal cortex enter the hippocampus proper, from which the hypothalamus and thalamus are innervated. Thalamocortical projections complete a loop back to the cingulate. This recurrent circuit forms a major component of the *limbic system.*[1]

The functions of the cingulate gyrus and related limbic lobe are heteromodal and extremely complex. Some aspects of these functions have been demonstrated by electrical stimulation studies performed in surgery[2] and by positron-emission tomographic studies in human volunteers.[3] Alteration in blood pressure, heart and respiratory rate, dilation of the pupils, and piloerection and in more complex responses, such as fear, anxiety, and pleasure, have all been observed following stimulation of the cingulate cortex. Positron-emission tomographic studies of volunteers exposed to painful stimuli have demonstrated that the anterior portion of the cingulate cortex is the one area of cortex consistently activated in response to nociceptive (painful) stimuli.[3]

Based on connectivity, as well as stimulation and ablation studies, a unified description of cingulate cortical function has been developed.[4] This region of cortex appears to integrate sensory information from association portions of neocortex and the limbic system. By attaching a motivational relevance to the stimuli based on the bias set by the intrapersonal and extrapersonal sensorium, cingulate cortex can direct attention to specific stimuli through its extensive intracortical connections and, through its limbic system output to the hypothalamus, it can also engage the endocrine and autonomic nervous systems in the overall response.

CLINICAL DEFICIT

Damage to the cingulate gyrus can present as akinesia (lack of response), apathy (lack of attention or concern), mutism, incontinence, or indifference to pain. Cingulectomies have been performed to treat patients in intractable pain[5] and with psychotic and neurotic conditions.[6] A form of contralateral neglect syndrome has also been observed after unilateral lesions of the cingulate cortex in rhesus monkeys.[7]

PIRIFORM CORTEX

The piriform cortex is found on the inferior surface of the temporal lobe. From an evolutionary perspective, it is older than the more lateral and superior neocortex, having only three cytologically definable layers, compared to the six layers found in the neocortex. The piriform cortex represents the most inferomedial border of the cerebrum. It is best seen on the inferior surface of the brain, where it covers most of the parahippocampal gyrus (Fig. 9-2). As such, the mantle of piriform cortex overlies portions of the hippocampus and amygdala. A distinctive feature of the piriform cortex is that it contains the cortical representation of the olfactory system.

190

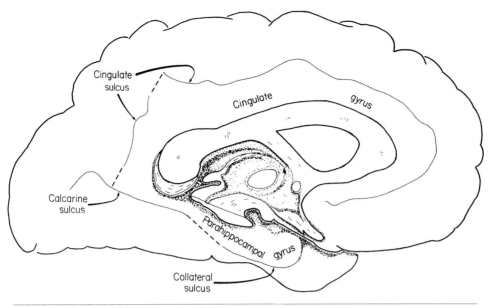

Figure 9-1. Medial view of brain outlining the limbic lobe composed of the cingulate and parahippocampal gyri.

Figure 9-2.
This ventral view of the brain illustrates the piriform cortex covering the parahippocampal gyrus. The photograph (*above*) illustrates the location of the anterior perforated substance (APS), mamillary bodies (MB), optic chiasm (OC), and olfactory tract (OLF). The companion line drawing (*below*) illustrates the location of the lateral olfactory tract (LOT) and the two regions of the piriform cortex: uncus and entorhinal cortex.

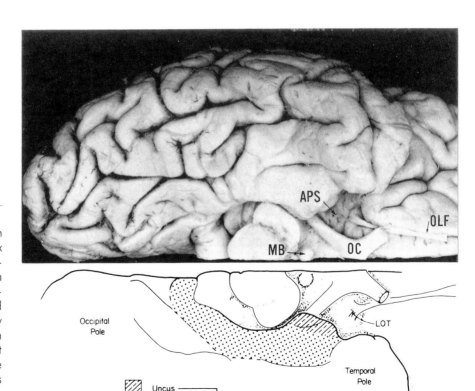

Olfactory Cortex

The olfactory bulb is located at the rostral tip of the olfactory tract and receives primary afferent fibers from bipolar neurons in the portions of the nasal epithelium. As the olfactory tract approaches the ventral forebrain, it divides into medial and lateral striae (see Fig. 9-2). Between the stria is the anterior perforated substance, a region richly supplied with vasculature. The medial stria crosses the midline to innervate the contralateral olfactory bulb. The lateral olfactory stria enters the medial aspect of the ipsilateral temporal lobe and its fibers spread out through a portion of the piriform cortex. That portion of piriform cortex receiving axons directly from neurons in the olfactory bulb is called the *primary olfactory cortex.* The remainder of the piriform cortex receives projections not from the bulb, but from primary olfactory cortex. Therefore, this region is called the *secondary olfactory cortex.* The primary olfactory cortex corresponds approximately to the region of the uncus, a protuberance on the medial aspect of the temporal lobe, whereas the secondary olfactory cortex approximates the entorhinal area (see Fig. 9-2).

CLINICAL DEFICIT

Damage or irritation to the medial aspect of temporal lobe, including the olfactory cortex, can present as complex partial seizures with preceding olfactory hallucinations.[8] Patients experience cacosmia, the sensation of unpleasant or foul odors, especially preceding the onset of the seizure.

Uncus

A large bulge, the uncus, is present on the medial aspect of the temporal lobe. It is created by the almond-shaped nucleus, the amygdala, lying under the surface of the parahippocampal gyrus. A thin veneer of piriform cortex overlies the amygdala. This cortex receives primary olfactory axons from the olfactory bulb; as such, it represents the primary olfactory cortex. Major projections from the primary olfactory cortex reach the amygdala; others reach the secondary olfactory cortex (entorhinal area) as well as possibly the hypothalamus.[9]

CLINICAL DEFICIT

Unilateral lesions of the uncus are not well documented in the clinical literature; bilateral lesions damage the amygdala and can result in the Kluver-Bucy syndrome (see p. 195). Another clinical significance of the uncus involves its physical location. Expansion of the cerebral hemisphere due to edema or a lesion can push the uncus ventromedially onto the third cranial nerve and brain stem, resulting in third nerve palsy (see Chap. 6).

Entorhinal Area

The entorhinal area (sometimes called the entorhinal cortex) is the visible portion of the parahippocampal gyrus when examined from an inferior view (see Fig. 9-2). Laterally, it is bordered by the collateral sulcus; the optic tract and brain stem form the medial border. A thin veneer of piriform cortex overlies the entorhinal area. It receives information from the olfactory cortex and association areas in frontal, parietal, and temporal cortex and sends information directly to the hippocampus. The entorhinal area is closely tied to the functions of the hippocampus, which involve various forms of memory and emotional behavior.

CLINICAL DEFICIT

Because of their close juxtaposition, damage to or irritation of entorhinal cortex is difficult to distinguish from that of the hippocampus; consequently, they will be considered in the discussion of the hippocampus.

HIPPOCAMPUS

The medial aspect of the temporal lobe (parahippocampal gyrus) folds inward to form the hippocampus (Fig. 9-3). This C-shaped structure arches around the rostral end of the brain stem. The rostral pole of the hippocampus abuts the amygdala in the temporal lobe; its caudal pole ends in a fiber tract, the fornix. This tract curves superiorly and rostrally to course under the corpus callosum and then descends rostral to the thalamus, finally terminating in the mamillary bodies of the hypothalamus. The fornix contains many afferent and efferent connections of the hippocampus.[10]

The hippocampus is a folded sheet of cerebral cortex. It has a trilayered organization, composed of a central layer of pyramidal cells, with sheets of fibers on either side. The pyramidal cell layer is differentiated into four longitudinal stripes called CA1, CA2, CA3, and CA4, with a ridge of small granule cells forming the outer border of CA4. This granule cell layer is called the *dentate gyrus.*

The major afferent connections reaching the hippocampus arise in the ipsilateral amygdala, claustrum, septal area, numerous regions of the hypothalamus and thalamus, and the ipsilateral entorhinal cortex. This latter structure receives projections from the major association portions of parietal, frontal, and temporal neocortex. The hippocampus also receives fibers from several chemically defined pathways in the brain stem. Fibers arising in the ventral tegmental nucleus (VTA; see Plate 20) contain dopamine, those coming from the raphe nuclei (RaNu; see Plate 18) contain

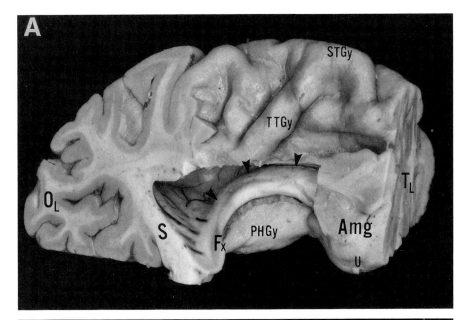

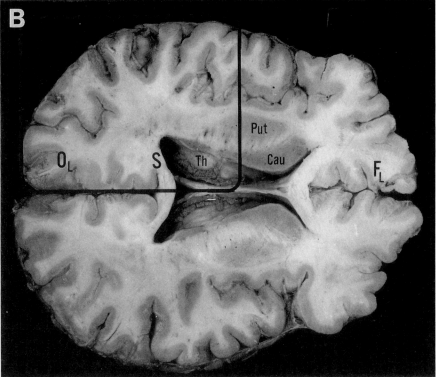

Figure 9-3. A view of the temportal lobe (from above) with the thalamus and brain stem removed. The inferior horn of the lateral ventricle has been opened by removing its roof. The rostral aspect of the temporal lobe (T_L) has been removed. The medial edge of the parahippocampal gyrus (PHGy) is seen as it turns upward to merge with the hippocampus (*arrowheads*). The thin ridge coursing parallel to the hippocampus is the fimbria; at the caudal end of the hippocampus, the fimbria becomes the fornix (Fx). The mass of tissue rostral to end of the hippocampus is the amygdala (Amg). The ventral and medial surfaces of the amygdala form the uncus (U) and are covered by the thin velum of piriform cortex. Amg, amygdala, Fx, fornix; O_L, occipital lobe; PHGy, parahippocampal gyrus; STGy, superior temporal gyrus; T_L temporal lobe; TTGy, transverse temporal gyrus; U, uncus, Put, putamen; Cau, caudate; S, splenium of corpus callosum; F_L, frontal lobe; Th, thalamus.)

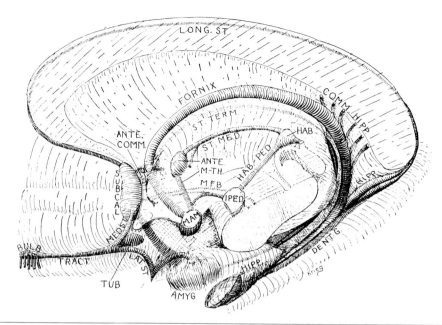

Figure 9-4. A diagram of the hippocampus, fornix, and thalamic nuclei involved in the limbic circuits as seen from the ventromedial surface of the brain. Amyg, amygdala; Ante Comm, AC, anterior commissure; Ante, anterior nucleus of thalamus; Bulb, olfactory bulb; Comm Hipp, hippocampal commissure; DentG, dentate gyrus; Diag Bd, diagonal band; Hab, habenula; Hab-ped, habenulopeduncular tract; Hipp, hippocampus; Iped, interpeduncular nucleus; LatSt, lateral olfactory stria; Long St, longitudinal stria; Mam, mammillary body; MedSt, medial olfactory stria; MFB, medial forebrain bundle; M-th, mammillothalamic tract; StMed, stria medullaris; StTerm, stria terminalis; Subcal, subcallosal gyrus; Tract, olfactory tract; Tub, olfactory tubercle. (Kreig W, Functional neurocanatomy. 2nd ed. Toronto: Blakiston, 1953:345)

serotonin; and those from the locus coeruleus (LC; see Plate 15) release norepinephrine.

The fornix represents a major efferent pathway for the hippocampus (Fig. 9-4). Fibers in the fornix innervate the septal area, hypothalamus, and portions of the thalamus. Based on its connections, it appears that the hippocampus assembles sensory information as processed in the neocortex and forms an output to the rostral end of the brain stem.

The hippocampal formation is a target of several cerebral pathologies.[10] The region of the hippocampus called CA1, also known as the *Sommer sector,* is particularly sensitive to anoxia and ischemia.[11] Loss of cells in this region may play a role in the anterograde amnesia that follows prolonged periods of anoxia, consequent to cardiorespiratory arrest.[12] The most consistent site of cellular degeneration in temporal lobe epilepsy is also in the Sommer sector (CA1). In some cases, the loss of cells from this portion of the hippocampus is quite striking. Finally, extensive loss of neurons and excessive accumulation of neurofibrillary tangles can occur in the CA1 region in Alzheimer's disease.

CLINICAL DEFICIT

The most striking deficit resulting from bilateral damage to the medial aspect of the temporal lobe in humans is amnesia.[11–16] Memory for events predating the incident is intact (retrograde memory); however, there is limited or no ability to form new memory traces (anterograde amnesia). Restricted lesions in monkeys[17] and humans[12] have demonstrated that these memory losses can be obtained by damage to the hippocampus and/or its overlying entorhinal cortex. Pure lesions of the amygdala did not produce these memory deficits.[18]

Unilateral lesions of the hippocampus also produce memory dysfunctions. However, the specific type of deficits is lateralized. Lesions of the temporal lobe of the dominant side result in language-related memory losses, whereas those of the nondominant temporal lobe present with deficits in retaining nonverbal patterns, such as geometric or tonal patterns.[19]

Recently, it has been demonstrated that the hippocampal damage resulting from the ischemia of cardiac arrest is delayed by as much as 24 hours postinsult.[11] This is considerably longer than the time taken for damage to appear in other areas in the brain. The delay time between insult and damage in the hippocampus may offer an opportunity for therapeutic intervention.

AMYGDALA

At the rostral end of the hippocampus, deep to the piriform cortex, is an almond-shaped mass of cells called the amygdala. When it is viewed externally, it forms a bump known as the uncus (see Fig. 9-3). Some of the afferent connections to the amygdala come from the olfactory cortex. The amygdala also receives sensory information concerning the external environment from the frontal, parietal, and temporal association neocortex as well as viscerosensory information from the nucleus of the solitary tract and the dorsal motor nucleus of the vagus. The major output of the amygdala occurs through the ventral amygdalofugal pathway and the stria terminalis. Using these tracts, projections from the amygdala pass to the prefrontal and premotor cortex, the hypothalamus, the septal area, and the dorsomedial nucleus of the thalamus as well as to many brain stem nuclei, including the dorsal motor nucleus of the vagus.

The amygdala is part of the limbic system circuitry relating the neocortex to the autonomic control portions of the brain. It is involved in modulating neuroendocrine functions and autonomic effector mechanisms. It appears to play a role in complex patterned behavior—such as ingestion, aggression, reproduction—and in the processes of memory and learning.[20]

CLINICAL DEFICIT

Damage to the medial aspect of the temporal lobe can present as the temporal lobe syndrome of amnesia. The extent to which the amygdala is involved in this amnesia has long been debated. Monkeys receiving isolated lesions of the amygdala performed well on a battery of memory tests[18] that were severely compromised in monkeys having isolated lesions of the hippocampus[21] or entorhinal cortex.[17] Although these observations tend to minimize the function of the amygdala, it appears likely that this structure plays other roles in the memory process. Sophisticated

testing of memory loss in primates with lesions carefully restricted to the amygdala demonstrates that the affected component relates to polysensory input. Animals with bilateral amygdaloectomies could make associations dependent on one sensory modality but faulted in recall associations contingent on input from two or more sensory systems.[22]

Bilateral damage to the amygdala and surrounding temporal lobe in humans and other primates produces the *Kluver-Bucy syndrome.* Initially dubbed "psychic blindness," after its more salient sign, the disease involves the following characteristics[23]:

- **Psychic blindness.** Inability to recognize common objects in the face of normal visual fields; in humans this takes the form of visual agnosia (most likely this results from damage to the surrounding temporal lobe).
- **Oral tendencies.** Most objects encountered are examined by mouth and smell.
- **Hypermetamorphosis.** A compulsion to attend and react to every visual stimulus, regardless of its significance.
- **Emotional changes.** A marked diminution of behavior associated with anger or fear; all objects are approached without caution.
- **Sexual behavior.** A striking increase in the amount of auto-, homo-, and heterosexual behavior.
- **Dietary habits.** Compulsive and indiscriminate eating of any food offered.

This syndrome has been re-created, in part, in a human following bilateral temporal lobe surgery to alleviate intractable epilepsy.[24] Spontaneous expression of Kluver-Bucy syndrome has arisen in patients subsequent to inflammatory or degenerative processes affecting the temporal lobes. In a cohort of 12 patients expressing the syndrome, causative factors included head trauma, Alzheimer's and Pick's disease, and herpes encephalitis.[25]

Discrete lesions of the *temporal cortex* or *amygdala* were capable of producing specific signs of Kluver-Bucy syndrome.[26] Most of the behavioral signs could be elicited subsequent to amygdaloectomy with the exception of visual agnosia, which is probably developed from damage to the inferior temporal lobe.

UNIT B

Case Study 9-3

A 33-year-old man with hallucinations and amnesia

A 33-year-old, unemployed migrant worker was brought to the emergency room by police who found him wandering the streets and rubbing his nose. He was quite confused and disoriented, complaining of smelling burning odors and seeing large people and trucks in the emergency room. The patient could give no information on his activities for the last 3 hours.

Past Medical History

The patient denied any recent or past history of trauma, and there were no indications of trauma (bruises, swelling, or discoloration) on his head or body.

General Physical Examination

This was a young man of good physical condition, who appeared his stated age. He was confused and disoriented, with noticeable defects in memory. Because of his memory dysfunction, his correct age was not known until obtained at a later date from his last place of employment. His chest was clear to auscultation and palpation; the abdomen was soft, with no masses or tenderness. Lymph nodes were not palpable in axilla or groin. Blood pressure, pulse, temperature, and respirations were normal.

Neurologic Examination

Mental Status.   At the time of admission the patient was cooperative, yet confused and disoriented with respect to time and place. He could not state his name or age but could describe and name the farm where he had last worked; otherwise he could supply only a few details of his past life. He had experienced periods of global amnesia during the past 24 hours and described numerous visual and olfactory hallucinations. He was able to follow two- and three-step commands accurately but could not repeat the commands by memory after a delay of 5 minutes. His speech and comprehension of language were appropriate; however, he was unable to read. He could recite the first 10 letters in the alphabet with one or two mistakes. He could write several words such as *cat* or *dog* and could copy written words but was unable to read words that he had copied. He could do simple one- and two-digit calculations. He was unable to identify colors and could not provide the name for many common objects, such as *door* or *window,* but he could describe these objects and state their use.

Cranial Nerves.   Optic discs were clear, with sharp borders; a pronounced deficit in the upper right visual field was present. Jaw-jerk and gag reflexes were normal, facial expressions were complete and symmetric, palate and uvula elevated symmetrically, and the tongue protruded on the midline.

Motor Systems.   His motor system was intact throughout his body, with normal deep tendon reflexes and no loss of strength.

Sensation.   Pinprick, temperature, vibratory, and proprioceptive sensation were intact through his body and face.

Follow-up

The patient was admitted to the hospital for observation. After 24 hours the visual and olfactory hallucinations decreased. Two days later he was discharged to a the local community shelter for assistance. Examination 2 weeks later revealed that the defect in forming recent memories had cleared; however, he still could not recall events from 24 hours prior to his admission through the end of his first week of discharge. He was capable of supplying his name and some details from his life, but still could not recall his age. He could do simple arithmetic calculations. However, the alexia and a pronounced anomia for visual objects and colors was observed to persist.

196

QUESTIONS

1. Does the patient exhibit a language or memory deficit or an alteration in consciousness or cognition?

2. Are signs of cranial nerve dysfunction present?

3. Are there any changes in motor functions, such as reflexes, muscle tone, movement, or coordination?

4. Are any changes in sensory functions detectable?

5. At what level in the central neuraxis is this lesion most likely located?

6. Is the pathology focal, multifocal, or diffuse in its distribution within the nervous system?

7. What is the clinical–temporal profile of this pathology: acute or chronic; progressive or stable?

8. Based on your answers to the previous two questions, decide whether the symptoms in this patient are most likely caused by a vascular accident, a tumor, or a degenerative or inflammatory process.

9. If you feel this is the result of a vascular accident, what vessels are most likely involved?

► DISCUSSION
Limbic Lobe Vasculature

The medial aspect of the temporal lobe borders on a large cistern surrounding the midbrain, called the *ambient cistern* (Fig. 9-5). Coursing around the brain stem within the cistern are several major cerebral vessels, two of which routinely supply penetrating branches to the temporal lobe. These are the anterior choroidal arteries and the posterior cerebral artery.

ANTERIOR CHOROIDAL ARTERY

The anterior choroidal artery arises from the internal carotid artery between the stems of the posterior communicating and anterior cerebral arteries (see Chap. 6). In a few instances (12%), the artery arises from the middle cerebral artery. It supplies the optic tract and lateral aspect of the thalamus (portions of the lateral geniculate nucleus) before penetrating the medial aspect of the temporal lobe to supply the hippocampus, amygdala, and portions of the basal ganglia and internal capsule. Penetrating branches from this artery also reach the midbrain to supply the cerebral

peduncle, substantia nigra, and red nucleus. The normal and pathologic anatomy of the anterior choroidal arteries is reviewed by Goldberg.[27]

CLINICAL DEFICIT
Damage to this artery can present as contralateral hemianesthesia, homonymous hemianopsia, and hemiplegia. The clinical presentation of this picture is rare because of the extensive anastomotic network surrounding this artery.[28] The visual dysfunction stems from the branches of the anterior choroidal artery to the lateral geniculate nucleus in the thalamus. The homonymous defect consists of superior and inferior visual field loss with sparing of a horizontal strip through the center of the visual field.[29]

POSTERIOR CEREBRAL ARTERY

The posterior cerebral artery arises at the terminus of the basilar artery in the interpeduncular fossa. After passing around the cerebral peduncles, the posterior cerebral sweeps laterally to reach the medial aspect of the temporal lobes. In this passage, it gives off the thalamogeniculate and posterior choroidal arteries supplying the posterolateral thalamus and posterior

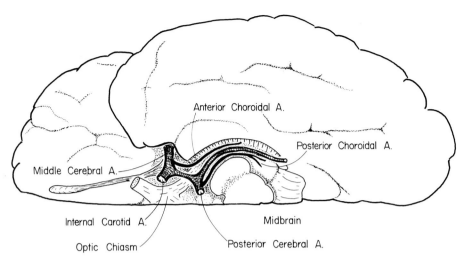

Anterior Choroidal A.

Posterior Choroidal A.

Middle Cerebral A.

Internal Carotid A.

Optic Chiasm

Midbrain

Posterior Cerebral A.

Figure 9-5.
Ventral view of the brain illustrates the ambient cistern surrounding the brain stem and its arterial components.

limb of the internal capsule. Callosal branches of the posterior cerebral artery supply the splenium of the corpus callosum, and cortical branches supply portions of the temporal, occipital, and inferior parietal lobes. Its penetrating branches perfuse the piriform cortex and underlying hippocampus and amygdala. Margolis and colleagues[30] review in detail the normal anatomy and radiology of the posterior cerebral artery; its pathology is reviewed by Newton and colleagues.[31]

CLINICAL DEFICIT

The deficits resulting from damage to the cortical distribution of the posterior cerebral artery were discussed in Chapter 8. These include contralateral homonymous hemianopsia, visual neglect, visual agnosias, and visual hallucinations.

Damage to penetrating branches of the posterior cerebral artery has a wide range of presentations.[32] These include contralateral hemiplegia (damage to the internal capsule), homonymous hemianopsia (damage to the optic radiations), memory defects (damage to the hippocampus and entorhinal cortex), and visual hallucinations (damage to the secondary visual cortex). If the branches to the splenium of the corpus callosum and surrounding occipital white matter are damaged, the patient can exhibit alexia without agraphia, as well as several forms of anomia.[29]

Memory dysfunctions can result from unilateral lesions in the territory of the posterior cerebral artery, An infarction of this artery on the dominant (left) side in a 55-year-old, right-handed man destroyed the medial aspect of the temporal lobe, hippocampus, fornix, splenium of the corpus callosum, and portions of rostral and medial occipital lobe as well as the ventroposterior lateral nuclei in the thalamus. The patient displayed an alexia without agraphia and color anomia, a right hemianopia, a loss of sensory input from the right hand, a transient recent memory loss,

and a more protracted but still transient topographic memory loss.[33]

► Bibliography

Adams RD, Victor M. The limbic lobes and the neurology of emotion. In: Principles of neurology. New York: McGraw-Hill, 1989: Chap. 25.

Barr ML, Kiernan JA. Olfactory system. In: The human nervous system: an anatomical viewpoint. Philadelphia: JB Lippincott, 1988, Chap. 17.

Barr ML, Kiernan JA. Limbic system. In: The human nervous system: an anatomical viewpoint. Philadelphia: JB Lippincott, 1988, Chap. 18

Biller J. Vascular syndromes of the cerebrum. In: Brazis PW, Masdeu JC, Biller J, eds. Localization in clinical neurology. Boston: Little, Brown, 1990; Chap. 20.

Daube JR, Ragan TJ, Sandok BA, Westmoreland BF. The vascular system. In: Medical neurosciences. Boston: Little, Brown, 1986; Chap. 11.

Daube JR, Ragan TJ, Sandok BA, Westmoreland BF. The supratentorial level. In: Medical neurosciences. Boston: Little, Brown, 1986, Chap. 15.

Haines DE. Neuroanatomy: an atlas of structures, sections, and systems. Baltimore: Urban & Schwarzenberg, 1987, Figs. 3-5 through 3-7.

Masdeu JC. The localization of lesions affecting the cerebral hemispheres. In: Brazis PW, Masdeu JC, Biller J, eds. Localization in clinical neurology. Boston: Little, Brown, 1990; Chap. 19:361–428.

Nieuwenhuys R, Voogd J, van Huijzen C. The human central nervous system. Berlin: Springer-Verlag, 1988:293–363.

► References

1. Papez JW. A proposed mechanism of emotion. Arch Neurol Psychiatr 1937;38:725.
2. Baleydier C, Mauguiere F. The duality of the cingulate gyrus in monkey: neuroanatomical study and functional hypothesis. Brain 1980;103:525.
3. Roland P. Cortical representation to pain. Trends Neurosci 1992;15:3.

4. Mesulam M-M. A cortical network for directed attention and unilateral neglect. Ann Neurol 1981;10:309.

5. Crosby EC, Schnitzlein HN. Comparative correlative neuroanatomy of the vertebrate telencephalon. New York: Macmillan, 1982:820.

6. Adams RD, Victor M. Principles of neurology. New York: McGraw-Hill Information Services, 1989.

7. Watson RT, Heilman KM, Cauthen JC, King FA. Neglect after cingulectomy. Neurology 1973;23:1003.

8. Strobos RJ. Mechanisms in temporal lobe seizures. Arch Neurol 1961;5:36.

9. Price J. Olfactory system. In: Paxinos G, ed. The human nervous system. San Diego: Academic Press, 1990:979–998.

10. Amaral DG, Insausti R. Hippocampal formation. In: Paxinos G, ed. The human nervous system. San Diego: Academic Press, 1990:711–755.

11. Petito CK, Fledmann E, Pulsinelli WA, Plum F. Delayed hippocampal damage in humans following cardiorespiratory arrest. Neurology 1987;37:1281.

12. Zola-Morgan S, Squire LR, Amaral DG. Human amnesia and the medial temporal lobe region: enduring memory impairment following a bilateral lesion limited to field CA1 of the hippocampus. J Neurosci 1986;6:2950.

13. Cummings JL, Tomisyasu U, Read S, Benson F. Amnesia with hippocampal lesions after cardiopulmonary arrest. Neurology 1984;34(5):679.

14. Penfield W, Mathieson G. Memory. Arch Neurol 1974;31:145.

15. Scoville WB, Milner B. Loss of recent memory after bilateral hippocampal lesions. J Neurol Neurosurg Psychiatr 1957;20:11.

16. Duyckaerts C, Derouesne C, Signoret JL, Gray F, Escourolle R, Castaigne P. Bilateral and limited amygdalohippocampal lesions causing a pure amnesic syndrome. Ann Neurol 1985;18(2):314.

17. Zola-Morgan S, Squire LR, Amaral DG, Suzuki WA. Lesions of perirhinal and parahippocampal cortex that spare the amygdala and hippocampal formation produce severe memory impairment. J Neurosci 1989;9:4355.

18. Zola-Morgan S, Squire LR, Amaral DG. Lesions of the amygdala that spare adjacent cortical regions do not impair memory or exacerbate the impairment following lesions of the hippocampal formation. J Neurosci 1989;9:1922.

19. Masdeu JC. The localization of lesions affecting the cerebral hemispheres. In: Brazis PW, Masdeu JC, Biller J, eds. Localization in clinical neurology. Boston: Little, Brown, 1990:361–428.

20. de Olmos JS. Amygdala. In: Paxinos G, ed. The human nervous system. San Diego: Academic Press, 1990:583–710.

21. Zola-Morgan S, Squire LR, Amaral DG. Lesions of the hippocampal formation but not lesions of the fornix or the mammillary nuclei produce long-lasting memory impairment in monkeys. J Neurosci 1989;9:898.

22. Mishkin M, Appenzeller T. The anatomy of memory. Sci Am 1987;256(6):80.

23. Kluver H, Bucy PC. "Psychic blindness" and other symptoms following bilateral temporal lobectomy in Rhesus monkeys. Am J Physiol 1937;119:352.

24. Terzian H, Ore G. Syndrome of Kluver and Bucy reproduced in man by bilateral removal of the temporal lobes. Neurology 1955;5:373.

25. Lilly R, Cummings JL, Benson F, Frankel M. The human Kluver-Bucy syndrome. Neurology 1983;33:1141.

26. Horel JA, Keating EG, Misantone LJ. Partial Kluver-Bucy syndrome produced by destroying temporal neocortex or amygdala. Brain Res 1975;94:347.

27. Goldberg HI. The anterior choroidal artery. In: Newton TH, Potts DG, eds. Radiology of the skull and brain: angiography. St Louis: CV Mosby, 1974:1628–1658.

28. Hennerici M, Aulich A, Freund H-J. Carotid system syndromes. Hdbk Clin Neurol 1988;53(9):291.

29. Biller J. Vascular syndromes of the cerebrum. In: Brazis PW, Masdeu JC, Biller J, eds. Localization in clinical neurology. Boston: Little, Brown, 1990.

30. Margolis MT, Newton TH, Hoyt WF. The posterior cerebral artery: gross and roentgenographic anatomy. In: Newton TH, Potts DG, eds. Radiology of the skull and brain: angiography. St Louis: CV Mosby, 1974:1551–1579.

31. Newton TH, Hoyt WF, Margolis MT. The posterior cerebral artery: pathology. In: Newton TH, Potts DG, eds. Radiology of the skull and brain: angiography. St. Louis: CV Mosby, 1974:1580–1627.

32. Caplan LR. Posterior cerebral artery syndromes. Hdbk Clin Neurol 1988;53(9):409.

33. Geschwind N, Fusillo M. Color-naming defects in association with alexia. Arch Neurol 1966;15:137.

10 CEREBRAL HEMISPHERES: BASAL GANGLIA

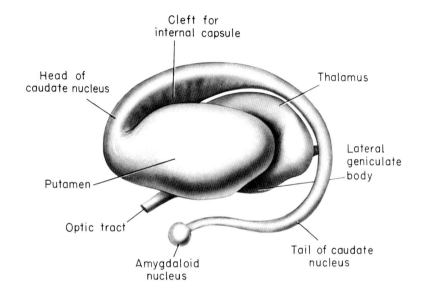

Cleft for internal capsule

Head of caudate nucleus

Thalamus

Putamen

Lateral geniculate body

Optic tract

Tail of caudate nucleus

Amygdaloid nucleus

► Introduction

The basal ganglia consist of several interconnected nuclei located deep to the cerebral cortex and rostral, dorsal, and lateral to the thalamus. Rostrally, these nuclei wrap around the anterior limb of the internal capsule; caudally, they form a thin, curved tail extending along the inferior horn of the lateral ventricle into the temporal lobe.

A major source of afferent fibers to the basal ganglia is the cerebral cortex; particularly extensive connections arise in the association areas of the frontal and parietal lobes. Projections from the basal ganglia, directed to thalamus and brain stem, influence the motor control regions of the brain, such as the motor cortex, as well as modulate behavior and cognition through connections with the prefrontal cortex.[1,2] The basal ganglia play a significant role in scaling the intensity of movements, and possibly, the intensity of cognitive responses.[3,4] Their blood supply is derived from penetrating branches of the anterior, middle, and posterior cerebral arteries as well as those of the anterior choroidal artery.

In this chapter the individual components of the basal ganglia will be studied, along with the connections and proposed functions. A neural circuit passing through the basal ganglia will be described and an attempt made to relate this circuit to specific neurologic disease processes. The vasculature of the basal forebrain will be studied and several clinicopathologic cases will be presented.

GENERAL OBJECTIVES

1. To learn the locations, connections, and functions of the major nuclei in the basal ganglia
2. To learn the clinically detectable deficits associated with destruction of these nuclei or specific components of their neural circuitry
3. To use the information gathered in the preceding objectives to localize the extent of cerebral damage based on the patient's presenting neurologic signs and symptoms

INSTRUCTIONS

In this chapter you will be presented with one or more clinical case studies. *Each study will be followed by a list of questions that can best be answered by using a knowledge of regional and functional neuroanatomy and by referring to outside reading material.* Following the questions will be a section devoted to structures from a specific region of the central nervous system. Before attempting to answer the questions, compile a list of the patient's neurologic signs and symptoms, then examine the structures and their functions and study their known clinical deficits. After becoming familiar with the material, reexamine the list of neurologic signs and symptoms and formulate answers to the questions. Be aware that some of the questions can have multiple responses or require information beyond the scope of this manual. It may be necessary to obtain material or advice from additional resources, such as specialty texts, a medical dictionary, or clinical personnel.

MATERIALS

1. Human brains sectioned in the frontal and horizontal planes
2. A human brain cut in the midsagittal plane

UNIT A

Case Study 10-1

A 34-year-old male with labile emotions and a movement disorder

This is a 34-year-old, right-handed laborer in a paper and pulp company who was referred to the company physician by his floor supervisor. He had been employed, in good standing, by the company for 16 years; however, recently his work habits and personality had undergone a progressive change. He had become extremely emotional, yelling at his fellow workers and making unusually rude and sexual comments to the office staff. He had also begun arriving late and frequently got confused on the job, leaving tasks unfinished. In addition, he had begun to move his hands and arms strangely. At first insidious, these random movements now interfered with his work. He appeared clumsy, frequently dropping tools and occasionally stumbling when walking. The supervisor suspected alcoholism and requested the physician's evaluation to determine if it was safe to have him remain working around heavy industrial equipment.

Family History

At the time of first examination, he was living with his wife and two children, who were 15 and 16 years of age. His mother was alive and in good health. His father had died at age 38 in an accident at the paper company plant 18 years before but had been in good health until that time. The maternal and paternal grandparents were dead. The paternal grandfather had died at 43 years of age; he had not seen a physician but was described by the family as

202

having gone "daffy" and died of the "shakes," which they had attributed to his excessive drinking.

Past Medical History

The patient had left public school at the age of 18 after completing the 10th grade and obtained a job at the paper company. He had not seen a physician previously, and the only records available were those of the grade school nurse, which were unremarkable. He admitted to a 25-pack-year history of smoking and to having consumed two to three (16 oz) cans of beer per day.

General Physical Examination

The patient was a well-nourished, well-hydrated, muscular adult male appearing the stated age, with poor hygiene. Head was normocephalic. Funduscopic examination revealed no evidence of exudate, hemorrhage, or papilledema. There was no cervical, supraclavicular, or inguinal lymphadenopathy. The thyroid was positioned on the midline without masses or nodules. He had a regular heart rate and rhythm without gallops or murmurs and carotid pulsations were clear. The lungs were clear to auscultation and percussion. The abdomen was soft, without masses, tenderness, rigidity, or rebound. Peripheral pulses were intact (+2/4) at the radial, femoral, popliteal, dorsales, and tibialis. There was no peripheral edema. Genitalia showed a circumcised penis with testes descended bilaterally. A soft, reducible mass was present in the right inguinal ring. Rectal examination showed sphincter tone intact without fissures, tags, or stenosis. Prostate was grade II without nodules or tenderness, and the stool was guiac negative.

Neurologic Examination

Mental Status. The patient was awake but seemed disoriented with respect to time and place. He was irritable and responded inconsistently to questions. He was able to add and subtract single-digit numbers but could not divide or multiply. He could follow most two-step commands but not three-step commands. Speech, comprehension, and memory were appropriate for his education.

Cranial Nerves. He had a full range of eye movements and complete visual fields. Pupils were equal and reactive to light, both direct and consensual. His hearing was normal in both ears. His facial expressions were full and symmetric. The corneal, jaw-jerk, and gag reflexes were intact. The palate elevated symmetrically and the tongue protruded on the midline. His shoulders elevated symmetrically.

Motor Systems. Strength was 5/5 in the upper and lower extremities; coordination appeared intact but was hard to assess because of the involuntary motion. Tone in the limbs appeared slack, when not in motion. Deep tendon reflexes were +2/4 symmetric in all limbs; however, tendon taps were pendular. A continuous writhing motion was present in his hands and arms. This consisted of jerky, quick motions about the wrist and slower, wandering motions in the arm. He could not stop these motions on command and frequently tried to hide the more obvious ones by combining the motion with other, more purposeful arm movements. He also had jerky movement in his feet and legs that interfered with his gait, causing him to lose balance occasionally and contributing to his drunken appearance. He denied the existence of the involuntary movements, claiming he was nervous about being in a doctor's office. His wife was not sure when the movements began, but claimed that he had been making them for at least 9 months. She also stated that he did not have any involuntary motion when asleep.

Sensation. Cutaneous sensory functions were intact throughout the body; proprioception was intact in all limbs.

QUESTIONS

1. Does the patient exhibit a language or memory deficit or an alteration in consciousness or cognition?

2. Are signs of cranial nerve dysfunction present?

3. Are there any changes in motor functions, such as reflexes, muscle tone, movement, or coordination?

4. Are any changes in sensory functions detectable?

5. At what level in the central neuraxis is this lesion most likely located?

6. Is the pathology focal, multifocal, or diffuse in its distribution within the nervous system?

7. What is the clinical–temporal profile of this pathology: acute or chronic; progressive or stable?

8. Based on your answers to the previous two questions, decide whether the symptoms in this patient are most likely caused by a vascular accident, a tumor, or a degenerative or inflammatory process.

9. If you feel this is the result of a vascular accident, what vessels are most likely involved?

10. What are the possible links between the patient's mental status and his motor control?

11. Describe the pathophysiology of this disease in terms of the possible neural circuitry involved.

Case Study 10-2

A 67-year-old with bradykinesia, tremor, and rigidity

A 67-year-old, right-handed, retired city worker was brought to you by his wife because of "shaking" and "weakness." The wife reported that not only did his hands shake, but there had been changes in his personality. She also complained that he had become very slow or "weak" in his movements and often sat motionless with an expressionless face. He had difficulty getting up and moving about the house. She admitted that this had been going on for over a year and was getting worse, but she had resisted seeking treatment since she felt that he had just grown lazy after retirement. He had recently suffered several falls, one of which had resulted in a skin laceration on his forehead. She was seeking a physician at this time because he had started to make "funny noises with his mouth."

Past Medical History

At the time of examination the patient had been retired for 2 years; until now he had been in good health except for an appendectomy at age 18. He had three children, who were living independently; none had attended college.

General Physical Examination

This was an alert, cooperative, well-hydrated, and well-nourished individual, oriented for place and time and appearing his stated age. He was seated quietly and did not offer much information during the examination, letting his wife provide most of the history. Optic discs were clear with sharp borders. Chest was clear to auscultation and percussion. Blood pressure was normal; peripheral pulses were intact; respirations and temperature were normal. Abdomen was soft to palpation, with no masses or tenderness present. Skin was of normal texture and turgor; a recent skin laceration, 2 cm in length, was present on his forehead.

Neurologic Examination

Mental Status.   The patient was alert, oriented for time and place, and cooperative. Memory and knowledge were appropriate for his age. Speech was clear and meaningful, but soft and low in volume; his comprehension of language was good. He was capable of writing, but his letters were noticeably reduced in size when compared with a previous sample of 10 years ago provided by his wife.

Cranial Nerves.   His range of movement for the extraocular eye muscles was full, and visual fields were complete to confrontation. The corneal, jaw-jerk, and gag reflexes were intact; palate and uvula elevated symmetrically; tongue protruded midline; and shoulder shrug was symmetric. A three-per-second resting tremor was present in the orofacial musculature that diminished on speaking and swallowing, or when he opened his mouth. There was a detectable high-frequency hearing loss, more in the right ear than in the left.

Motor Systems.   His strength was intact, and deep tendon reflexes were normal in all extremities. He had a three-per-second tremor in both upper and lower extremities that was ameliorated with movement and returned upon resting. There was cogwheel rigidity upon passive movement of the limbs. He had no dysmetria or past-pointing present in any extremity. With his arms extended, the tremor diminished and there was no pronator drift. The tremor returned when his arms were relaxed. His gait was slow, with many shuffling steps. Postural reflexes were compromised; if given an abrupt push, he retropulsed, with many short steps and was at risk for falling. The patient could not stand from a seated position in a low, soft-padded chair, but he could, after one or two attempts, rise from a higher chair with a stiffer seat.

Sensation.   Cutaneous sensation and proprioception were intact throughout the body and face.

QUESTIONS

1. Does the patient exhibit a language or memory deficit or an alteration in consciousness or cognition?

2. Are signs of cranial nerve dysfunction present?

3. Are there any changes in motor functions, such as reflexes, muscle tone, movement, or coordination?

4. Are any changes in sensory functions detectable?

5. At what level in the central neuraxis is this lesion most likely located?

6. Is the pathology focal, multifocal, or diffuse in its distribution within the nervous system?

7. What is the clinical–temporal profile of this pathology: acute or chronic; progressive or stable?

8. Based on your answers to the previous two questions, decide whether the symptoms in this patient are most likely caused by a vascular accident, a tumor, or a degenerative or inflammatory process.

9. If you feel this is the result of a vascular accident, what vessels are most likely involved?

10. Describe the pathophysiology of this disease in terms of the possible neural circuitry involved.

Case Study 10-3

A 54-year-old woman with a hemiparesis of rapid onset resolving into a movement disorder

This was a 54-year-old, right-handed housewife who developed hemiparesis and hemiparesthesia of rapid onset in the right arm and leg 9 months earlier. Subsequently, the paresis and sensory deficit resolved over a 3-month interval; however, an involuntary, flinging motion of the right arm and a writhing, jerky motion of the right leg slowly developed during this time. She is in considerable distress, since the involuntary motions of her extremity disrupted her gait and postural station and thus incapacitated her in her daily routines. She admitted to severe social embarrassment because of the involuntary motion.

Past Medical History

Her past medical history was positive for hypertension, smoking, and alcohol consumption. Nine months previously, she had suffered a cerebrovascular event that left her with hemiparesis and hemibody sensory loss on the right side. Language and cognition were not noticeably affected in this event.

General Physical Examination

The patient was an alert, well-hydrated, but underweight female, appearing older then the stated age. Signs of exhaustion and distress were evident, and she was of anxious demeanor. Her optic discs were clear and had sharp borders; visual acuity was normal. Her neck was supple, with no bruits. Her blood pressure, heart rate, and respirations were slightly elevated. Her chest was clear to percussion, and the abdomen was soft, with no masses or tenderness. The remainder of the examination was precluded because of the excessive involuntary limb motion.

Neurologic Examination

Mental Status.   This is an alert, oriented, and cooperative female in considerable emotional distress. Language, comprehension, reading, and memory were appropriate.

Cranial Nerves.   Testing was complicated by the violence of her involuntary motion in the upper extremity. She had a full range of eye movements, pupils were equal and reactive to light, and accommodation was intact. The corneal and gag reflexes were intact; jaw-jerk was normotensive. Her hearing was equal in both ears. Her tongue protruded on the midline.

Motor Systems. Muscle strength and reflexes were normal in both extremities on the left but were difficult to test definitively on the right because of the the continuous and violent involuntary motion. The movement in the upper extremity consisted of violent flinging motions superimposed on a continuous writhing jerky movement. The lower extremity demonstrated the continuous writhing motion with only brief jerks. Occasionally, the jerky motion in the lower extremity became violent. Attempts to reduce the motion in either extremity by physical restraint were unsuccessful. She could move the right extremities on command in between the involuntary motions. Gait was severely compromised by the flinging of the upper extremity. Although she did not experience an embarrassment of postural reflexes, the upper-extremity motion was continually pulling her off station. The involuntary movement of the right extremities was ameliorated with sleep but returned upon waking.

Sensation. Vibratory sensation and pinprick were intact on the left; to the extent that it could be tested, both modalities were equivocal on the right.

QUESTIONS

1. Does the patient exhibit a language or memory deficit or an alteration in consciousness or cognition?

2. Are signs of cranial nerve dysfunction present?

3. Are there any changes in motor functions, such as reflexes, muscle tone, movement, or coordination?

4. Are any changes in sensory functions detectable?

5. At what level in the central neuraxis is this lesion most likely located?

6. Is the pathology focal, multifocal, or diffuse in its distribution within the nervous system?

7. What is the clinical–temporal profile of this pathology: acute or chronic; progressive or stable?

8. Based on your answers to the previous two questions, decide whether the symptoms in this patient are most likely caused by a vascular accident, a tumor, or a degenerative or inflammatory process.

9. If you feel this is the result of a vascular accident, what vessels are most likely involved?

10. What is the most common etiology of this disease?

11. In this patient, would you have expected to see language dysfunction with hemiparesis and sensory loss such as present in the initial pathology?

12. Describe the pathophysiology of this disease in terms of the possible neural circuitry involved.

207

► DISCUSSION
Basal Ganglia Structures

The basal ganglia are located deep to the cerebral cortex and surround the rostral border of the internal capsule. They can be divided into three groups of nuclei based on phylogeny; fortunately, these divisions also reflect structural and functional boundaries. The oldest portion is the **archistriatum** (called the amygdala) and is involved in modulating emotions and memory associations; it has been discussed in Chapter 9. The intermediate-aged portion of the basal ganglia is the **paleostriatum** (called the globus pallidus) and represents a link between the younger parts of the basal ganglia and the thalamus. The youngest portion is called the **neostriatum** and is composed of the caudate and putamen; these nuclei receive projections from the ipsilateral cerebral cortex and communicate with the ipsilateral thalamus through the globus pallidus. The paleostriatum and neostriatum are involved in controlling the activity of the somatic motor system as well as cognitive and behavioral systems.[1–4]

A variety of other terminologies are used for structures in the basal ganglia (Fig. 10-1). The caudate nucleus and putamen are referred to as the **striatum** or **dorsal striatum,** the globus pallidus is called the **pallidum** or **dorsal pallidum,** and the putamen and globus pallidus together are called the **lentiform nucleus.** Collectively, all these structures are referred to as the **corpus striatum.**

Several additional structures are often included in the general term *basal ganglia* because of their intimate connections and interlocking functions. These are the **subthalamic nucleus** and **substantia nigra** (Fig. 10-2). Each of these forms reciprocal connections with portions of the corpus striatum.

Recently, two other regions in the forebrain have been included in the term *basal ganglia*.[5,6] The nucleus accumbens, located ventral and medial to the striatum, was recognized as resembling the caudate and putamen in terms of parallel neural connections and neurochemistry; it has thus been named the **ventral striatum.** For similar reasons, the precommissural septum has been called the **ventral pallidum** in reference to the globus pallidus, a structure with which it is continuous.

CAUDATE AND PUTAMEN

The caudate nucleus consists of a large, globular *head* located lateral and anterior to the internal capsule, a tapering *body,* and a long, thin *tail* (see Fig. 10-2). The body of the caudate arches over the thalamus laterally, coursing alongside the body of the lateral ventricle (see Plates 21 to 25) and extends into the temporal lobe as the tail of the caudate. At the rostral pole of the temporal lobe, the tail merges with the amygdala.

The putamen is a disk-shaped nucleus on the lateral border of the basal ganglia (see Fig. 10-2 and Plates 21 to 25). Medially, it is bounded by the globus pallidus and internal capsule. At its anterior extreme, it is continuous with the head of the caudate nucleus; along its length it is partially separated from the caudate by fascicles of the internal capsule. The striated appearance given these two structures by the penetrating fibers is responsible for their conjoint name, *corpus striatum* (see Fig. 10-1).

The caudate and putamen contain very similar neuronal circuits.[2] Both receive glutaminergic fibers from areas in the ipsilateral neocortex. These fibers end on cholinergic and GABAergic neurons. GABAergic fibers from the caudate-putamen innervate the ipsilateral globus pallidus and a closely associated structure, the reticular portion of the substantia nigra. The close association of the caudate and putamen and the parallel organization of their neuronal circuits and neurochemistry explain the often used term *caudoputamen* when referencing these structures.

Despite the similarity in neuronal organization, current thought suggests that portions of the caudate and putamen play different roles in the activity of the brain. The rostral caudate appears closely related to the prefrontal cortex and is involved in controlling behavioral and cognitive functions.[1] The putamen is closely related through its connections to premotor and motor cortex and influences the motor operation of distal limb musculature.[7]

CLINICAL DEFICIT
Lesions in the caudate or putamen, or degeneration of their neurons can lead to hyperkinetic states of movement such as **chorea** (a rapid, jerky, aimless, and

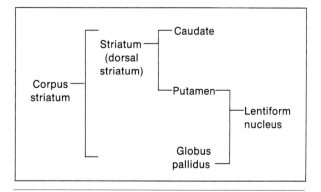

Figure 10-1. A table of terminology used for the corpus striatum.

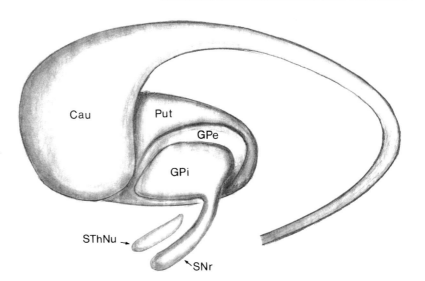

Figure 10-2.
Stylized drawing of the medial aspect of the basal ganglia. (Cau, caudate; GPe, external segment of globus pallidus; GPi, internal segment of globus pallidus; Put, putamen; SNr, reticular portion of substantia nigra; SThNu, subthalamic nucleus.)

constant motion of the limbs), **athetosis** (a slow, sinuous motion of the limbs), and **dystonia** (slow, sustained, contorting postures). In addition, behavioral and cognitive changes can accompany the loss of normal caudate and putamen output.

The separate functions of portions of the caudate and putamen may be reflected in differing neurologic presentations.[8] Lesions restricted to the putamen have resulted in motor dysfunction in the contralateral limbs (reviewed in Kanazawa[9]); behavioral defects have been associated with caudate lesions.[3] These behavioral defects are characterized by apathy, disinhibition, or a major affective disturbance.

GLOBUS PALLIDUS

The wedge-shaped globus pallidus is trapped between the putamen laterally and the internal capsule medially (see Fig. 10-2 and Plates 22 to 25). A lateral medullary lamina of fibers separates the globus pallidus from the putamen, and a vertically oriented, thin, fibrous sheet, called the medial medullary lamina, divides this nucleus into internal and external segments. The caudal portion of the internal segment is in close association with the reticular portion of the substantia nigra, with which it shares many similarities in neuronal organization.

Both segments of the globus pallidus receive GABAergic projections from the caudate and putamen (see Fig. 10-3); however, there are intrinsic differences in these projections. The GABAergic fibers to the internal segment also contain a neuropeptide, substance P; those projecting to the external segment contain enkephalin.

The external portion of the globus pallidus has an inhibitory projection onto the ipsilateral subthalamic nucleus that uses GABA as its neurotransmitter. The internal portion has an inhibitory projection, also using GABA as a neurotransmitter, onto several ipsilateral thalamic nuclei. These include ventrolateral and portions of the ventroanterior nuclei (see Fig. 10-3), centromedian nucleus, and dorsomedial nucleus.

The GABAergic/substance-P-containing fibers between corpus striatum and internal segment are part of a *direct pathway* through the basal ganglia[2] involving the striatum, internal segment of globus pallidus, and thalamus, which will be described later. The GABAergic/enkephalin-containing neurons between corpus striatum and external segment are part of an *indirect pathway* through the basal ganglia. This latter pathway involves striatum, external segment of globus pallidus, subthalamic nucleus, internal segment of globus pallidus, and thalamus. The organization and function of these connections will be presented in the section on neuronal circuits (see p. 213).

CLINICAL DEFICIT

Lesions in portions of the globus pallidus lead to a profound hypokinesia, somewhat similar to Parkinsonian rigidity but without the associated tremor. Stereotaxically placed lesions in the globus pallidus have been used by neurosurgeons to ameliorate unwanted body motions.[10] Profound rigidity and catatonic posture is also associated with severe degeneration of the globus pallidus as seen in anoxic states such as carbon dioxide or carbon disulfide intoxication, respiratory failure, and pure nitrogen inhalation.[11]

SUBTHALAMIC NUCLEUS

The subthalamic nucleus is a thin, elongated wedge of gray matter located medial to the globus pallidus and ventral to the thalamus (see Figs. 10-2 and 10-3; Plates 21 and 22). Laterally, it is bounded by the internal capsule and medially, by the lenticular fasciculus. It receives inhibitory (GABAergic) fibers from the external portion of the globus pallidus and sends excitatory (glutaminergic) projections to the internal segment of the globus pallidus. Thus, the subthalamic nucleus provides a source of excitation to the internal

segment of the globus pallidus that can be modulated by the external segment. The significance of this arrangement will be discussed in the section on neuronal circuits (p. 213).

CLINICAL DEFICIT

Lesions of the subthalamic nucleus result in ballistic motions on the side contralateral to the lesion. Lateralized ballistic motions are referred to as hemiballistic and are defined as a violent, flinging, uncontrolled movement of the limb. The most common cause of these lesions is cerebrovascular accidents.[12] Lesion of the subthalamic nucleus in a primate with experimentally induced parkinsonian symptoms can ameliorate the motor disturbances.[13]

SUBSTANTIA NIGRA

The substantia nigra is located in the midbrain but extends rostrally to lie in close association with the globus pallidus (see Figs. 10-2 and 10-3; Plates 19 to 21). Ventrolaterally, it is bounded by the cerebral peduncle, and dorsomedially, by the red nucleus. The substantia nigra is divided into two segments: the pars compacta and pars reticulata. The neurons of the compact portion contain melanin, a by-product of the production of dopamine. Axons from these cells innervate the ipsilateral caudate and putamen, forming the nigrostriatal pathway. The pars reticulata shares similarities in its neural circuits with that of the internal portion of the globus pallidus and is thought to represent a caudal extension of that nucleus (see Figs. 10-2 and 10-3).

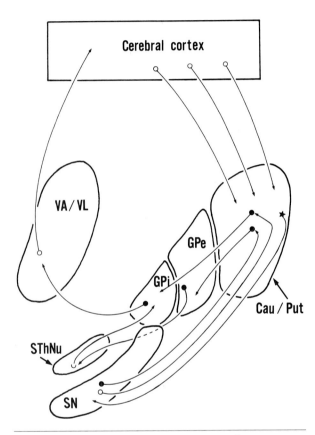

Figure 10-3. The basic organization of connections involving the basal ganglia. The mainstream pathway for motor signals to the spinal cord descends from motor cortex. The basal ganglia and associated pathways appear as a loop starting in the cerebral cortex, passing through the corpus striatum and thalamus, then returning to cerebral cortex. Several side loops through subthalamus and substantia nigra are also present. (Cau, caudate; GPe, external segment of globus pallidus; GPi, internal segment of globus pallidus; Put, putamen; SN substantia nigra; SThNu, subthalamic nucleus; VA/VL, ventroanterior and ventrolateral nuclei of thalamus.)

CLINICAL DEFICIT

Destruction of the dopamine-containing cells in the pars compacta of the substantia nigra can result in parkinsonian signs and symptoms on the contralateral half of the body. Bilateral degeneration of the dopamine-producing cells can result in bilateral expression of parkinsonism.

Recently, certain synthetic heroins, sold as street drugs, have been demonstrated to be neurotoxic for the dopamine cells of the substantia nigra.[14] Attention was directed to these compounds when young adults in northern California developed profound parkinsonism after using the synthetic heroin. The active ingredient in the street drug is a neurotoxin named 1-methyl-4-phenyl-,2,3,6-tetrahydropyridine (MPTP). This compound is currently being used to induce a parkinson model system for study in primates.

NUCLEUS ACCUMBENS

The nucleus accumbens is located in the small area bounded by the base of the septum, the ventral aspect of the internal capsule, and the third ventricle. It is continuous dorsally with the caudate and putamen. It is called the ventral striatum, since it has close parallels with the dorsal striatum in neurochemistry and connectivity. The nucleus accumbens receives cortical projections from the cingulate and temporal gyri and from the piriform lobe. It has projections to the precommissural septum as well as other regions of the brain.

PRECOMMISSURAL SEPTUM

Several named cell groups are located in the vicinity of the anterior commissure. Ventrally, this area is continuous with the internal segment of the globus pallidus, with which it shares a similar neurochemistry and parallel connectivity. In reference to these relationships, the precommissural nuclei are collectively referred to as the ventral pallidum. Projections to the ventral pallidum arise in the ipsilateral ventral striatum (nucleus accumbens). Its efferent axons reach the ipsilateral dorsomedial nucleus of the thalamus. Thus, the ventral pallidum, like its dorsal counterpart, the globus pallidus, is a gateway from portions of the striatum to the thalamus.

► Connections of the Basal Ganglia

The connections of the nuclei within the basal ganglia are very complex. However, an appreciation of their arrangement is necessary to understand their function in the motor system, as well as the pathophysiology of numerous disease states affecting the motor system.

AFFERENT PROJECTIONS TO THE BASAL GANGLIA

There are three main sources of projections to the basal ganglia: neocortex, thalamus, and brain stem.

Corticostriate Fibers

The caudate and putamen receive glutaminergic fibers from most of the ipsilateral neocortex (Figs. 10-3 and 10-4). These projections are arranged in an or-
derly fashion creating a cortical map laid out over caudate and putamen (corpus striatum). The premotor cortex and supplementary motor cortex are represented in the putamen while prefrontal and posterior parietal cortex project to the caudate.[1] Through these projections, the striatum is informed of activity in most portions of the neocortex.

Thalamostriate Fibers

The intralaminar nuclei of the thalamus project to the ipsilateral striatum. Many of the ascending somatic sensory pathways that pass through thalamus to the neocortex give off collateral fibers to the intralaminar nuclei. In addition, these nuclei receive projections from various regions of the brain stem reticular formation that are privy to ascending fibers from the spinal cord. Consequently, through direct (spino-intralaminar) and indirect (spino-reticular-intralaminar) projections, caudate and putamen are informed of external events affecting the somatic sensory system.

Brain Stem Afferents

The striatum receives diffuse projections of fibers from several areas of the brain stem. Some of these projections have been identified based on their neuropharmacology. The midbrain raphe nuclei provide serotinergic axons to striatum; the substantia nigra provides dopaminergic axons. These later, nigrostriatal axons will be further discussed on pp. 212–213.

INTERNAL CONNECTIONS OF THE BASAL GANGLIA

The internal connections of the basal ganglia can be divided into two groups. The first group is composed of pathways that connect the striatum to the ipsilateral globus pallidus; the second includes a series of reciprocal loops between the striatopallidal complex and the substantia nigra and the subthalamic nucleus.

Striatopallidal Connections

The striatum, which receives fibers from neocortex and thalamic intralaminar nuclei, projects axons to the globus pallidus (Fig. 10-3). The striatopallidal fibers are GABAergic and provide an inhibitory influence on both the internal and external portion of the globus pallidus. These fibers are arranged in a topographic array; thus, globus pallidus receives a precise

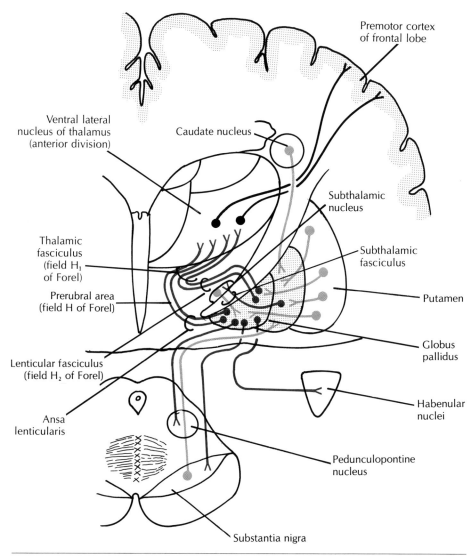

Figure 10-4.   A diagram of the major afferent and efferent fiber tracts of the globus pallidus. (Barr ML, Kiernan JA. The human nervous system: an anatomical viewpoint. Philadelphia: JB Lippincott, 1988:213)

map of striatal neuronal activity. A distinctive feature helps to separate GABAergic neurons that project to the internal segment from those that project to the external segment of the globus pallidus. Those with axons terminating in the internal segment contain the neuropeptide substance P, as well as GABA. Those terminating in the external segment produce (colocalize) enkephalin with GABA. These two cell populations represent two separate pathways for the flow of information out of the basal ganglia; a **direct path** involving the GABA/substance P fibers and an **indirect pathway** involving the GABA/enkephalinergic cells (this will be discussed further on pp. 213–215).

Striatonigral and Pallidonigral Fibers

The substantia nigra receives axons from the striatum (striatonigral) and globus pallidus (pallidonigral). At this writing, it is known that the striatonigral fibers produce neuropeptides, but the chemistry of the pallidonigral fibers remains largely unknown.[15]

Nigrostriatal Fibers

Dopaminergic neurons in the compact portion of the substantia nigra give rise to a projection to the corpus striatum called *nigrostriatal fibers*. Recent evidence suggests that these fibers inhibit those striatal neurons projecting to the external segment of globus pallidus (the GABA/enkephalin fibers of the indirect pathway) while exciting those striatal neurons projecting to the internal segment (the GABA/substance P fibers of the direct pathway). Thus, the nigrostriatal fibers can shift the balance between the direct and indirect pathways to favor that of the direct (see discussion on pp. 213–215).[2]

Subthalamopallidal and Pallidosubthalamic Fibers

The subthalamic nucleus forms reciprocal connections with the globus pallidus. The pallidosubthalamic fibers, producing GABA, originate in the external segment of the globus pallidus, while subthalamopallidal fibers, producing glutamate, terminate in the internal segment of the globus pallidus.[15] This arrangement is considered part of the indirect pathway through the basal ganglia circuit.[2]

EFFERENT CONNECTIONS OF THE BASAL GANGLIA

There are two major efferent pathways from the basal ganglia: projections to the ipsilateral thalamus, which then influence the neocortex, and projections to the tegmentum of the midbrain, which eventually influence motor nuclei in the brain stem.

Pallidothalamic Fibers

In humans, the largest output from the basal ganglia is directed to ventrolateral, ventroanterior, and centromedian nuclei of the thalamus; subsequently, these nuclei influence portions of motor, premotor, supplementary motor, and prefrontal cortex. The thalamic projections arise in the internal segment of the globus pallidus. Two pathways are used to reach the thalamus from the internal segment (see Fig. 10-4). Some fibers pass under the inferior border of the internal capsule and then curve superiorly to enter the ventroanterior thalamus; this pathway is called the **ansa lenticularis** (Plates 23 to 25; Fig. 10-4). The second pathway involves fibers that pass directly through the internal capsule and enter the ventrolateral thalamus; these fibers are called the **lenticular fasciculus** (Plates 22 and 23; Fig. 10-4). Both pathways come into close juxtaposition at the medial border of the zona incerta and, in this region, are called the **thalamic fasciculus** (see Chap. 7). The pallidotha-

lamic projections produce GABA and have an inhibitory influence on the neurons of the thalamus.

Pallidotegmental Fibers

In addition to the thalamic fibers, the globus pallidus sends axons into the brain stem. These fibers leave the globus pallidus with those of the lenticular fasciculus; however, instead of curving superiorly into the thalamus, they turn inferiorly and pass into the midbrain, terminating in the nucleus tegmenti pedunculopontis (Fig. 10-4). This latter structure is a large nucleus in the midbrain tegmentum that is wrapped around the dorsolateral border of the decussation of the superior cerebellar peduncle. From the tegmental nucleus, projections pass to the brain stem region involved in motor control (vestibular and reticular formation areas). Using the pallidotegmental connection, the basal ganglia mediate control over brain stem motor function. Although this connection is important in the control of motor pathways for nonprimate species, it has been overshadowed by the pallidothalamic fibers in primates.

► Neuronal Circuits in the Basal Ganglia

Although the basal ganglia may seem like a plethora of interconnected structures, there is an underlying, fundamental pattern for the passage of information through these nuclei. Each of the various functions of the basal ganglia are represented by parallel connections or neural circuits (Fig. 10-5). These connections pass through differing portions of striatum, pallidum, and thalamus.

A generic neural circuit will be described for these pathways through the basal ganglia, and four specific examples will be provided. The significance of these parallel circuits is that they share the same neurochemistry (as described for the generic circuit) and therefore can be expected to have related responses to fluctuation in neurotransmitter levels and to degenerative neuronal pathologies.

GENERIC CIRCUIT

The generic circuit is organized as a large loop, beginning in the cerebral cortex and passing through the corpus striatum, thalamus, and back to cerebral cortex (see Figs. 10-3 and 10-5). Two separate

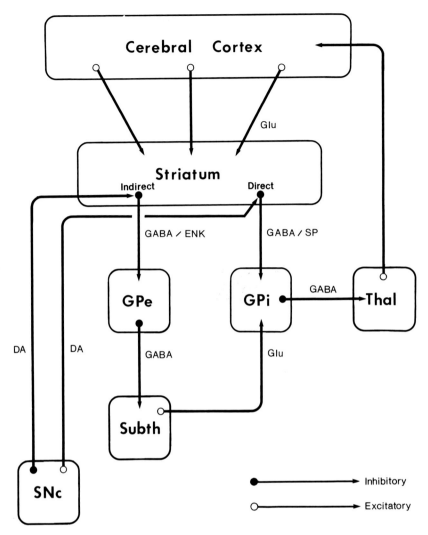

Figure 10-5.
A schematic diagram of a generic neuronal circuit involving the basal ganglia. Open circles are excitatory neurons; closed circles are inhibitory. (Modified from Alexander GF, Crutcher MD. Functional architecture of basal ganglia circuits: neural substrates of parallel processing. Trends Neurosci 1990;13:266–271)

routes—direct and indirect—are used in the passage of information through the corpus striatum.

The generic neuronal circuit for the basal ganglia is illustrated in Figure 10-5. It begins with glutaminergic (excitatory) fibers projecting from cerebral cortex to striatum. Two essentially antagonistic pathways leave the striatum to reach the internal segment of the globus pallidus. The **direct pathway** involves GABAergic/substance-P-containing fibers that directly innervate the internal segment of the pallidum. The **indirect pathway** features a loop passing from striatum to external pallidal segment, to subthalamus, and finally, onto internal pallidal segment. In this latter pathway, striatal GABAergic/enkephalinergic fibers provide an inhibitory innervation to the external segment of the pallidum. In turn, GABAergic fibers from the external segment provide an inhibitory innervation to the subthalamic nucleus. The indirect pathway ends

with an excitatory, glutaminergic projection from the subthalamic nucleus to the internal segment of the globus pallidus. Significantly, both pathways converge, with opposing effects, on the internal pallidal segment. Thus, a balance is struck in the internal segment between the inhibitory influence of the direct pathway and the excitatory influence of the indirect pathway. The outcome is a dynamic modulation of the pallidothalamic pathways.

GABAergic neurons of the internal segment project axons through the ansa lenticularis or the lenticular fasciculus to reach the thalamus. These axons exert an inhibitory influence on the thalamic targets. From the thalamus, projections are returned to the cerebral cortex using glutaminergic fibers; thus, thalamic input is excitatory to cortex.

A significant feature of the two-pathway circuit through the corpus striatum is that the *inhibitory out-*

put of the internal segment of the pallidum is controlled by the balance between the direct pathway (inhibitory) and the indirect pathway (excitatory). The output of the internal segment controls the activity of thalamus and, subsequently, portions of cerebral cortex. Both direct and indirect pathways are influenced by the nigrostriatal (dopaminergic) axons; however, there is a differential effect. Within the striatum, dopamine fibers inhibit the GABAergic neurons of the indirect pathway while exciting those of the direct pathway. *Thus, the substantia nigra can modulate the balance between these two pathways.*

In summary, the two striatal pathways have an antagonistic effect on the output of the internal segment and, acting through the thalamus, differentially modulate this neural activity of cerebral cortex. According to the model, increased activity in the direct pathway *or* decreased activity in the indirect pathway will result in diminished output of the internal segment. Since the internal segment is inhibitory to thalamus, the result is a **disinhibition** of thalamus, which is then free to send more activity to cortex; as such, the patient experiences a **hyperactive state.** The reverse situation occurs when the activity of the direct pathway is de-

creased *or* that of the indirect pathway is increased. The internal segment becomes more active and consequently supplies more **inhibition** to the thalamus, which then supplies less excitation to the cerebral cortex. The result is that the patient experiences **hypoactivity.**

MOTOR CIRCUIT

The motor form of the generic basal ganglia circuit is illustrated in Figure 10-6**A**. The corticostriatal projections arise in the somatic sensory, supplementary, premotor, and motor cortex; their striatal termination is in the putamen. The thalamic target for these projections is the ventrolateral nucleus, which then projects back to supplementary motor cortex.

CLINICAL DEFICIT
Using the model for neuronal organization provided, it is possible to reexamine the signs and symptoms of movement disorder consequent to lesions of basal ganglia damage. Loss of the dopaminergic fibers from the substantia nigra will lower the activity of the direct pathway and increase (through disinhibition) the

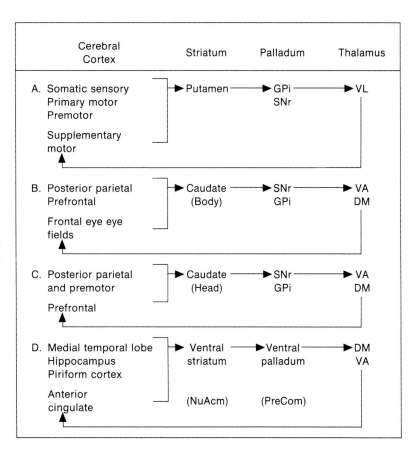

Figure 10-6.
Table illustrates the various circuits passing through the corpus striatum (DM, dorsomedial thalamic nucleus; GPi, internal segment of globus pallidus; NuAcm, nucleus accumbens; PreCom, precommissural area; SNr, pars reticulata of substantia nigra; VA, ventroanterior thalamic nucleus; VL, ventrolateral thalamic nucleus.) (Modified from Alexander GE, DeLong MR, Strick Pl. Parallel organization of functionally segregated circuits linking basal ganglia and cortex. Ann Rev Neurosci 1986;9:357)

activity of the indirect pathway. The net result is that the internal segment provides a stronger inhibition of thalamus. This could contribute to the bradykinetic state experienced by Parkinson's patients.

Degeneration of the GABAergic/enkephalinergic neurons of the striatum, such as occurs in Huntington's chorea, decreases the outflow from striatum to the external segments of the pallidum, diminishing activity in the indirect pathway. The balance is tipped in favor of the direct pathway, and consequently, the internal segment of globus pallidus expresses decreased inhibition on the thalamocortical unit. The thalamus, minus its palladial inhibition, is allowed to operate at a higher level of activity, and the cerebral cortex receives more information. This could account for the hyperkinetic state experienced by Huntington's patients.

A rigid form of Huntington's chorea has been described. The patient presents with bradykinesia instead of chorea, limb rigidity with cogwheeling on passive movement, and a masked face. Although initially this presents similar to Parkinson's disease, it is due to degeneration of the corpus striatum and can occur in families with Huntington's disease. Recently, it has been demonstrated that GABAergic projections from the striatum to both internal and external segments of the globus pallidus have degenerated in the rigid form of Huntington's.[16] Putting this observation into the circuit diagram of the basal ganglia (see Fig. 10-5), one can conclude that the internal segment is receiving only excitatory input from the subthalamic nucleus. Consequently, it is strongly inhibiting the thalamus, and the patient experiences bradykinesia similar to the situation in Parkinson's disease.

Cerebrovascular accidents that damage the subthalamic nucleus on one side would be expected to remove the excitation from that structure to the internal segment of the pallidum (decrease activity in the indirect pathway). As a consequence, the internal segment would not be able to inhibit the thalamocortical unit; thus, the thalamus would release too much activity to the cerebral cortex. The hyperkinetic state experienced by the patient would be confined to the contralateral side of the body. This mechanism could explain the hemiballistic motion expressed by patients subsequent to vascular lesions of the subthalamic nucleus.

OCULOMOTOR CIRCUIT

A specific circuit in the basal ganglia is related to control of eye movement,[1] called the oculomotor circuit (see Fig. 10-6**B**). The corticostriatal fibers arise in the posterior parietal and prefrontal cortex and the frontal eye fields; they terminate in the body of the caudate. The ventroanterior and dorsomedial thalamic nuclei receive the pallidothalamic fibers from the internal segment of the globus pallidus. Thalamocortical projections are directed back to the frontal eye fields. This circuit functions to control the movement of the extraocular eye muscles.

ASSOCIATION CIRCUIT

A circuit through basal ganglia involving the association areas of cerebral cortex has been defined (see Fig. 10-6**C**). Called the association circuit, it appears to function in modulating cognitive and behavioral processes.[1] The corticostriatal projections arise in the prefrontal, premotor, and posterior parietal cortex and terminate in the head of the caudate nucleus. The thalamic targets of this circuit are the ventroanterior and dorsomedial nuclei, two structures that project to the prefrontal cortex.

CLINICAL DEFICIT

In a recent study, the case histories of a cohort of 18 patients with identifiable lesions confined to the caudate nucleus were examined.[17] Several of the patients had no detectable motor signs, others experienced hemiparesis that was transient. The most notable defects involved behavioral and cognitive dysfunction such as abulia, restlessness, hyperactivity, neglect (contralateral), language abnormalities, and poor memory. These findings support the contention that the basal ganglia circuit passing through the caudate is involved in scaling behavioral and cognitive functions in much the same way that the putamenal circuit scales motor activity.

LIMBIC CIRCUIT

A circuit through the basal ganglia also involves components of the limbic system (see Fig. 10-6**D**; Chap. 9). The cortical sources of projections to the striatum are cingulate gyrus, piriform lobe, and portions of the temporal gyri. The striatal target for these projections is nucleus accumbens (ventral striatum). The pallidal target of projections from the accumbens is the precommissural septal area (ventral pallidum) extending caudally into parts of the internal segment of globus pallidus. The thalamic area involved in this circuit is a portion of the dorsomedial nucleus, which has the cingulate gyrus as its cortical target, thus completing the circuit.

UNIT B

Case Study 10-4

A 75-year-old man with postural movement disorder
subsequent to a cerebrovascular accident

This was a 75-year-old, right-handed male with tonic posturing motions of the left upper extremity that developed subsequent to a resolving spastic paralysis. He presented for an annual checkup, 2 years following a cerebrovascular event.

Past Medical History

He was a Jewish scholar who emigrated from eastern Poland to the United States after the World War II. He had been in good health until 2 years before, when he suffered a cerebrovascular accident of rapid onset that left him with spastic paralysis and sensory paresthesia in the left extremities. At that time his strength in the left limbs was 2/5 and his deep tendon reflexes were elevated at +4/4. No language or cognitive deficit was recorded at the time of the first presentation.

General Physical Examination

This was an alert, oriented, and cooperative man. He was well nourished and well hydrated and appeared his stated age. He had the male-pattern baldness. His optic discs were clear, with sharp borders. Visual acuity was normal with his glasses. His neck was supple; a slight bruit was present over the right carotid. His chest was clear to percussion and abdomen was soft to palpation, with no tenderness or masses. His heart rate, blood pressure, and respirations were physiologic. His peripheral pulses were intact at the wrists and ankles. His skin was warm and moist, with good turgor.

Neurologic Examination

Mental Status. He was alert, oriented for time and place, and cooperative. He gave a precise history. Memory was appropriate; speech, writing, and reading (English, Polish, and Hebrew) were intact. He could list all the presidents in order and recite passages from the Torah verbatim.

Cranial Nerves. He had a full range of eye movements, and visual fields were intact. His hearing was significantly diminished, especially for the high frequencies, more so in the right ear than in the left. The corneal and jaw-jerk reflexes were intact; facial expression was symmetric and appropriate to the situation. The gag reflex was intact; palate, uvula, and tongue were symmetric in position. He had slightly diminished sensation to vibratory sense on the left side of his face.

Motor Systems. Strength was 5/5, and deep tendon reflexes were +2/4 for both extremities on the right. Strength was mildly reduced (4/5) for the upper limb on the left, and deep tendon reflexes were slightly elevated (+3/4). The lower limb on the left had reduced strength (3/5) and increased deep tendon reflexes (+3/4). An involuntary, posturing movement was present in the left limbs that had not been detected in his first presentation, poststroke. In the upper limb, the movement consisted of slow, writhing postural changes, including pronounced flexion of the wrist, and phalangeal–metacarpal joints. With the upper limbs held horizontally extended, the left limb wandered in position continuously. Occasional, sudden jerky movements of the upper limb occurred. The lower left limb displayed slow postural movements that interfered with his gait. The movement disorder was somewhat masked by the more pronounced residual paralysis in the lower left limb.

217

The involuntary motion ceased when the patient slept, returning when he awoke. Past-pointing and dysmetria were not present on either side. Pronator drift did not appear to be present, but this was difficult to evaluate on the left side because of the wandering motion in the upper limb. With the upper limbs extended anteriorly and held in a fixed position, a 10-Hz tremor was present in the right arm, but not in the left. This movement in the right limb was ameliorated when the arm was relaxed to the adducted portion. The tremor could be seen in his writing, particularly if he held his hand off of the paper's surface as he wrote.

Sensation. Response to pinprick, vibratory stimuli, and position sense was normal on the right side of his body and only slightly reduced on the left side.

QUESTIONS

1. Does the patient exhibit a language or memory deficit or an alteration in consciousness or cognition?

2. Are signs of cranial nerve dysfunction present?

3. Are there any changes in motor functions, such as reflexes, muscle tone, movement, or coordination?

4. Are any changes in sensory functions detectable?

5. At what level in the central neuraxis is this lesion most likely located?

6. Is the pathology focal, multifocal, or diffuse in its distribution within the nervous system?

7. What is the clinical–temporal profile of this pathology: acute or chronic; progressive or stable?

8. Based on your answers to the previous two questions, decide whether the symptoms in this patient are most likely caused by a vascular accident, a tumor, or a degenerative or inflammatory process.

9. If you feel this is the result of a vascular accident, what vessels are most likely involved?

10. What is the significance of the 10-Hz tremor experienced by this patient?

► DISCUSSION
Basal Ganglia Vasculature

The basal ganglia and internal capsule receive a complex blood supply derived from several sources that ultimately originate from the anterior circulation. Two major suppliers of the corpus striatum, the medial and lateral striate vessels, arise from the proximal portions of the anterior and middle cerebral arteries (Fig. 10-7). The third source, the anterior choroidal artery, is derived directly from the internal carotids.[18] Given the intense anastomosis of vessels in the basal ganglia, it is not yet possible to associate specific signs and symptoms of neurologic damage with specified vessels.

MEDIAL STRIATE VESSELS

The internal carotid artery ascends to the level of the basal forebrain, where it bifurcates into the anterior and middle cerebral arteries. The proximal por-

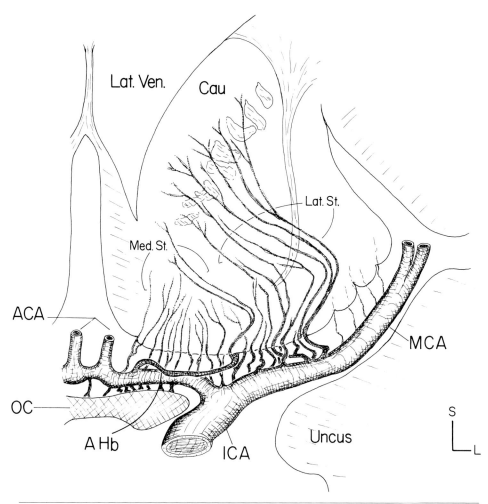

Figure 10-7. Diagram of a coronal section through the head of the caudate nucleus illustrates the medial and lateral striate arteries. The medial striate arteries enter the brain through an area called the anterior perforated substance. (ACA, anterior cerebral arteries; AH$_b$, Heubner's artery; Cau, caudate nucleus; ICA, internal carotid artery; L, lateral; Lat. St., lateral striate arteries; Lat. Ven., lateral ventricles, anterior horn; MCA, middle cerebral artery; Med. St., medial striate arteries; OC, optic middle cerebral artery; Med. St., medial striate arteries; OC, optic chiasm; S, superior.) (Modified from Seeger W. Atlas of topographical anatomy of the brain and surrounding structures. New York: Springer-Verlag, 1978)

tions of these arteries present a horizontal surface coursing directly inferior to the anterior perforated substance (see Fig. 10-7). It is from this dorsal surface of this vessel that the medial striate arteries arise. They are derived from the proximal stem of both the anterior and the middle cerebral artery (see Fig. 10-7). The ventral side of the proximal portion of the anterior cerebral artery gives rise to short branches that perfuse the optic nerve, chiasm, and tracts (see Fig. 10-7).

The medial striate arteries consist of three to six vascular channels penetrating the basal forebrain.[19] Most are quite small and only reach the external segment of the globus pallidus. One large vessel stands out in radiographs, the recurrent artery of Heubner (AH$_b$ in Fig. 10-7), which usually arises from the anterior cerebral artery, courses laterally and then superiorly to reach the anteromedial aspect of the head of the caudate, anterior portion of the putamen, globus pallidus, and a portion of the anterior limb of the internal capsule (see Fig. 10-7).

LATERAL STRIATE VESSELS

These vessels arise from the proximal segment of the middle cerebral artery.[19] After entering the forebrain these vessel make a long, graceful arc, curving from inferolateral to superomedial across the corpus striatum (see Fig. 10-7). They supply substantia innominata, putamen, and globus pallidus as well as the anterior and posterior limb of the internal capsule. Anteriorly, these vessels anastomose with the medial striate vessels; posteriorly, they anastomose with the anterior choroidal artery.

ANTERIOR CHOROIDAL ARTERY

The anterior choroidal arterial tree arises from the internal carotid in most cases, but it can spring off of the middle cerebral artery as well. As the anterior choroidal winds its way around the cerebral peduncle in the ambient cistern (see Chap. 6), it gives off penetrating branches into the base of the cerebrum. These branches reach the posterior portion of the globus pallidus, putamen, and genu of the internal capsule. The anatomy and pathology of the anterior choroidal artery is reviewed by Goldberg.[20]

CLINICAL DEFICIT

Vascular lesions of the basal ganglia have varying presentations, depending on the portion of the structure damaged. Unfortunately, lesion location and symptomatology have not been well correlated to date. Small infarctions confined to the caudate and/or putamen can present with choreiform motion,[21,22] behavior and cognitive dysfunction.[17] Focal dystonia has been reported as a presenting complaint in a lacunar infarction confined to the lenticular nucleus.[23] Hemidystonia can result from vascular lesions in the caudate nucleus, lentiform nucleus (particularly the putamen), or thalamus.[24] Hemiballism and hemichorea have occurred in a patient with a small lesions in the putamen.[25]

Lesions that extend into the internal capsule can present with an initial pure hemiparesthesia or pure hemiparesis that subsequently resolves into a movement disorder. The initial hemiplegia masks the movement disorder, but as the plegia resolves, the involuntary motions are expressed. These are called posthemiplegic movement disorders. A frequent movement disorder to follow lesions of the internal capsule is athetosis, a slow, writhing series of postural adjustments. It most likely represents interruption of the pallidothalamic fibers as they pass through the capsule. Dysarthria can also accompany involvement of the internal capsule in the lesion.[26]

► Bibliography

Adams RD, Victor M. Principles of neurology. New York: McGraw-Hill, 1989; Chap. 4.

Barr ML, Kiernan JA. Corpus striatum. In: The human nervous system: an anatomical viewpoint. Philadelphia: JB Lippincott, 1988; Chap. 12.

Barr ML, Kiernan JA. Motor systems. In: The human nervous system: an anatomical viewpoint. Philadelphia: JB Lippincott, 1988; Chap. 23.

Brazis PW, Masdeu JC, Biller J. Localization in clinical neurology. Boston: Little, Brown, 1990, Chap. 18.

Daube JR, Ragan TJ, Sandok BA, Westmoreland BF. Medical neurosciences. Boston: Little, Brown, 1986, Chap. 9.

Haines DE. Neuroanatomy: an atlas of structures, sections, and systems. Baltimore: Urban & Schwarzenberg, 1987, Figs. 4-5 to 4-13, 4-16 to 4-22, and 5-29 to 5-36.

Nieuwenhuys R, Voogd J, van Huijzen, C. The human central nervous system. Berlin: Springer-Verlag, 1988:258–278.

► References

1. Alexander GE, DeLong MR, Strick PL. Parallel organization of functionally segregated circuits linking basal ganglia and cortex. Ann Rev Neurosci 1986;9:357.

2. Alexander GF, Crutcher MD. Functional architecture of basal ganglia circuits: neural substrates of parallel processing. Trends Neurosci 1990;13:266.

3. Mendez MF, Adams NL, Lweandowski KS. Neurobehavioral changes associated with caudate lesions. Neurology 1989;39: 349.

4. Laplane D, Levasseur M, Pillon B, et al. Obsessive-compulsive and other behavioural changes with bilateral basal ganglia lesions a neuropsychological, magnetic resonance imaging and positron tomography study. Brain 1989;112:699.

5. Heimer L, Wilson RD. The subcortical projections of the allocortex. Similarities in the neural associations of the hippocampus, the piriform cortex, and neocortex. In: Santini M, ed. Golgi centential symposium: perspectives in neurology. New York: Raven Press, 1976:177–193.

6. Alheid GF, Heimer L, Switzer RC. Basal ganglia. In: Paxinos G, ed. The human nervous system. San Diego: Academic Press, 1990:483–582.

7. Liles SL. Activity of neurons in putamen during active and passive movements of wrist. J Neurophysiol 1985;53:217.

8. Rafal RD, Posner MI, Walker JA, Friedrich FJ. Cognition and the basal ganglia. Brain 1984;107:1083.

9. Kanazawa I. Clinical pathophysiology of basal ganglia disease. Hdbk Clin Neurol 1986;49(5):65.

10. Jellinger K. Degenerations and exogenous lesions of the pallidum and striatum. Hdbk Clin Neurol 1968;6:631.

11. Jellinger K. Exogenous lesions of the pallidum. Hdbk Clin Neurol 1986;49(5):465.

12. Fahn S. Huntington disease and other forms of chorea. In: Rowland LP, ed. Merrit's textbook of neurology. Philadelphia: Lea & Febiger, 1989:647–652.

13. Bergman H, Wichmann T, DeLong MR. Reversal of experimental parkinsonism by lesions of the subthalamic nucleus. Science 1990;249:1436.

14. Ballard PA, Tetrud JW, Langston JW. Permanent human parkinsonism due to 1-methyl-4-phenyl-1,2,3,6-tetrahydropyridine (MPTP): seven cases. Neurology 1985;35:949.

15. Graybiel AM. Neurotransmitters and neuromodulators in the basal ganglia. Trends Neurosci 1990;13:244.

16. Albin RL, Reiner A, Anderson KD, Penney JB, Young AB. Striatal and nigral neuron subpopulations in rigid Huntington's dis-

ease: implications for the functional anatomy of chorea and rigidity-akinesia. Ann Neurol 1990;27:357.

17. Caplan LR, Schmahmann JD, Kase CS, et al. Caudate infarcts. Arch Neurol 1990;47:133–143.

18. Gillilan LA. The arterial and venous blood supplies to the forebrain (including the internal capsule) of primates. Neurology 1968;18:653.

19. Leeds NE. The striate (lenticulostriate) arteries and the artery of Heubner. In: Newton TH, Potts DG, eds. Radiology of the skull and brain: angiography. St Louis: CV Mosby, 1974:1527–1539.

20. Goldberg HI. The anterior choroidal artery. In: Newton TH, Potts DG, eds. Radiology of the skull and brain: angiography. St Louis: CV Mosby, 1974:1628–1658.

21. Goldblatt D, Markesbery W, Reeves AG. Recurrent hemichorea following striatal lesions. Arch Neurol 1974;31:51.

22. Saris S. Chorea caused by caudate infarction. Arch Neurol 1983;40:590.

23. Russo LS. Focal dystonia and lacunar infarction of the basal ganglia. Arch Neurol 1983;40:61.

24. Marsden CD, Obeso JA, Zarranz JJ, Lang AE. The anatomical basis of symptomatic hemidystonia. Brain 1985;108:463.

25. Kase CS, Maulsby G, deJuan E, Mohr JP. Hemichorea--hemiballlism and lacunar infarction in the basal ganglia. Neurology 1981;31:452.

26. Kase CS. Middle cerebral arterial syndromes. Hdbk Clin Neurol 1988;53(9):353.

ANSWERS TO CASE QUESTIONS

CHAPTER 1
INTRODUCTION TO NEUROANATOMY

► Case No. 1-1

1. ***Does the patient exhibit a language or memory deficit or an alteration in consciousness or cognition?***

   Yes. The alterations occurred in a specific chronology: When the patient first presented, he was conscious and capable of giving a history; he proceeded to lose consciousness over the next 4 hours and never recovered. His speech was described as dysarthric; however, since he was capable of comprehensible speech (he gave a coherent history), this dysarthria could be the result of damage to the fibers mediating cortical control over the brain stem rather than to the mantle of the cerebral cortex. It is also possible that it relates to damage to the peripheral nervous system or larynx, but this is unlikely, since the history does not involve trauma.

2. ***Are signs of cranial nerve dysfunction present?***

   Yes. He presented with an eye movement disorder. He was incapable of willful conjugate vision into the left hemisphere, yet his eyes could be deflected into that hemisphere using the doll's eye maneuver. This suggests that the suprasegmental systems may be defective but that the segmental-level systems in the brain stem are still functional. This is confirmed by the bilateral response to light seen in the pupils. The asymmetry of the pupils may reflect a partial Horner's syndrome resulting from pressure on the hypothalamus. The loss of the doll's eye maneuver after 6 hours suggests that the upper brain stem segmental circuits have been damaged in this evolving process.

3. ***Are there any changes in motor functions, such as reflexes, muscle tone, movement, or coordination?***

   Yes. He experienced left flaccid paralysis (decreased reflexes), interrupted by periods of clonic and tonic movements (increased reflexes) in the leg and arm. The periodic alterations in reflexes suggest damage in progress in the suprasegmental circuits above the spinal cord level on the right side of the brain. Later in the progress of this event, he began decorticate and then decerebrate posturing; these suggest severe damage to the cerebral cortex initially, followed by compromised function in the upper brain stem.

4. ***Are any changes in sensory functions detectable?***

   Yes. Sensory reduction occurred on the left face and cornea, suggesting that damage has occurred either at the level of the ipsilateral (left) trigeminal complex in the brain stem or above, in the contralateral (right) thalamus or cerebral cortex

5. ***At what level in the central neuraxis is this lesion most likely located?***

   The sensory and motor deficits are consistent with an initial lesion occurring in the right supratentorial fossa, producing a buildup in pressure that eventually compromised function in the infratentorial fossa. The loss of volitional eye movement to the left and sensation from the left face suggests damage has been done to the lateral portion of the frontal and parietal lobes on the right. The progression of events to include the loss of upper and then lower brain stem functions most likely reflects increasing intracranial pressure in the infratentorial compartment with the concomitant rupture of small penetrating blood vessels supplying the brain stem.

6. ***Is the pathology focal, multifocal, or diffuse in its distribution within the nervous system?***

   The initial process is focal in the sense that the lesion began as a discrete process localized within the right cerebral hemisphere but has grown larger with time, to engage structures in the infratentorial fossa.

7. ***What is the clinical–temporal profile of this pathology: acute or chronic; progressive or stable?***

   It is of rapid onset (acute) and progressive, since the neurologic sequelae continued to develop over an 8-hour period.

8. ***Based on your answers to the previous two questions, decide whether the neurologic symptoms in this patient are most likely caused by a vascular accident, a tumor, or a degenerative or inflammatory process.***

   The rapid onset and progressive nature suggest that an initial intracranial vascular event has continued, becoming a space-occupying lesion as extravasated blood accumulates.

9. ***If you feel this is the result of a vascular accident, what vessels were most likely involved?***

   A branch of the middle cerebral artery is most likely involved, since this artery supplies the lateral aspect of the frontal cortex. The underlying process involves the spontaneous rupture of a relatively small branch of the artery deep within either the basal ganglia or the thalamus. The ruptured vessel, now spurting blood at arterial pressure, continues to leak, thus causing an accumulating mass of blood within these vital structures

10. ***Is the initial damage in this patient occurring within the epidural space, within the subarachnoid space, or intracerebrally?***

    The profile of rapid onset and subsequent evolving neurologic sequelae best fits an intracerebral vascular accident.

224

11. *Are the patient's neurologic sequelae due to the initial damage or to other processes?*

The initial event produced the signs and symptoms of supratentorial damage due to an arterial bleed. Subsequent evolution of the process involved increased intracranial pressure and further vascular accidents in the infratentorial compartment.

12. *What does the progress of events in this patient's demise reveal concerning the hierarchy of the central nervous system?*

The loss of consciousness marks the shutdown of the cerebral cortex. This releases brain stem and spinal cord circuits, such as the oculocephalic reflex and decorticate and decerebrate posturing. Loss of the oculocephalic reflex and relaxation of decerebrate posturing mark the destruction of the upper brain stem. This releases control of the cardiovascular and respiratory systems, resulting in fluxions of vital signs. Loss of vital signs marks the demise of the lower brain stem. Each of these steps demonstrates the demise of a level in the hierarchy of the central nervous system.

Comment

This progression of events is called rostral-to-caudal demise,[1] and reflects the hierarchy of function in the central nervous system. As noted earlier, the initiation of symptoms stemmed from an arterial rupture, likely related to the patient's history of hypertension. The patient first experienced focal losses at the cerebral level, while the brain stem reflexes remained intact. As the bleeding continued, he gradually lost consciousness, brain stem reflexes were compromised, and spinal cord reflexes became altered. This reflects the increasing effect of the accumulated mass of blood, probably accompanied by some early cerebral swelling (cerebral edema) and resultant increased intracranial pressure. The ultimate consequence of this increased intracranial pressure is transtentorial (uncal) herniation with distortion of the upper brain stem. When this occurs, small secondary hemorrhages occur in the upper brain stem (Duret hemorrhages). Finally, he died because of respiratory embarrassment as the lower portions of the brain stem were exposed to the effects of increasing intracranial pressure.

CHAPTER 2
SPINAL CORD

► Case Study 2-1

1. *Does the patient exhibit a language or memory deficit or an alteration in consciousness or cognition?*

This patient was awake, alert, and oriented; his language capability was appropriate, except for the slow, slurred speech. This is a motor defect and can be accounted for by damage to the lower motoneurons innervating the tongue, jaw, or pharynx and larynx. It does not necessarily indicate a supratentorial lesion.

2. *Are signs of cranial nerve dysfunction present?*

Yes. The weakened tongue musculature with fasciculations, suggesting damage to the hypoglossal nucleus or nerve, is a cranial nerve dysfunction. The presence of fasciculations suggests that this is a lower motor neuron or segmental level process that is occurring to the hypoglossal nucleus or nerve in this patient.

3. *Are there any changes in motor functions such as reflexes, muscle tone, movement, or coordination?*

Elevated reflexes are present in the lower extremity and depressed reflexes are present in the upper extremity. Signs of upper motoneuron damage in the control of the lower extremity indicate suprasegmental-level dysfunction and suggest central nervous system involvement in the pathology; the presence of

lower motoneuron signs in the upper extremity is a sign of segmental-level dysfunction and could result from damage to the ventral horn of the spinal cord or peripheral neuropathy.

4. *Are any changes in sensory functions detectable?*

This pathology seems to have attacked only motor elements in the nervous system. Thus, it is not likely that the lower motoneuron signs in the arm arise from peripheral nerve lesions, since they would be expected to involve sensory as well as motor components. Nor is it likely that this person is suffering a transection of the spinal cord (transverse myelitis), since sensory deficits would also be expected in such a case.

5. *At what level in the central neuraxis is this lesion most likely located?*

The major site of pathology appears to reside in the spinal cord and lower brain stem. Within these regions, the pathology appears to be confined to the motoneurons. With evidence of increased reflexes in the lower extremity, this suggests that further pathology may be present within the upper motoneurons or corticospinal tract.

6. *Is the pathology focal, multifocal, or diffuse in its distribution within the nervous system?*

The pathology for this disorder is diffuse in that it is bilateral and symmetric in distribution and involves multiple sites along the neuraxis. (For a description of term *diffuse* as used in neurologic presentations, see Daube and colleagues.[2])

7. What is the clinical–temporal profile of this pathology: acute or chronic; progressive or stable?

The process is chronic (with a 9-month history of weakness); it is also getting worse—hence, it is progressive.

8. Based on your answers to the previous two questions, decide whether the symptoms in this patient are most likely caused by a vascular accident, a tumor, or a degenerative or inflammatory process.

The progressive and chronic nature of this process is not compatible with a vascular accident, and the diffuse character of the lesion makes a tumor unlikely. A degenerative process is most likely, although toxins or other metabolic insults cannot be entirely ruled out

9. If you feel this is the result of a vascular accident, what vessels were most likely involved?

See answer 8.

10. What is the significance of the muscular fasciculations in this patient?

Muscular fasciculations are considered a sign of damage to the lower motor neuron or its axon. They most likely represent agonal discharges occurring in the axon stump connected to the muscle.[3]

11. How can obvious motor deficits be present at a given segmental level while sensory function seemingly remains unimpaired?

Sensory and motor channels are carried in close juxtaposition in the spinal nerves; however, as they enter the spinal cord, the dorsal (sensory) root splits apart from the ventral (motor) root. Once inside the spinal cord these channels are maintained separately. The membranes of different classes of neurons have distinct proteins on their outside surfaces, thus enabling immunosubstances and viruses to distinguish specific nerve cell types and to target specific pathways for attack.

12. What is the significance of the tremor observed in this patient?

The tremor observed in this patient is most likely of the benign essential type and is not directly related to the rest of the patient's neurologic presentation.

13. What spinal cord neurons are degenerating in this patient?

The alpha-motoneurons of the ventral horn of the spinal cord are degenerating in this patient.

Comment

The presence of progressive weakness and fasciculations in the absence of any sensory deficits strongly suggests that this case represents amyotrophic lateral sclerosis (motor neuron disease). This progressive degenerative disease of unknown etiology produces damage to the lower motoneurons with resultant progressive paralysis. Sensory modalities remain intact. Upper motoneurons are commonly involved, and in initial stages, increased deep tendon reflexes can be noted. As weakness and skeletal muscle atrophy increase, reflexes decrease in intensity and are eventually lost. Cognition remains intact throughout the course of this disease.

► Case Study 2-2

1. Does the patient exhibit a language or memory deficit or an alteration in consciousness or cognition?

Most of the deficits of language and cognition in this patient relate to the effects of alcohol intoxication and not to the traumatic injury.

2. Are signs of cranial nerve dysfunction present?

Cranial nerve functions are intact.

3. Are there any changes in motor functions such as reflexes, muscle tone, movement, or coordination?

The right lower extremity exhibits flaccid paralysis with absent deep tendon reflexes. The distal portion of the right upper extremity also presents with paralysis and loss of deep tendon reflexes. The presence of the scapulohumeral (C_{4-6}), biceps (C_{5-6}), and brachioradialis (C_{5-6}) reflexes suggests that the lesion is below C_6. This is confirmed by the diminution of reflexes at the triceps (C_{7-8}), wrist (C_{6-8}), and fingers (C_7-T_1).

4. Are any changes in sensory functions detectable?

Pain and temperature sensation are lost on the left side below the level of C_8. Discriminative touch and vibratory sense are lost on the right side of the body below C_8

5. At what level in the central neuraxis is this lesion most likely located?

The well-defined sensory level is the clue to the level in the spinal cord; it suggests that the lesion is localized between cord segmental levels C_7 and C_8.

6. Is the pathology focal, multifocal, or diffuse in its distribution within the nervous system?

This is a discrete focal lesion involving a single level of the spinal cord and the pronounced laterality in the patient's signs indicates that the lesion is restricted to one side (the right).

7. What is the clinical–temporal profile of this pathology: acute or chronic; progressive or stable?

Clearly, this lesion is acute, relating to the physical severing of half of the spinal cord due to the knife wound he received in the bar. The damage is stable and nonprogressive.

8. **Based on your answers to the previous two questions, decide whether the symptoms in this patient are most likely caused by a vascular accident, a tumor, or a degenerative or inflammatory process.**

Based on the patient's history, this is a traumatic process.

9. **If you feel this is the result of a vascular accident, what vessels were most likely involved?**

The primary cause of the pathology is nonvascular in nature.

10. **On follow-up, why is the patient's strength diminished on the right side when his deep tendon reflexes in these limbs are hyperactive?**

The spinal shock has worn off and the patient is expressing suprasegmental-level dysfunction or an upper motoneuron lesion. The knife has cut the right side of the spinal cord in the cervical enlargement; consequently, the limbs on the right side of the body have lost cortical and brain stem control over their spinal circuits. With the spinal circuits still active, the patient experiences elevated deep tendon reflexes, elevated muscle tone (spasticity), and loss of volitional control.

11. **Why were pain and temperature sensation lost on the left, whereas discriminatory touch and vibratory sense were lost on the right side of the body?**

Pain and temperature sensation are carried in large part by the anterolateral system, and its fibers cross the midline at the segmental level. Discriminative touch is handled by fibers in the dorsal column system (and dorsolateral fasciculus), whose fibers remain uncrossed until they reach the dorsal column nuclei in the caudal medulla. Thus, a lesion of one side of the spinal cord sections the pain and temperature fibers from the contralateral side and the discriminative touch fibers from the ipsilateral side.

12. **What is the significance of the presence of a Babinski sign?**

The sign of Babinski indicates the corticospinal tract or its cells of origin in the cerebral cortex have suffered damage. However, this observation alone does not tell you where the damage has occurred along the course of the corticospinal tract.

Comment

Central nervous system trauma and alcohol are frequent companions. Unfortunately, as this case illustrates, the long-term effects of this mixture often lead to catastrophic consequences. With careful neurologic examination, the anatomic site of a lesion of this type should be relatively easy to localize.

► Case Study 2-3

1. **Does the patient exhibit a language or memory deficit or an alteration in consciousness or cognition?**

Cognitive function and language are described as intact and appropriate and, as we will see, supratentorial structures remain unaffected in this disorder.

2. **Are signs of cranial nerve dysfunction present?**

Cranial nerve functions remain intact.

3. **Are there any changes in motor functions, such as reflexes, muscle tone, movement, or coordination?**

The major finding relates to the prominent atrophy, areflexia, and muscular fasciculations seen in the upper extremities, which implicate involvement of lower cervical and upper thoracic region motoneurons or their associated peripheral nerves (segmental-level dysfunction). Mild weakness and increased deep tendon reflexes are noted in the lower extremities, suggesting involvement of descending corticospinal tracts (suprasegmental-level dysfunction). The presence of elevated tendon reflexes and weakness strongly implies a central nervous system involvement in the lesion.

4. **Are any changes in sensory functions detectable?**

There is a characteristic capelike distribution of loss of temperature and pinprick sensation that extends out to the fingertips. Other sensory modalities remain intact. This implicates involvement of the pain and temperature fibers as they cross the midline in the ventral decussation. The posterior lateral funiculi remain unaffected at this stage of the disease. The absence of clinical signs below the upper extremities suggests that the anterolateral system is not involved in the lesion at the time of this examination.

5. **At what level in the central neuraxis is this lesion most likely located?**

The segmental level motor system damage and the distribution of the sensory loss suggest that this lesion involves the spinal cord at its lower cervical and upper thoracic levels.

6. **Is the pathology focal, multifocal, or diffuse in its distribution within the nervous system?**

The pathology is focal but extends across the midline and seems to extend for several segments along the longitudinal axis of the spinal cord.

7. **What is the clinical–temporal profile of this pathology: acute or chronic; progressive or stable?**

This pathology is progressive, with the history noting onset of weakness and sensory loss 3 years in duration.

8. **Based on your answers to the previous two questions, decide whether the symptoms in this patient are most likely caused by a vascular accident, a tumor, or a degenerative or inflammatory process.**

A focal progressive lesion suggests a process related to the presence of a tumor. This is true in this case if one considers the term *tumor* to imply a mass lesion (as opposed to a neoplasm). The case described is an example of syringomyelia and represents the effects of a slowly growing fluid-filled cyst, or syrinx, within the substance of the spinal cord.[4]

9. **If you feel this is the result of a vascular accident, what vessels were most likely involved?**

The pathology is nonvascular in nature.

10. **What features distinguish between flaccid and spastic paralysis?**

Both forms of paralysis present with diminished strength. Flaccid paralysis is typified by diminished deep tendon reflexes, hypotonic muscles, muscle fasciculations, and decreased resistance to passive motion; it indicates segmental-level dysfunction and can arise from central or peripheral lesions. Spastic paralysis features elevated deep tendon reflexes, hypertonic muscles, and increased resistance to passive motion; it indicates suprasegmental-level dysfunction, strongly suggesting central nervous system involvement.

11. **Which extremities in this patient illustrate signs of suprasegmental-level damage?**

Lower extremities have elevated deep tendon reflexes.

12. **Which extremities in this patient illustrate the signs of segmental-level damage?**

Upper extremities have decreased deep tendon reflexes with muscular fasciculations.

13. **How can the discriminative senses be intact in this patient while the nociceptive and thermal senses are diminished?**

These two sensory modalities can be separated, since they are processes through different channels (tracts), in different locations in the spinal cord. Discriminative senses are handled through the dorsal column system (and dorsolateral fasciculus) in the dorsal portion of the cord, and the nociceptive senses are carried in the anterolateral tract located in the anterolateral portion of the spinal cord.

Comment

This represents the classic presentation of a patient with the curious lesion referred to as syringomyelia (*syrinx,* in Greek, means "pipe" or "tube"). The disease involves the cavitation of the spinal cord, usually arising in the lower cervical portion of the cord with progressive expansion (proximally and distally) of a cystic structure within the substance of the cord. The cyst in typically located just ventral to the central canal and damages the ventral crossing fibers (pain and temperature) and the anterior horns (motoneurons), thus producing the classic symptoms described earlier. The nature of the cavitation remains poorly understood.

► Case Study 2-4

1. **Does the patient exhibit a language or memory deficit or an alteration in consciousness or cognition?**

He was awake and oriented with clear and meaningful speech. He was capable of giving a good history, suggesting unimpaired cognition.

2. **Are signs of cranial nerve dysfunction present?**

Cranial nerve functions appear to be intact.

3. **Are there any changes in motor functions, such as reflexes, muscle tone, movement, or coordination?**

There was a loss of muscle tone in the lower extremity, suggesting segmental-level damage to the ventral horn motoneurons or the peripheral nerves. Presence of altered muscle reflexes throughout the lower but not the upper extremity argues against a peripheral neuropathy or end organ disease.

4. **Are any changes in sensory functions detectable?**

There is a well-defined loss of sensation below T_{10}, which is restricted to pinprick and thermal sensation, suggesting damage to the anterior and lateral portion of the spinal cord. Preservation of vibratory and proprioceptive senses suggests the dorsal columns and dorsolateral fasciculus are intact.

5. **At what level in the central neuraxis is this lesion most likely located?**

The complete loss of sensation below T_{10}, coupled with the diminished tendon reflexes in the lower extremity, indicates a lesion of the spinal cord involving multiple segments below T_{10}. The preservation of dorsal column and dorsolateral fasciculus functions suggests the lesion is in the ventral portion of the cord.

6. **Is the pathology focal, multifocal, or diffuse in its distribution within the nervous system?**

Although this presentation is bilaterally symmetric, the well-defined sensory level suggests the lesion is restricted to a focal portion of the spinal cord.

7. **What is the clinical–temporal profile of this pathology: acute or chronic; progressive or stable?**

This pathology is of acute onset with a 2-day progression, after which it stabilized.

8. **Based on your answers to the previous two questions, decide whether the symptoms in this patient are most likely caused by a vascular accident, a tumor, or a degenerative or inflammatory process.**

The acute onset suggests a vascular accident in the spinal cord; the short progression to a stationary condition would indicate an infarction rather than a bleeding event.

9. **If you feel this is the result of a vascular accident, what vessels were most likely involved?**

The anterior spinal artery supplies the ventral and lateral portion of the spinal cord, and its infarction would affect the anterolateral tract and ventral horn, possibly including the corticospinal system. It would leave the dorsal columns and dorsolateral fasciculus largely intact.

10. **Provide an explanation for the sensory dissociation present below T$_{10rt}$.**

The vascular territory compromised by occlusion of the anterior spinal artery has affected the anterior white commissure and the anterolateral system; thus, pain and thermal sensation have been lost below T$_{10}$. The dorsal column system and dorsolateral fasciculus, containing the proprioceptive sense and discriminative touch, are serviced by the posterior spinal system and have survived this occlusive event.[4]

11. **What type of paralysis is being expressed in the lower extremity of this patient and what is its source?**

Muscle tone and reflexes were absent in the lower extremity; this is flaccid paralysis. It is derived from segmental-level damage to the ventral horn cells due to occlusion of the anterior spinal artery.

Comment

Infarction of the spinal cord is a relatively rare condition and almost always involves loss of anterior spinal artery supply. The underlying causes may reflect severe aortic atherosclerosis and/or dissection of an aortic aneurysm.

CHAPTER 3
MEDULLA

► Case Study 3-1

1. **Does the patient exhibit a language or memory deficit or an alteration in consciousness or cognition?**

The patient was awake and oriented, with appropriate memory and meaningful, clear speech.

2. **Are signs of cranial nerve dysfunction present?**

The patient had a full range of eye movements; however, he experienced diplopia and nystagmus on left lateral gaze. This suggests damage to the vestibular apparatus, nerve, or nucleus on the right side (peripheral vestibular syndrome). The mild loss of hearing bilaterally is most likely an age-related phenomenon. The ptosis and miosis in the right eye would also be consistent with a lesion occurring in the right dorsolateral quadrant of the medulla affecting the descending autonomic pathways from hypothalamus and brain stem to spinal cord (Horner's syndrome). The loss of pain from the right side of the face and loss of right corneal reflex could indicate trigeminal nerve or spinal trigeminal nucleus and tract damage on the right. It also could indicate damage to the ventral trigeminothalamic tract on the left; however, this is unlikely, since all other cranial nerve signs localize to the right side of the medulla. The hoarseness experienced by the patient could have arisen from compromised function of the vagal nuclei (nucleus ambiguus).

3. **Are there any changes in motor functions, such as reflexes, muscle tone, movement, or coordination?**

There are no changes in muscle reflexes; however, the patient did experience ataxia in the extremities on the right. This could indicate damage to the right side of the cerebellum or any of its three peduncles. The inferior cerebellar peduncle passes through the dorsolateral medulla in close juxtaposition with the spinal trigeminal nucleus and tract and the vestibular and cochlear nuclei and tracts. This peduncle carries the spinocerebellar axons from the extremities, and damage to it will present as ataxia, such as that seen in this patient.

4. **Are any changes in sensory functions detectable?**

The loss of pain sensation in the right face has been discussed; the patient also experienced decreased pain sensation from the left side of the body. This situation is known as alternating analgesia and is pathognomonic for lesions occurring in the dorsolateral medulla.

5. **At what level in the central neuraxis is this lesion most likely located?**

The involvement of cranial nerves suggests that the damage lies in the vicinity of the posterior cranial fossa. The specific involvement of cranial nerves VIII, IX, and X indicates the involvement of the medulla. The loss of pain sensation, despite preserved vibratory sense (medial lemniscus) and normal reflexes (pyramidal tract), suggests that the lesion is positioned laterally in the medulla (see Plates 8 to 13). The loss of nociception from the ipsilateral face and the contralateral body also strongly suggests a lesion in the lateral portion of the medulla or lateral medullary syndrome.

6. **Is the pathology focal, multifocal, or diffuse in its distribution within the nervous system?**

The process is focal, since the presentation is strongly lateralized and all the affected structures can be found in a circumscribed region of the lateral medulla.

7. ***What is the clinical–temporal profile of this pathology: acute or chronic; progressive or stable?***

    The hard neurologic signs are of rapid onset (acute); however, they were preceded by headaches over a period of several weeks.

8. ***Based on your answers to the previous two questions, decide whether the symptoms in this patient are most likely caused by a vascular accident, a tumor, or a degenerative or inflammatory process.***

    The rapid onset of neurologic signs and lack of additional progression indicate an infarctive vascular accident; this is consistent with the patient's prior history of hypertension.

9. ***If you feel this is the result of a vascular accident, what vessels were most likely involved?***

    The lateral medullary syndrome can result from occlusion of the vertebral artery or of one of its branches, such as the posterior inferior cerebellar artery (see Plates 8 to 13).

10. ***Explain the loss of pain and temperature sensation from the left side of the body but the right side of the face.***

    In the lateral medullary region, the anterolateral tract, carrying pain and temperature sensation from the contralateral side of the body, courses in close juxtaposition with the spinal trigeminal nucleus and tract, which carry pain and temperature sensation from the ipsilateral side of the face (see Plates 8 to 14). A lesion in this region, affecting these two structures, produces an alternating analgesia such as that present in this patient.

11. ***Explain the loss of pain sensation but not touch from the right side of the face.***

    Discriminative touch is processed in the chief sensory trigeminal nucleus of the pons; the sensation of pain and temperature are processed primarily in the spinal trigeminal nucleus of the medulla. A lesion in one tract will not necessarily compromise function in the other.

12. ***Offer an explanation for the presence of ataxia in the right extremities.***

    The ataxia experienced by this patient most likely stems from irritation or damage affecting the right inferior cerebellar peduncle in the medulla. This structure is carrying proprioceptive information from the spinal cord to the cerebellum (spinocerebellar tracts).

13. ***Damage to what medullary structure can account for the patient's (a) dizziness, (b) deviation of the uvula, or (c) hoarseness?***

    The dizziness most likely stems from irritation of the vestibular nerve or nuclei; deviation of the uvula from damage to the nucleus ambiguus or its radiations, which provide motor innervation to the muscles of the soft palate (levator veli palatini muscle and the musculus uvulae); and the hoarseness also stems from damage to the nucleus ambiguus, which provides motor innervation to the muscles of the pharynx and larynx.

Comment

The lateral medullary syndrome is a classic neurologic syndrome related to circumscribed (lacunar) infarction in a small, wedge-shaped area of the lateral medulla just dorsal to the inferior olivary nucleus. Although the posterior inferior cerebellar artery provides the blood supply for this region, careful dissection of a number of cases has revealed that the majority are related to localized occlusion of the vertebral artery itself.[5]

► Case Study 3-2

1. ***Does the patient exhibit a language or memory deficit or an alteration in consciousness or cognition?***

    This patient was awake, alert, and oriented; his language capability was appropriate, except for dysarthric speech. The dysarthria can be accounted for by damage to the lower motoneurons (segmental level) or their axons innervating the tongue, jaw, or pharynx and larynx and does not necessarily indicate a supratentorial lesion.

2. ***Are signs of cranial nerve dysfunction present?***

    The patient's tongue deviates to the left on attempted protrusion, suggesting damage to the left hypoglossal nucleus or nerve. The fasciculations present in the tongue help to confirm a segmental-level (lower motoneuron) lesion

3. ***Are there any changes in motor functions, such as reflexes, muscle tone, movement, or coordination?***

    He had elevated deep tendon reflexes and weakness in both right extremities, indicating a suprasegmental-level (upper motoneuron) lesion of the cerebral cortex or descending corticospinal tracts. This is confirmed by the presence of a Babinski response.

4. ***Are any changes in sensory functions detectable?***

    All sensory systems tested were intact.

5. ***At what level in the central neuraxis is this lesion most likely located?***

    The involvement of the hypoglossal nucleus/nerve suggests that damage occurred in or around the posterior cranial fossa. The presence of suprasegmental-level signs is pathognomonic for a central lesion; this information, combined with the hypoglossal paralysis, indicates a lesion of the medulla within the posterior cranial fossa (see Plates 8 and 9). The involvement of the corticospinal tracts indicates a medially placed lesion, and the lack of sensory deficits argues that the lesion is restricted to the ventromedial extreme of the medulla and has not damaged the medial lemniscus (see Plates 8 and 9). The lack of detectable damage to the medial lemniscus also suggests that this lesion involves the hypoglossal nerve and not the hypoglossal nucleus.

6. **Is the pathology focal, multifocal, or diffuse in its distribution within the nervous system?**

The lesion is focal, since it is unilateral and restricted to a circumscribed region of the medulla.

7. **What is the clinical–temporal profile of this pathology: acute or chronic; progressive or stable?**

The neurologic signs are of rapid onset (acute)

8. **Based on your answers to the previous two questions, decide whether the symptoms in this patient are most likely caused by a vascular accident, a tumor, or a degenerative or inflammatory process.**

The rapid onset of neurologic signs and lack of additional progression indicate a vascular accident most likely of an infarctive nature.

9. **If you feel this is the result of a vascular accident, what vessels were most likely involved?**

The signs and symptoms suggest involvement of the pyramid and the emerging hypoglossal fibers (see Plates 8 and 9). This area of the brain stem is perfused by the lateral branches of the anterior spinal artery caudally and median branches of the vertebral artery rostrally.

10. **Explain the presence of a cranial nerve palsy on the left side of the patient while extremity palsies were expressed on the right.**

The hypoglossal nerve exits the brain stem in close proximity to the pyramidal tract. This nerve innervates the muscles of the tongue on the ipsilateral side, whereas the pyramidal tract controls body musculature on the contralateral side. A unilateral lesion affecting these two structures produces alternating hemiplegia; the deficit is expressed in the ipsilateral cranial nerve functions and the contralateral body musculature. When the hypoglossal nerve is involved, this presentation is called inferior alternating hemiplegia. Similar syndromes occur involving the corticospinal tract and the abducens nerve of the pons (middle alternating hemiplegia) or the oculomotor nerve of the midbrain (superior alternating hemiplegia).

Comment

This is an extremely rare infarctive lesion referred to as medial medullary syndrome. When it occurs, it is generally related to occlusion of the vertebral artery with inadequate collateral flow from adjacent branches of the circle of Willis.

CHAPTER 4
PONS

► Case Study 4-1

1. **Does the patient exhibit a language or memory deficit or an alteration in consciousness or cognition?**

This patient was awake, alert, and oriented; his language capability was appropriate, except for dysarthria. This deficit can be accounted for by damage to the lower motoneurons or their peripheral nerves innervating the muscles of the tongue, face, jaw, or pharynx and larynx (segmental-level lesion) and hence does not necessarily indicate a supratentorial lesion.

2. **Are signs of cranial nerve dysfunction present?**

The patient experienced lateral gaze palsy to the left; this can result from supranuclear lesions in the right frontal eye fields of the cerebral cortex, the right corticonuclear fibers in the brain stem, the left paramedian pontine reticular formation (see Plate 14), or the left abducens nucleus; it cannot be accounted for by a lesion of the left abducens nerve alone. The response of the eyes to the doll's head maneuver and to caloric testing suggested that the segmental-level connections of this system involving the abducens nucleus are in-

tact. A left hemifacial paralysis (entire left side of the face) was present, indicating segmental-level damage to the facial nerve or nucleus on the left. Note that the paramedian pontine reticular formation is in close juxtaposition with the facial nucleus and the radiations of its nerve in the pons (see Plate 14). All other cranial nerve functions appeared intact.

3. **Are there any changes in motor functions, such as reflexes, muscle tone, movement, or coordination?**

There were elevated deep tendon reflexes in the right extremities, suggesting a suprasegmental-level (upper motoneuron) lesion, such as in the cerebral cortex or anywhere along the descending corticospinal tract; this notion was supported by the presence of a Babinski sign on the right.

4. **Are any changes in sensory functions detectable?**

All sensory systems tested were intact.

5. **At what level in the central neuraxis is this lesion most likely located?**

The cranial nerve involvement suggested the lesion was in or around the posterior cranial fossa. The suprasegmental-level signs (spastic paresis) of the extremities were pathognomonic for a lesion in the central nervous system. The left-sided hemifacial paralysis and left lateral gaze palsy suggested damage had occurred within the inferior pons on the left side.

6. ***Is the pathology focal, multifocal, or diffuse in its distribution within the nervous system?***

This lesion appeared to be unilateral and confined to the pontine region, suggesting it was not diffuse. The involvement of the facial nucleus or its radiations, the paramedian pontine reticular formation or its cortical afferent fibers, and the corticospinal tract could result from a focal lesion of one or several lateral penetrating arteries.

7. ***What is the clinical–temporal profile of this pathology: acute or chronic; progressive or stable?***

It was of rapid onset (acute) with stable follow-up.

8. ***Based on your answers to the previous two questions, decide whether the symptoms in this patient are most likely caused by a vascular accident, a tumor, or a degenerative or inflammatory process?***

The profile of this event was of rapid onset, with no significant progression, suggesting an infarctive vascular accident that has stabilized.

9. ***If you feel this is the result of a vascular accident, what vessels were most likely involved?***

The anterolateral or lateral penetrating vessels of the basal artery supply the territory of concern in this case.

10. ***Damage to what fiber tracts could produce right-sided weakness and hyperreflexia?***

Damage to the left corticospinal tract above its decussation at the cervicomedullary junction and to the right lateral corticospinal tract below the level of the pyramidal decussation could produce these symptoms. In this case it appeared to be the left corticospinal tract in the pons, based on the involvement of the cranial nerves.

11. ***Damage to what structure(s) could cause loss of volitional conjugate vision to the left without diplopia?***

Loss of volitional conjugate vision to the left can result from damage to several structures: the right frontal eye fields of cerebral cortex, the right corticonuclear fibers, the left paramedian pontine reticular formation, and the left abducens nucleus. Based on the doll's head and caloric testing, the abducens nucleus appeared to be intact in this patient.

12. ***Damage to what structure(s) could cause drooling from the left side of the mouth, left facial weakness, and inability to close the left eye completely?***

The left facial nerve or facial nucleus could result in these neurologic signs; damage to the corticonuclear fibers to the facial nucleus would not be expected to weaken the orbicularis oculi muscles significantly, because they receive bilateral corticonuclear input.

13. ***What are the possible explanations for the patient's failure to perform the finger-to-nose test on the right?***

The patient is unable to perform the test most likely because of the paralysis expressed in the right limbs as a result of damage to the left corticospinal tract in the pons. From this information it is not possible to evaluate the condition of the left pontine nuclei or left middle cerebellar peduncle.

Comment

Clinically, this is a most unusual case that is introduced primarily to demonstrate clinicopathologic relationships within certain regions of the pons. It is referred to as Foville's syndrome and presents with hemifacial paralysis, lateral gaze palsy, and crossed hemiparesis. It is due to an infarction of the long circumferential branches (lateral penetrating) of the basilar artery in the inferior pons.

In actual clinical practice most lesions involving the pons produce rapid alteration of consciousness (*i.e.,* involvement of the reticular activating system) and other vital functions and thus result in profound deterioration of neurologic function, which precludes subtle differentiation of regional distinctions in this area of the brain stem. The more typical infarctive lesion involving the pons is produced by ischemia in the distribution of the medial perforating arteries to produce midline pontine cystic infarctive lesions (so-called lacunar infarcts), which may either be silent or produce weakness related to involvement of descending corticospinal tracts. Lateral perforating artery occlusion in the pons is most unusual.

► Case Study 4-2

1. ***Does the patient exhibit a language or memory deficit or an alteration in consciousness or cognition?***

He is awake and oriented, with appropriate memory and language abilities.

2. ***Are signs of cranial nerve dysfunction present?***

He has a complete left hemifacial paralysis. He also has a hemianalgesia on the left side of his face and a partial hemianalgesia on the right side; this latter finding could result from damaging the spinal trigeminal tract or nucleus on the right (which is unlikely with the left-sided facial paralysis) or damaging the trigeminothalamic fibers on the left, after they had crossed the midline. The partial hemianalgesia is consistent with damage to the trigeminothalamic tract, because at this level it has a diffuse distribution.

3. **Are there any changes in motor functions, such as reflexes, muscle tone, movement, or coordination?**

Muscle strength and reflexes are normal in all limbs. He does, however, have ataxia in both extremities on the left; this could indicate damage in the left cerebellar hemisphere or its peduncles. The middle cerebellar peduncle is in close juxtaposition to the facial nucleus and nerve.

4. **Are any changes in sensory functions detectable?**

He has markedly diminished pinprick and thermal sense from the right side of the face, arm, trunk, and leg and the left side of his face. This suggests damage to the anterolateral, spinal trigeminal, and trigeminothalamic systems; these systems course in close proximity throughout the brain stem. However, below the pons, trigeminal representation is ipsilateral, whereas anterolateral representation is contralateral. At the pontine level, trigeminal representation, in the ventral trigeminothalamic tract, crosses to become contralateral, placing it in register with the anterolateral system. This man has damage to the anterolateral tract, spinal trigeminal nucleus or tract, and trigeminothalamic tract all on the left side of the brain stem.

5. **At what level in the central neuraxis is this lesion most likely located?**

The hemibody loss of pain and thermal sense suggests a central, rather than a peripheral, event. The damage most probably has occurred at or above the pontine level, since pain and thermal sense have been lost from the same side of the body. The involvement of the facial nucleus or its radiations argues for the caudal pontine level. The involvement of the middle cerebellar peduncle (ataxia) is consistent with this location.

6. **Is the pathology focal, multifocal, or diffuse in its distribution within the nervous system?**

The structures involved in this lesion—anterolateral system, ventral trigeminothalamic tract, facial nucleus or radiations, and middle cerebellar peduncle—are in close juxtaposition in the pontine brain stem; thus, the lesion appears to be focal.

7. **What is the clinical–temporal profile of this pathology: acute or chronic; progressive or stable?**

The event is of rapid onset (acute) and has stabilized.

8. **Based on your answers to the previous two questions, decide whether the symptoms in this patient are most likely caused by a vascular accident, a tumor, or a degenerative or inflammatory process.**

The acute, focal nature of this event suggests a vascular accident in the pons.

9. **If you feel this is the result of a vascular accident, what vessels were most likely involved?**

This event appears to have occurred in the lateral pons; the involvement of the facial nucleus or radiations makes this a lateral inferior pontine syndrome. The possible arterial sources for this lesion are the lateral branches of the basilar artery or the penetrating branches of the anterior inferior cerebellar artery.

Comment

As we noted in the comments to Case Study 4-1, examples of discrete lesions of this type are extremely uncommon in the pontine region. This case displays rather precise localization related to knowledge of structure and function in this complex area of the brain.

CHAPTER 5
CEREBELLUM

► Case Study 5-1

1. **Does the patient exhibit a language or memory deficit or an alteration in consciousness or cognition?**

Language function, cognition, and level of consciousness appear intact; the patient is capable of giving a coherent history.

2. **Are signs of cranial nerve dysfunction present?**

Nystagmus may indicate cranial nerve dysfunction; however, it may also reflect pathology in the cerebellar hemisphere itself. Clinically, nystagmus is not a particularly helpful localizing sign. All other cranial nerve functions tested seem to be intact.

3. **Are there any changes in motor functions, such as reflexes, muscle tone, movement, or coordination?**

Muscle reflexes remain intact and symmetric; the patient is normotensive. However, there are noticeable changes in the coordination of muscle groups. Although he has normal strength in his limbs, the timing of muscle contractions is faulty. Past-pointing, dysdiadochokinesia, dysmetria, and ataxia are the clinical signs of timing errors in muscle contractions.

4. **Are any changes in sensory functions detectable?**

Sensation also remains unaffected in this person.

233

5. **At what level in the central neuraxis is this lesion most likely located?**

Evidence of impaired finger-to-nose and heel-to-shin testing, inability to perform alternating movements in the right hand properly, broad-based gate, nystagmus on right lateral gaze, and a tendency to veer to the right (timing errors in muscle contractions) all suggest unilateral cerebellar hemisphere involvement (on the right side). The pathology appears confined to the cerebellum as cranial nerve, strength, and sensory function remain intact.

6. **Is the pathology focal, multifocal, or diffuse in its distribution within the nervous system?**

The unilateral signs and symptoms displayed in this patient, as described earlier, can result from a focal lesion of the cerebellum.

7. **What is the clinical–temporal profile of this pathology: acute or chronic; progressive or stable?**

The patient's symptoms have been of long duration and are continuing to worsen; the lesion is chronic and has had a progressive course.

8. **Based on your answers to the previous two questions, decide whether the symptoms in this patient are most likely caused by a vascular accident, a tumor, or a degenerative or inflammatory process.**

A focal lesion of this type with a chronic progressive course strongly suggests that the lesion is a tumor.

9. **If you feel this is the result of a vascular accident, what vessels were most likely involved?**

The pathology is of a nonvascular nature.

10. **What events can cause papilledema?**

Papilledema results from increase intracranial pressure such as can occur from a mass expanding lesions (tumor); it can also result from systemic hypertension.

11. **What is the significance of the absence of Romberg's sign? Is it consistent with the rest of the motor test?**

The absence of the Romberg sign suggests that the patient's neurologic signs do not originate in faulty sensory information (sensory ataxia) alone. Cerebellar damage can produce instability that is present, whether or not the eyes are open. Since it is the cerebellum that is damaged in this patient, one would not expect the signs to get significantly worse with sensory deprivation, such as closing the eyes.

Comment

This case represents the effects of a progressively expanding mass lesion in the right lateral hemisphere of the cerebellum. Half of all neoplasms in the brain represent metastatic spread to the nervous system of malignant lesions elsewhere in the body. Accordingly, one must first consider the possibility that this case represents a cerebellar metastasis from an occult primary. In view of this patient's relatively young age (36 years) this seems less likely, although certainly possible. Of primary neoplasms occurring in this region in a man of this age one should consider a cerebellar hemangioblastoma as the most likely diagnosis.

► Case Study 5-2

1. **Does the patient exhibit a language or memory deficit or an alteration in consciousness or cognition?**

The patient shows no deficit of language, consciousness, or cognition; her prolonged response time to questioning may be due to the amount of pain she is experiencing.

2. **Are signs of cranial nerve dysfunction present?**

There are no indications of cranial nerve dysfunction.

3. **Are there any changes in motor functions, such as reflexes, muscle tone, movement, or coordination?**

Muscle reflexes and strength are intact and symmetric. The patient is experiencing timing errors in the contraction of axial musculature (truncal ataxia); thus, she was unable to maintain posture while seated. This process seems to spare the limb muscles, since she did not exhibit past-pointing if her torso was supported and she only relied on her limb muscles.

4. **Are any changes in sensory functions detectable?**

Sensory function remains intact in the body and face.

5. **At what level in the central neuraxis is this lesion most likely located?**

The presence of timing errors in muscle contraction in the face of preserved sensorium in this case strongly suggests a cerebellar lesion. Supratentorial structures are intact, as are motor, sensory, and cranial nerve functioning. The lack of lateralizing signs, the presence of truncal ataxia, and increased intracranial pressure (blurred optic disks, headaches) suggest midline cerebellar involvement.

6. **Is the pathology focal, multifocal, or diffuse in its distribution within the nervous system?**

Although her neurologic signs are bilateral, she does not show any loss in sensory function. This argues against most diffuse processes. Her signs and symptoms can be accounted for by a focal lesion (or closely positioned multifocal lesions), extending across the midline in the cerebellum.

7. **What is the clinical–temporal profile of this pathology: acute or chronic; progressive or stable?**

The signs and symptoms experienced in this patient are of long duration and are worsening; the lesion is chronic and progressive in nature.

8. ***Based on your answers to the previous two questions, decide whether the symptoms in this patient are most likely caused by a vascular accident, a tumor, or a degenerative or inflammatory process.***

The focal, chronic, and progressive nature suggest the lesion represents a tumor occupying the midline cerebellum.

9. ***If you feel this is the result of a vascular accident, what vessels were most likely involved?***

The pathology is of a nonvascular nature.

10. ***What are some of the criteria for differentiating between limb and truncal ataxia?***

Limb ataxia presents with past-pointing, decomposition of movements, and slowing of rapid alternating motion; this ataxia is usually lateralized. Truncal ataxia involves postural instability when seated and affects axial muscle groups bilaterally. Both types of ataxia can produce gait dysfunctions.

11. ***What are some of the pathophysiologic mechanisms of nystagmus, and what is the diagnostic significance of nystagmus?***

Nystagmus can occur from damage to the temporal bone, vestibular nerve, vestibular nuclei and pathways, medial longitudinal fasciculus, cerebellum, and other regions in the brain stem. Nystagmus can take multiple, different forms: It can lateralize, being prominent only on lateral gaze, or it can be in the form of up- or down-beat nystagmus. It can also be rotary or bobbing, occurring equally in either direction. Lateral gaze nystagmus to one side is considered an indication of vestibular nerve or nuclear involvement. Up- and downbeat as well as rotary nystagmus can localize to the cerebellum; otherwise, nystagmus is considered to be a poor value as a localizing sign in clinical neurology.

Comment

This case represents the classic presentation of a relatively common childhood brain tumor, the medulloblastoma. This tumor arises in the midline cerebellum and typically fills the fourth ventricle. It is a particularly aggressive lesion that can grow rapidly and even spread along the cerebrospinal fluid pathways with multiple implants. It is commonly treated aggressively with surgery, chemotherapy, and radiation, but in most cases the tumor eventually recurs.

► Case Study 5-3

1. ***Does the patient exhibit a language or memory deficit or an alteration in consciousness or cognition?***

He is awake and oriented to time and place.

2. ***Are signs of cranial nerve dysfunction present?***

He has a left-beating nystagmus on left lateral gaze. This is a nystagmus with the fast (saccadic) phase to the left. Nystagmus can suggest damage to the vestibular

nerve or nuclei or damage to the cerebellum. The left pupil is smaller than the right, suggesting a mild Horner's syndrome. This is supported by the enlarged palpebral fissure on the left. The mild paresis of the lower right facial muscles suggests a supranuclear (suprasegmental) lesion involving the corticonuclear fibers to the facial nucleus.

3. ***Are there any changes in motor functions, such as reflexes, muscle tone, movement, or coordination?***

Strength and reflexes were physiologic in all extremities. However, he does have errors in timing muscle contractions in the left extremities. These take the form of ataxia, dysmetria, and intention tremor in the left arm and of a left pronator drift. These are signs of damage to the cerebellum or its peduncles.

4. ***Are any changes in sensory functions detectable?***

There was a loss of pinprick sensation of the right side of his body and face, suggesting damage to the anterolateral and trigeminothalamic tracts as they course together above the level of the medulla. All other sensory functions in this body seemed intact.

5. ***At what level in the central neuraxis is this lesion most likely located?***

The presence of timing errors in limb muscles on the left points to a lesion of the cerebellar hemisphere of the left. Based on cranial nerve dysfunction, the involvement of the brain stem in this lesion is obvious. Right-sided supranuclear facial paresis and associated loss of pinprick sensation from the right face and body point to damage in the mid- to upper pons on the left.

6. ***Is the pathology focal, multifocal, or diffuse in its distribution within the nervous system?***

The restriction of damage to a limited region of the cerebellum and brain stem as well as the lateralization of the neurologic signs suggests a focal lesion.

7. ***What is the clinical–temporal profile of this pathology: acute or chronic; progressive or stable?***

This processes had an acute onset and seems to have stabilized by the time of the interview.

8. ***Based on your answers to the previous two questions, decide whether the symptoms in this patient are most likely caused by a vascular accident, a tumor, or a degenerative or inflammatory process.***

The acute onset and stabilization with residual ataxia, dysmetria, and intention tremor are consistent with a cerebellar infarction occurring within the territory of one of the major cerebellar arteries.

9. ***If you feel this is the result of a vascular accident, what vessels were most likely involved?***

Separating the involvement of the different cerebral arteries is difficult at best. Each can present with nystagmus of various types; each can result in ataxia. Vertigo is less common with superior cerebellar arterial infarction than with either of the posterior cerebellar arteries.[6] In addition, intention tremor occurs more often with infarctions within the territory of the superior cerebellar artery than with the other two sources.[6] For these reasons, this is *most likely* an infarction within the territory of the superior cerebellar artery. This notion is supported by the specific cranial nerve signs. Supranuclear facial paresis, in register analgesia (body and face of the same side), and preserved hearing functions are indicative of superior cerebellar artery involvement. Alternatively, had the patient exhibited facial hemiparesis, alternating analgesia, and defective hearing, it would have been plausible to suggest anterior inferior cerebellar artery involvement in the lesion.

10. ***What are the neurologic signs and symptoms that would help differentiate infarction in any of the three cerebellar arterial systems?***

    I. Superior cerebellar artery
      A. Cerebellar territory
        1. Limb and gait ataxia
        2. Abnormal saccades
        3. Up-beating nystagmus
      B. Brain stem territory
        1. Transient chorea
        2. Loss of pain and temperature sensation from the contralateral face and body

        3. Horner's syndrome
        4. Contralateral supranuclear palsy
    II. Anterior inferior cerebellar artery
      A. Cerebellar (and middle cerebellar peduncle) territory
        1. Ataxia
        2. Dysmetria
      B. Brain stem territory
        1. Ipsilateral hemifacial palsy
        2. Ipsilateral multimodal trigeminal sensory loss
        3. Ipsilateral Horner's syndrome
        4. Analgesia over the contralateral body
        5. Deafness or tinnitus
        6. Lateral gaze palsy
        7. Vertigo, nausea, vomiting
        8. Nystagmus
    III. Posterior inferior cerebellar artery
      A. Cerebellar territory
        1. Rotary dizziness
        2. Nausea, vomiting
        3. Imbalance
        4. Nystagmus (horizontal and in both directions)
        5. Ataxia and dysmetria[7]
      B. Brain stem territory
        1. Infarction in the brain stem territory of the inferior posterior cerebellar artery presents with the signs and symptoms of a lateral medullary lesion (see Chap. 3).

CHAPTER 6
MIDBRAIN

► Case Study 6-1

1. ***Does the patient exhibit a language or memory deficit or an alteration in consciousness or cognition?***

She has not experienced any altered states of consciousness or syncopal episodes. She is alert and oriented, with articulate speech and memory. She was capable of giving a good history.

2. ***Are signs of cranial nerve dysfunction present?***

She has an external strabismus on the right side, with a drooping eyelid, suggesting a palsy of the third cranial nerve or nucleus. The normal pupil in this eye at first seem contrary to the presentation; however, the fascicles of the autonomics course medial to the general efferent fibers in the trajectory of the third nerve and could have been spared in this lesion. She also has a mild supranuclear defect in the facial nerve. This could be caused by irritation or injury of the corticonuclear fibers to the facial nucleus. The expression of this deficit is on the left, since the corticonuclear fibers to the facial nucleus have still not crossed at the midbrain

level. The third-nerve involvement suggests the locus of damage lies in the midbrain or along the third nerve; the preservation of the pupillary reflex indicated a central rather than a peripheral nerve lesion.

3. ***Are there any changes in motor functions, such as reflexes, muscle tone, movement, or coordination?***

There was a slight increase in the deep tendon reflexes of the lower extremity. This suggests that the corticospinal tract fibers have been irritated, possibly by edema in the surrounding tissue. In agreement with this assumption is the presence of a Babinski sign on the left and the loss of abdominal reflexes, also on the left. Although these signs could develop from a lesion of the corticospinal tract anywhere along its course, their occurrence along with third-nerve palsy suggests a central lesion of the midbrain affecting the corticospinal fibers in the cerebral peduncle.

4. ***Are any changes in sensory functions detectable?***

The lack of sensory loss is consistent with a midbrain lesion, since it is in this region of the brain stem that the sensory lemnisci move furthest away from the corticospinal tract.

5. At what level in the central neuraxis is this lesion most likely located?

A safe conclusion, given the preceding discussion, is that the lesion has involved the midbrain. The oculomotor palsy in the face of no sensory loss argues for a ventromedial position of the lesion rather than a dorsolateral one.

6. Is the pathology focal, multifocal, or diffuse in its distribution within the nervous system?

The signs and symptoms appear to be lateralized, suggesting that the lesion is focal in nature. This is supported by the observation that the oculomotor palsy and altered spinal reflexes can originate from a circumscribed region of the midbrain.

7. What is the clinical–temporal profile of this pathology: acute or chronic; progressive or stable?

This is of sudden onset (acute), and it appears to be stable.

8. Based on your answers to the previous two questions, decide whether the symptoms in this patient are most likely caused by a vascular accident, a tumor, or a degenerative or inflammatory process.

The rapid onset, stable nature, and focal distribution suggest a small infarction of the midbrain.

9. If you feel this is the result of a vascular accident, what vessels were most likely involved?

Plate 20 illustrates the curved nature of the anteromedial and anterolateral branches of the basilar artery. A perfusion deficit in either of these clusters of branches could compromise the function of the cerebral peduncle and radiation of the oculomotor nerve without damaging the major sensory lemnisci located more dorsolaterally on this section.

10. What brain stem structures, when damaged, can result in ptosis of the eyelid?

Ptosis can result from paralysis of the levator palpebrae and/or the tarsal muscles. Levator paralysis can result from damage to the oculomotor nucleus or nerve and forms a more extensive ptosis. Paralysis of the tarsal muscles can result from damage to the descending autonomic projections in the brain stem and spinal cord (Horner's syndrome).

11. Is the right eye paralysis consistent with the left-sided increase in deep tendon reflexes and Babinski sign?

The radiations of the third nerve pass in close juxtaposition to the corticospinal fibers in the cerebral peduncle. At this level the corticospinal fibers have not crossed the midline, so, when damaged, their deficit

will present on the contralateral side. This association of ipsilateral third-nerve palsy and contralateral spastic paresis is called superior alternating hemiplegia.

12. Is the loss of motor function consistent with the preservation of the sensorium?

The sensory lemnisci have moved dorsolaterally in the midbrain, whereas the corticospinal tracts have moved ventromedially (see Plates 18 to 20). At this level the separation between these tracts is the greatest of any position in the brain stem. As a consequence, it is possible to observe complete dissociation of sensory and motor function in small lesions of the midbrain.

► Case Study 6-2

1. Does the patient exhibit a language or memory deficit or an alteration in consciousness or cognition?

He is awake and oriented with appropriate memory and language abilities.

2. Are signs of cranial nerve dysfunction present?

The right eye is positioned down and out, with the pupil dilated compared to the left. This suggests damage to the oculomotor nucleus/nerve. All other cranial nerve functions were within normal limits.

3. Are there any changes in motor functions, such as reflexes, muscle tone, movement, or coordination?

A slight elevation of deep tendon reflexes was present on the left, compared to the right, suggesting some compromise of the corticospinal tract; this could be the result of tissue swelling the vicinity of the lesion. The intention tremor and ataxia in the left upper extremity indicated damage to the left cerebellum hemisphere or its peduncles. The dentothalamic fibers of the superior cerebellar peduncle decussate as they pass through the midbrain on their way to the thalamus (see Plate 19). Thus, damage to dentothalamic fibers after they cross the midline would present as ataxia on the side contralateral to the lesion.

4. Are any changes in sensory functions detectable?

The diminution of vibratory sense and proprioception on the left side of the body suggests damage to the left dorsal column system, right medial lemniscus, right thalamus, or somatic sensory cortex. To be consistent with the third-nerve involvement, the damage is most likely in the midbrain.

5. At what level in the central neuraxis is this lesion most likely located?

The sensory loss over one side of the body suggests that this is a central rather than a peripheral lesion. The oculomotor palsy directs attention to the midbrain. The medial lemniscus and dentothalamic fibers are in close proximity with the third nerve at this level of the brain stem (see Plates 19 and 20). All of these factors point toward a lesion occurring in the midbrain and involving, at least, its dorsolateral side.

6. **Is the pathology focal, multifocal, or diffuse in its distribution within the nervous system?**

   The lateralization of signs and symptoms suggest a focal lesion. The structures involved in this lesion (radiations of the third cranial nerve, medial lemniscus, and superior cerebellar peduncle) are in close juxtaposition in the midbrain (see Plates 19 and 20), supporting the notion that the lesion is focal.

7. **What is the clinical–temporal profile of this pathology: acute or chronic; progressive or stable?**

   The event is of rapid onset (acute) and has stabilized.

8. **Based on your answers to the previous two questions, decide whether the symptoms in this patient are most likely caused by a vascular** *accident, a tumor, or a degenerative or inflammatory process.*

   The acute, focal nature of this event suggests an infarctive event in the medial midbrain.

9. **If you feel this is the result of a vascular accident, what vessels were most likely involved?**

   The penetrating branches of the anterior choroidal artery, collicular arteries, and the posterior cerebral artery supply the area of concern in the lateral midbrain (see Plate 20). Infarction in this portion of the midbrain results in Benedikt's syndrome.

Comment

Benedikt's syndrome is another classical clinical syndrome that involves destruction of structures comprising the lateral aspect of the midbrain. The clinical presentation tends to be very stereotyped. Usually, Benedikt's syndrome is described without the involvement of the corticospinal tract. This patient, with the elevated deep tendon reflexes on the left and diminished strength on the left, is actually a slightly modified presentation of Benedikt's.

CHAPTER 7
THALAMUS

► Case Study 7-1

1. **Does the patient exhibit a language or memory deficit or an alteration in consciousness or cognition?**

   Although consciousness is not impaired, the patient shows considerable confusion and disorientation. The impairment of speech is likely related to supratentorial interruption of motor pathways involving the production of speech.

2. **Are signs of cranial nerve dysfunction present?**

   The patient shows a right homonymous hemianopia, indicating involvement of the optic tract, lateral geniculate nucleus, optic radiations, or visual cortex. The facial paralysis, described as a loss of movement during emotional expressions, suggests suprasegmental-level dysfunction rather than involvement of the cranial nerve VII nucleus or tract.

3. **Are there any changes in motor functions, such as reflexes, muscle tone, movement, or coordination?**

   The right-sided hemiparesis with a positive Babinski sign is indicative of upper motor (suprasegmental) impairment. This could reflect pressure from swelling on the internal capsule, especially since on follow-up the hemiparesis resolved in 6 weeks.

4. **Are any changes in sensory functions detectable?**

   Sensation is intact throughout the face and body except for proprioception of the right hand. This could reflect involvement of the medial lemniscus or of the ventroposterior lateral nucleus.

5. **At what level in the central neuraxis is this lesion most likely located?**

   The severely impaired cerebral function and the suprasegmental dysfunction involving the right extremities and facial musculature suggest that the lesion is supratentorial, either involving the left internal capsule and possibly the adjacent cortex and optic radiations or involving the anterolateral vascular territory of the thalamus. The presentation of confusion, neglect, paraphasia, and perseveration in the face of good repetition has been associated with lesions in the vicinity of the ventrolateral nucleus of the thalamus on the dominant side.[8] The presence of "emotion" facial paralysis has also been associated with supratentorial lesions in frontal cortex, thalamus, and basal ganglia.[9] The thalamic area associated with emotional facial expression lies in the anterolateral vascular territory. These observations, taken together, point to a thalamic lesion in the territory of the anterolateral vascular supply; however, cortical involvement cannot be ruled out.

6. *Is the pathology focal, multifocal, or diffuse in its distribution within the nervous system?*

The unilateral presentation of signs in this case suggest a focal lesion involving either thalamus or internal capsule, possibly both; however, multifocal lesions cannot be entirely ruled out.

7. *What is the clinical–temporal profile of this pathology: acute or chronic; progressive or stable?*

The onset of the pathology is acute, and the lesion appears stable.

8. *Based on your answers to the previous two questions, decide whether the symptoms in this patient are most likely caused by a vascular accident, a tumor, or a degenerative or inflammatory process.*

Because of the onset, course, and anatomic location, this disorder most likely is caused by a vascular lesion, such as an infarction.

9. *If you feel this is the result of a vascular accident, what vessels were most likely involved?*

The lesion is likely ischemic (infarctive) and could represent pathology involving portions of the distribution of the middle cerebral artery and posterior cerebral artery territories. However, in this particular case, the lesion was confined to rather extensive destruction of the anterolateral vascular territory of the thalamus[10] (see chart under Thalamic Blood Supply, Chap. 7). Because of the close relationship between cortical and thalamic functions, it can be difficult to make distinctions clinically in the location of cerebral infarctions in the supratentorial region.

10. *Destruction of what structures could account for the visual dysfunction seen in this patient?*

Damage to the optic tract on the lateral aspect of the thalamus, the lateral geniculate in the posterior thalamus, or the optic radiations as they leave the thalamus could all present with the visual dysfunction similar to that present in this patient. Damage to the visual area in the occipital lobe would most likely include some macular sparing and damage located in the optic radiations usually present with a quadrantanopia.

11. *Damage to what structures could account for the patient's paralysis?*

The decreased strength and increased deep tendon reflexes could be caused by damage to the internal capsule or cerebral cortex. If the vascular accident had occurred in the cerebral cortex, it would most likely have spared the foot, since this portion of the homunculus is served by the anterior cerebral artery. Discrete lesions of ventrolateral thalamus present with contralateral hypotonia, reduction in emotional expression, and transient neglect,[8] but they do not result in spastic paralysis.

12. *Damage to what thalamic structure(s) would provide an explanation for the impairment of memory?*

The mamillary bodies, mamillothalamic tract, parafascicular nucleus, and dorsomedial nucleus have been associated with memory functions, and their destruction has been reported with memory loss. Given the position of the lesion in this patient, the dorsomedial nucleus, its efferent axons, or the parafascicular nucleus is the most likely source of memory loss in this patient.

► Case Study 7-2

1. *Does the patient exhibit a language or memory deficit or an alteration in consciousness or cognition?*

The patient shows no evidence of an alteration of language, cognition, or consciousness. He did exhibit periods of rage, expressed at the hospital staff and physicians.

2. *Are signs of cranial nerve dysfunction present?*

The only cranial nerve dysfunction described is a bitemporal hemianopsia. This sign generally results from lesions impinging on the optic chiasm from the midline.

3. *Are there any changes in motor functions, such as reflexes, muscle tone, movement, or coordination?*

Muscle reflexes are intact and physiologic.

4. *Are any changes in sensory functions detectable?*

Sensory modalities, with the exception of vision, are intact throughout body and face.

5. *At what level in the central neuraxis is this lesion most likely located?*

The symptoms related to excessive thirst and polyuria (with a high volume of urine of a low specific gravity) all suggest hypothalamic dysfunction (diabetes insipidus) or possibly a lesion involving the posterior pituitary. The bitemporal hemianopsia suggests a midline lesion involving hypothalamus and optic chiasm. This observation is supported by the combination of loss of libido, short stature, poor thermoregulation, and erratic behavior.

6. *Is the pathology focal, multifocal, or diffuse in its distribution within the nervous system?*

Although the signs and symptoms of this patient are bilateral, they can be accounted for by a small lesion extending across the midline in a circumscribed region of the hypothalamus; thus, the lesion appears to be focal.

7. *What is the clinical–temporal profile of this pathology: acute or chronic; progressive or stable?*

The long-term loss of libido, repression of growth, and obesity coupled with his long history of diabetes insipidus suggests the course is chronic and progressive.

8. *Based on your answers to the previous two questions, decide whether the symptoms in this patient are most likely caused by a vascular accident, a tumor, or a degenerative or inflammatory process.*

The location, onset, and course of the illness all indicate that this is related to a tumor.

9. *If you feel this is the result of a vascular accident, what vessels were most likely involved?*

The pathology is nonvascular in nature.

10. *Destruction of what region(s) of the brain could result in obesity, excessive thirst, sexual dysfunction, and fluctuant temperature?*

A midline lesion of the hypothalamus can disturb the ventromedial hypothalamic nucleus, producing hyperphagia, and the paraventricular and supraoptic hypothalamic nuclei, diminishing the release of ADH and resulting in diuresis. The diminished sexual function is harder to explain; it may originate in the destruction of the arcuate nucleus (midline structure), resulting in the reduced levels of gonadotropin-releasing hormone.

11. *How can you explain the visual dysfunction in this patient?*

Expansion of the hypothalamic tumor ventrally would place pressure on the optic chiasm; the first fibers to falter would be the crossing tracts carrying the axons from the nasal retina with representation of the temporal visual field.

12. *Discuss the possible problems in "compliance" that this patient would have experienced had he lived.*

This is a broad discussion question, with no exact answer. The patient had not done much to take care of his health through the first 49 years of his life, so there is no compelling reason to suspect that he would be willing to begin at this time.

Comment

Although the clinical evidence presented makes it difficult to determine the specific origin of this tumor, the long history and prominent symptoms related to diabetes insipidus suggest that it arose in the midline hypothalamus. Although relatively uncommon, many kinds of tumors can arise in this location. Nevertheless, this tumor would likely grow slowly and produce pressure damage on the adjacent optic chiasm. In this setting, either a slow-growing astrocytoma (benign tumor of astrocytes) or an ectopic pinealoma would likely represent the pathologic diagnosis. Even for tumors of this type, the inordinately prolonged clinical history is unusual.

► Case Study 7-3

1. *Does the patient exhibit a language or memory deficit or an alteration in consciousness or cognition?*

In general, language, consciousness, and cognition are preserved. He does show, with special testing, a short-term visual memory deficit. There are two stages to the memory process: short term (seconds to minutes) and long term (hours to days). Short-term memory is a necessary step to obtain the long-term status. This patient had difficulty recalling design objects that were viewed several minutes before.

2. *Are signs of cranial nerve dysfunction present?*

Cranial nerve function remains intact.

3. *Are there any changes in motor functions, such as reflexes, muscle tone, movement, or coordination?*

The presence of myotonia and proximal muscle weakness undoubtedly relates to the patient's prior diagnosis of myotonic dystrophy. This is a form of muscular dystrophy that is unrelated to the patient's acute neurologic problem. (Students please note: Patients in teaching exercises typically have one and only one disorder. However, in real life, multiple conditions do appear, sometimes producing bizarre combinations of symptoms or masking symptoms that might otherwise be obvious. Just because you have a broken arm does not mean that you cannot catch a cold.) The finding of athetoid posturing of the left hand likely relates to ventrolateral thalamic involvement and is frequently called *thalamic hand.*

4. *Are any changes in sensory functions detectable?*

He has a prominent unilateral loss of pinprick, light touch, proprioception, vibration two-point discrimination, graphesthesia, and stereognosis. The involvement of the hemibody and face in this sensory loss argues against this being a cortical lesion and is consistent with representing a deafferentation of sensory input in the thalamus. Sensation can be perceived yet not interpreted precisely because of a lack of thalamic linkage to the neocortex. The abrupt boundary for sensory loss along the midline of the torso is also suggestive of a thalamic lesion.[11]

5. *At what level in the central neuraxis is this lesion most likely located?*

The loss of sensory input accompanied by the athetoid movements in the hand suggests that the lesion is localized to the posterior aspect of the thalamus involving sites for sensory input and relay to the cortex. Specifically, this would involve the ventroposterior and ventrolateral nuclei (see Plate 21). Also, the abrupt boundary for sensory loss along the midline of the torso is a characteristic of thalamic lesions, particularly those in the posterolateral vascular zone that involve the ventroposterior thalamic nuclei.

6. **Is the pathology focal, multifocal, or diffuse in its distribution within the nervous system?**

The lesion is focal, since it has prominent unilateral expressions and can be explained by damage to a circumscribed region of the thalamus, the posterolateral vascular zone.

7. **What is the clinical–temporal profile of this pathology: acute or chronic; progressive or stable?**

Based on the stated history, this problem is acute in onset and is stable in nature.

8. **Based on your answers to the previous two questions, decide whether the symptoms in this patient are most likely caused by a vascular accident, a tumor, or a degenerative or inflammatory process.**

This process relates to a vascular occlusion involving the supply of the posterior aspect of the thalamus.

9. **If you feel this is the result of a vascular accident, what vessels were most likely involved?**

This region is supplied by posterior choroidal and thalamogeniculate arteries, branches that arise off of the proximal posterior cerebral arteries (see Plate 21).

Comment

This case represents an example of a classical clinical syndrome referred to as *Dejerine-Roussy syndrome*. Originally described in 1906, it involves destruction of the ventrolateral posterior aspect of the thalamus, generally related to infarction of this region. The signs and symptoms are as described, although some cases may also experience a curious, and troubling, painful sensation related to the affected side of the body (so-called thalamic pain).

► Case Study 7-4

1. **Does the patient exhibit a language or memory deficit or an alteration in consciousness or cognition?**

The patient was disoriented, did not understand why she is in the hospital, and was agitated. She also had memory dysfunction and attempted to cover this through confabulation. Such signs typify damage to supratentorial structures. Her insomnia could be su-

pratentorial in origin; however, areas of the midbrain could also be involved.

2. **Are signs of cranial nerve dysfunction present?**

All cranial nerve functions appear to be intact.

3. **Are there any changes in motor functions, such as reflexes, muscle tone, movement, or coordination?**

The patient's strength and reflexes were normal.

4. **Are any changes in sensory functions detectable?**

No. All sensory systems tested were within normal range of limits.

5. **At what level in the central neuraxis is this lesion most likely located?**

The alterations in consciousness and memory functions suggest a supratentorial lesion. The triad of confusion, memory dysfunction, and insomnia have been reported as indicating the involvement of the anterior thalamus.[12] However, these deficits could also indicate involvement of the cingulate and prefrontal cortex. As an additional caveat, memory loss should be viewed with caution in any patient. Such loss can result from damage to the medial aspect of the temporal lobe. This is of special interest if the patient has experienced any periods of ischemia, since the temporal lobe (hippocampus) is easily affected by anoxia (see Chap. 9).

6. **Is the pathology focal, multifocal, or diffuse in its distribution within the nervous system?**

This question has become more difficult to answer with lesions in the supratentorial region. Infections or embolic showers can create numerous deficits, such as confusion, memory dysfunction, and insomnia. In addition, diffuse degeneration, such as that accompanying some forms of dementia, can present with this triad. The rapid onset of this process argues against dementia, degeneration, or infection. Lesions confined to the paramedian vascular territory of the thalamus have been reported to produce this triad in the face of no other localizing neurologic signs.[12]

7. **What is the clinical–temporal profile of this pathology: acute or chronic; progressive or stable?**

The presentation of agitation and confusion in this patient is of acute onset.

8. **Based on your answers to the previous two questions, decide whether the symptoms in this patient are most likely caused by a vascular accident, a tumor, or a degenerative or inflammatory process.**

The rapid onset with possible localization to one region of the thalamus favors a vascular origin to this process.

9. *If you feel this is the result of a vascular accident, what vessels were most likely involved?*

Based on studies by Castaigne and coworkers,[12] the triad of insomnia, confusion, and memory loss relate to an infarction in the paramedian territory of the thalamus. This involves the paramedian branches of the basilar artery that ascend into the thalamus along the midline.

10. *Is this patient exhibiting Alzheimer's syndrome? Why or why not?*

No. The rapid onset of the neurologic signs is not compatible with the degenerative nature of Alzheimer's disease.

CHAPTER 8
CEREBRAL HEMISPHERES: NEOCORTEX

► Case Study 8-1

1. *Does the patient exhibit a language or memory deficit or an alteration in consciousness or cognition?*

He has an aphasia characterized by decreased output and verbalizing with yes/no responses to most questions. However, he can understand written and spoken language. This constellation of signs suggests a motor (or Broca's) aphasia. It is seen in lesions of the inferior fronto-orbital cortex. This aphasia is also called *anterior aphasia* to distinguish it from the sensory (Wernicke's) aphasia seen in lesions *posterior* to the central sulcus. It is difficult to assess cognition and memory in this patient, given the severity of the language deficit; however, he does seem to recognize family members, suggesting some retrograde memory, and his ability to recognize hospital staff suggests that he retains some anterograde memory. Also, he is capable of following two- and three-step commands, suggesting that he still retains much of his memory and cognitive abilities.

2. *Are signs of cranial nerve dysfunction present?*

He has a weakness in the right lower quadrant of his face, suggesting a supranuclear (suprasegmental) lesion of the corticonuclear fibers to the facial nucleus. This can occur anywhere from the cerebral cortex to the upper border of the facial nucleus in the brain stem. The lack of any segmental-level cranial nerve signs coupled with the language deficit is most compatible with a supratentorial lesion (above the level of the midbrain).

3. *Are there any changes in motor functions, such as reflexes, muscle tone, movement, or coordination?*

There is an upper-limb hemiparesis with pronator drift. The hemiparesis is accompanied with a slight increase in deep tendon reflexes in the upper extremity. These signs are indicative of damage to the corticospinal tract. The sparing of the lower limb is compatible with the lesion occurring in the cerebral cortex.

4. *Are any changes in sensory functions detectable?*

Sensation to touch vibration, proprioception, and pain is decreased on the right arm and thigh. This could have occurred at any level where the medial lemniscus and anterolateral tract are in close juxtaposition (*e.g.,* the midbrain, thalamus, and cerebral cortex). The sparing of the lower limb is most compatible with the locus of damage occurring in the cerebral cortex.

5. *At what level in the central neuraxis is this lesion most likely located?*

The anterior (motor) aphasia, the sparing of the lower extremity in the hemiparesis, and the sensory loss are most compatible with the lesion being in the cerebral cortex. The sparing occurs since the lower extremity representation is serviced by a different blood supply from the upper extremity.

6. *Is the pathology focal, multifocal, or diffuse in its distribution within the nervous system?*

These unilateral signs could result from a focal lesion centered along the lateral precentral gyrus and spreading rostrally onto the premotor area of Broca. However, a multifocal event, such as a shower of emboli to the cerebral cortex, cannot be ruled out, although to be this confined in distribution is unlikely.

7. *What is the clinical–temporal profile of this pathology: acute or chronic; progressive or stable?*

The event is of rapid onset (acute), and it appears to be stable.

8. *Based on your answers to the previous two questions, decide whether the symptoms in this patient are most likely caused by a vascular accident, a tumor, or a degenerative or inflammatory process.*

The focal distribution with acute onset and stable nature suggests an infarctive vascular event.

9. *If you feel this is the result of a vascular accident, what vessels were most likely involved?*

The middle cerebral artery services the lateral aspect

of the cerebral hemispheres. The regions of the central sulcus and precentral gyrus are usually supplied by the upper division of the middle cerebral artery.

10. ***Is the sparseness of spontaneous speech consistent with the retention of comprehension?***

The portion of the cerebral cortex most often associated with comprehension of speech is Wernicke's area located at the parieto-occipitotemporal angle. This is supplied by the lower division of the middle cerebral artery. The motor area for speech is most often associated with the inferior fronto-orbital (Broca's) portion of cortex, supplied by the upper division of the middle cerebral artery. Given the separate blood supplies, it is possible to have isolated lesions in either of the two regions.

11. ***Explain the increased paresis in the upper extremity over that of the lower extremity.***

The representation of upper and lower extremities is supplied by different cerebral arteries. The upper extremity is supplied by the middle cerebral artery, and the lower extremity is supplied by the anterior cerebral artery. Disassociation of function can occur with cortical lesions in one or the other blood supplies. However, it should be noted that large lesions in the territory of the anterior cerebral artery can also damage the white matter under the precentral gyrus and produce deficits in the motor activity of the upper extremity and lower quadrant of the face (see Case Study 8–2).

► Case Study 8-2

1. ***Does the patient exhibit a language or memory deficit or an alteration in consciousness or cognition?***

Although he was awake and cooperative, he was disoriented. He demonstrated signs of a motor aphasia, except that he retained the ability to repeat carefully even complicated phrases. This is called *transcortical motor aphasia*. He also had poor comprehension of spoken or written language, a characteristic of a *transcortical sensory aphasia*. The combination of motor speech, poor comprehension, and repetition is then referred to as *mixed transcortical aphasia*. The transcortical aphasias are related to the supplementary sensory and motor portions of the cerebral cortex, located at the medial aspect of the central sulcus.

2. ***Are signs of cranial nerve dysfunction present?***

He had two possible signs of supranuclear lesions affecting the cranial nerves. His eyes tended to rest slightly to the left, suggesting a lesion of the left frontal eye fields or their corticonuclear fibers. The right lower quadrant of his face was mildly weak, suggesting a lesion or irritation of the cortical facial representation or its efferent fibers on the left.

3. ***Are there any changes in motor functions, such as reflexes, muscle tone, movement, or coordination?***

The patient showed signs of a right hemiparesis, more so in the leg than in the arm. The elevated deep tendon reflexes suggest that this is a supranuclear lesion. Such a lesion could occur at any level above the ventral horn of the spinal cord; however, the sparing of the arm over the leg is suggestive of a lesion in the leg representation at the cerebral cortical level. This is also consistent with the presence of the Babinski sign on the right. He also was incontinent for urine and feces and was aware of this problem. Incontinent with awareness can result from lesions to the anteromedial aspect of the cingulate gyrus.

4. ***Are any changes in sensory functions detectable?***

There seem to be changes in the sensorium; however, these are difficult to assess because of the patient's mental status and limited communication skills. Significantly, there is evidence of decreased sensory functions in the right leg, consistent with the altered muscle reflexes.

5. ***At what level in the central neuraxis is this lesion most likely located?***

The transcortical motor and sensory aphasias are known to occur in a halo surrounding the areas representing speech and comprehension, respectively. Damage to the area in between (frontoparietal junction, medially) results in a mixed transcortical aphasia. This, along with the selective change in muscle reflexes and sensorium from the leg, points to a lesion of the cerebral cortex (supratentorial lesion).

6. ***Is the pathology focal, multifocal, or diffuse in its distribution within the nervous system?***

The area associated with mixed transcortical aphasia is in close juxtaposition with the leg representation in the motor and sensory maps of frontal and parietal cortex. The neurologic signs are compatible with a focal lesion; however, a closely arranged series of multifocal events cannot be ruled out.

7. ***What is the clinical–temporal profile of this pathology: acute or chronic; progressive or stable?***

This event is of rapid onset and appears to have stabilized with a protracted period of unconsciousness.

8. ***Based on your answers to the previous two questions, decide whether the symptoms in this patient are most likely caused by a vascular accident, a tumor, or a degenerative or inflammatory process.***

The clinicotemporal profile is compatible with that of a supratentorial hemorrhage or infarction; however, based on the available clinical information, an infarctive lesion is much more likely.

9. If you feel this is the result of a vascular accident, what vessels were most likely involved?

The focal region of concern is supplied by branches of the anterior cerebral artery.

Comment

CT scan of the patient demonstrated a large infarction in the territory of the anterior cerebral artery, producing damage in the supplementary motor and sensory areas as well as in

the medial extreme of the central sulcus. Surgery performed on this patient demonstrated a ruptured aneurysm in the left anterior cerebral artery, producing a large infarcted zone distal to the aneurysm. Infarctions in the distribution of the anterior cerebral artery are typically related to thromboembolic occlusion rather than to thrombosis/ischemia underlying localized atherosclerosis. In this instance, the occlusion was likely related to inadvertent clipping of the anterior cerebral artery or to severe vasospasm of the vessels distal to the aneurysm.

CHAPTER 9
CEREBRAL HEMISPHERES: LIMBIC LOBE

► Case Study 9-1

1. Does the patient exhibit a language or memory deficit or an alteration in consciousness or cognition?

He experiences episodic loss of consciousness that coincide with his seizures. This is accompanied by automatic behaviors, olfactory hallucinations, and disoriented thoughts. At the time of the examination he is awake and oriented with respect to time and place and has appropriate language and memory functions.

2. Are signs of cranial nerve dysfunction present?

Cranial nerve functions were intact.

3. Are there any changes in motor functions, such as reflexes, muscle tone, movement, or coordination?

His motor system was intact.

4. Are any changes in sensory functions detectable?

There were no detectable deficits in somatic visual or auditory sensory functions; however, before the seizures he experienced olfactory hallucination consisting of foul odors.

5. At what level in the central neuraxis is this lesion most likely located?

The episodic loss of consciousness in the face of no cranial nerve, motor, or neosensory losses suggests a supratentorial event that has not affected the primary motor or sensory areas of the cerebral cortex. The olfactory hallucinations point to seizures that have originated from the temporal lobe on the right side; this is supported by the EEG findings.

6. Is the pathology focal, multifocal, or diffuse in its distribution within the nervous system?

The problem seems to involve periodic seizures that arise from an irritable focus in the right temporal lobe. Thus, a diffuse process is not likely; however, multifocal or clusters foci cannot be ruled out.

7. What is the clinical-temporal profile of this pathology: acute or chronic; progressive or stable?

The prime cause of the irritable focus in the temporal lobe may have been a traumatic experience; however, this is not provable with the available data. Consequently, it cannot be determined when this lesion began. It is obvious from the history that it is an ongoing process and thus chronic. The recent increase in the severity of the seizures suggests a progressive nature to the process (see comment). Posttraumatic seizures that occur within minutes to days after an event are usually transient. Delayed posttraumatic seizures can occur within 6 to 18 months of the event; as such, this group is not transient.

8. Based on your answers to the previous two questions, decide whether the symptoms in this patient are most likely caused by a vascular accident, a tumor, or a degenerative or inflammatory process.

In light of the history, this process most likely was initiated by a traumatic event. However, it could also arise from vascular degenerative, or toxic origins, or it could be a congenital process.[13]

9. If you feel this is the result of a vascular accident, what vessels were most likely involved?

It is not the result of a vascular accident. The seizure disorder displayed by this patient is likely related to disruption of the cerebral cortical architecture related to the healing of a superficial traumatic lesion (or lesions).

10. What is the source of the patient's olfactory hallucinations?

Irritation of the primary olfactory cortex near the focus of the lesion can cause the sensation of olfactory stimuli.

11. What is an aura? What is an automatism?

An aura is a hallucinatory sensory experience preceding the seizure. An automatism is a motor sequence executed automatically by the patient. It is not possible to suppress automatisms voluntarily.

12. *What is meant by consciousness? When is a patient considered unconscious?*

Clinically, consciousness is considered a state of functional activity in the brain. It is not an all-or-none event; instead, it is measured in degrees. A scale of consciousness has been defined for use in evaluating patients. Unconsciousness is not a well-defined clinical term. Five general levels of consciousness have been recognized: (a) alertness, (b) lethargy or somnolence, (c) obtundation, (d) stupor or semicoma, (e) coma.[14]

13. *Develop a short classification scheme for seizures.*

An internationally accepted scheme for the classification of seizures is available. See Delgado-Escueta.[15]

Comment

There are a wide range of underlying causes of seizures. An important clinical consideration is the age of the patient at the initiation of clinical symptomatology. Neonatal or childhood seizures may be related to metabolic derangements (such as hypoglycemia or hypocalcemia), congenital malformations, inherited metabolic defects, or meningitis. Adult-onset seizures may also reflect underlying hereditary disorders, infection (*e.g.,* brain abscess, viral encephalitis), and the remote effects or brain trauma. Approximately 5% of all cases of head trauma admitted to a hospital result in post-traumatic epilepsy. Many cases of epilepsy are of unknown etiology. Finally, in cases of seizures arising in later life (more than 50 years), intracerebral neoplasms (both primary brain tumors and metastatic lesions) represent a very common underlying etiology.

► Case Study 9-2

1. *Does the patient exhibit a language or memory deficit or an alteration in consciousness or cognition?*

He had a dense amnesia. He was disoriented with respect to time and place and did not know why he had been in the hospital or any of the history of his current illness. Yet his knowledge of events prior to his current illness was intact. This is particularly evident with sparing of some of his knowledge of American history, whereas he is unable to name the current president or to recall any of the recent (past 4 years) political events. This suggests preserved retrograde memory with loss of anterograde memory; hence, he is presenting with anterograde amnesia.

2. *Are signs of cranial nerve dysfunction present?*

The diminution of hearing is most likely age-related and not a product of his postsurgical anoxia.

3. *Are there any changes in motor functions, such as reflexes, muscle tone, movement, or coordination?*

He had a mild spastic paralysis expressed on the left, in both extremities. Although this could result from any location along the corticospinal tract, when it is coupled with the anterograde amnesia, it suggests that the anoxic event affected the motor cortex on the right.

4. *Are any changes in sensory functions detectable?*

There is a mild diminution of proprioception and vibratory sense in the left extremities, and he is experiencing paresthesias on the left as well. The sensory loss is in register with the motor dysfunction. This suggests that the postsurgical anoxic event involved both sides of the central sulcus on the right.

5. *At what level in the central neuraxis is this lesion most likely located?*

This lesion has produced severe anterograde amnesia, with mild lateralized sensory and motor losses. The amnesia suggests a supratentorial event. The colateralization of the motor and sensory loss suggests the area around the central sulcus or the cerebral cortex or internal capsule (supratentorial), since axons mediating these modalities are closely associated at this level.

6. *Is the pathology focal, multifocal, or diffuse in its distribution within the nervous system?*

The history of this patient includes several long periods of anoxia or hypoxia caused by cardiac arrest. Anoxia suggests a zone of ischemia has developed in response to the decreased perfusion. The presentation is consistent with several lesions developing throughout the cerebrum. The fact that he did not have a presurgical history of neurologic signs and symptoms suggests that the sensory and motor dysfunctions as well as the anterograde amnesia are related to one or more of the anoxic periods suffered during the surgery and recovery. The frontoparietal cortical junction of the right or the internal capsule on the right would account for the hard neurologic signs. Damage to several areas in the brain—midline thalamus, mamillothalamic tracts, entorhinal cortex, or hippocampus—is suspected of producing anterograde amnesia. However, recent reports have demonstrated that the hippocampus is very susceptible to anoxic periods, and its damage results in severe anterograde amnesia. Thus, the pathology appears to be multifocal ischemic zones developed consequent to anoxia of cardiopulmonary failure.

7. *What is the clinical–temporal profile of this pathology: acute or chronic; progressive or stable?*

The onset of the primary cause (anoxia) was acute; the problem has become stable and chronic.

245

8. ***Based on your answers to the previous two questions, decide whether the symptoms in this patient are most likely caused by a vascular accident, a tumor, or a degenerative or inflammatory process.***

The most likely explanation is an ischemic process occurring in the cerebrum consequent to anoxia, unrelated to any specific blood vessel.

9. ***If you feel this is the result of a vascular accident, what vessels were most likely involved?***

See answer to question 8.

10. ***What are the major regions of the central nervous system involved in memory?***

Almost all regions of the supratentorial cerebrum are involved in the processing or storage of memory. Areas with more salient roles in this process are the hippocampus, amygdala, entorhinal cortex, cingulate cortex, prefrontal cortex, and midline thalamus (dorsomedial nucleus, mamillothalamic tract, mamillary bodies, anterior nucleus).

11. ***What criteria will assist in distinguishing between retrograde and anterograde amnesia?***

Retrograde amnesia is loss of recall of events that predate a specific accident, whereas anterograde amnesia involves the loss of recall of events occurring since a specific event. Usually, anterograde amnesia will also present with a short period of retrograde memory loss centered around the precipitating accident.

Comment

There is growing interest in the neuroanatomic substrate of memory. Based primarily on clinical observation of patients with deficits in some aspects of memory functioning, the importance of the hippocampus, mamillary bodies, and midline thalamus has been recognized. It is increasingly clear that a complex function such as memory must employ many other areas of the brain, and one is cautioned about making specific statements regarding correlations of memory deficits to damage of isolated regions of the brain in any individual patient, as the extent of damage is generally rather widespread and diffuse.

► Case Study 9-3

1. ***Does the patient exhibit a language or memory deficit or an alteration in consciousness or cognition?***

He was confused and disoriented, with a marked inability to recall recent events—anterograde memory loss. He had also experienced periods of global amnesia in the past 24 hours. He could not recall his name or age but had some limited recall of the more distant past. He was alexic but not agraphic and had an ano-

mia for visual objects and colors. He could do simple calculations and follow two- and three-step commands.

2. ***Are signs of cranial nerve dysfunction present?***

He had a right homonymous hemianopia. His cranial nerve functions were otherwise intact.

3. ***Are there any changes in motor functions, such as reflexes, muscle tone, movement, or coordination?***

His motor system was intact.

4. ***Are any changes in sensory functions detectable?***

There were no detectable changes in somatic sensation. He did experience visual and olfactory hallucinations.

5. ***At what level in the central neuraxis is this lesion most likely located?***

The anterograde memory loss, alexia without agraphia, and color and object anomia all suggest a supratentorial lesion. This is supported by the presence of a homonymous visual field cut affecting the upper left. This deficit could be caused by a lesion anywhere between the optic chiasm and the cerebral cortex. However, since it is not a complete homonymous hemianopsia, it most likely is above the thalamus and on the right. The visual and olfactory hallucinations suggest damage to the temporal lobe.

6. ***Is the pathology focal, multifocal, or diffuse in its distribution within the nervous system?***

The left visual field cut and sensory hallucinations could arise out of a focal lesion of the right inferior temporal lobe. Alexia without agraphia is pathognomonic for the dominant occipital cortex involving the splenium of the corpus callosum. Involvement of the hippocampus (and entorhinal cortex) in this process could account for the anterograde memory loss.

7. ***What is the clinical–temporal profile of this pathology: acute or chronic; progressive or stable?***

The process was acute in onset and had apparently stabilized by the time of the examination.

8. ***Based on your answers to the previous two questions, decide whether the symptoms in this patient are most likely caused by a vascular accident, a tumor, or a degenerative or inflammatory process.***

The history is most compatible with a vascular event that has infarcted the inferior temporal lobe on the right, damaging the hippocampus and splenium of the corpus callosum as well.

9. ***If you feel this is the result of a vascular accident, what vessels were most likely involved?***

Branches of the anterior choroidal and posterior cerebral arteries supply this area. The anterior choroidal arteries are well covered with anastomosis. Thus, their

occlusion usually does not create large deficits. The branches of the posterior cerebral artery are the most likely culprits. This conclusion is supported by the involvement of the callosal branch of the posterior cerebral to the splenium of the corpus callosum.

CHAPTER 10
CEREBRAL HEMISPHERES: BASAL GANGLIA

► Case Study 10-1

1. ***Does the patient exhibit a language or memory deficit or an alteration in consciousness or cognition?***

The patient has experienced a change in mentation and in emotional state, yelling at fellow employees and making inappropriate comments to staff workers. He also is disoriented with respect to time and place and has become less dependable in the workplace. These changes in personal habits and behavior could reflect an organic disease process. However, the apparent lack of mathematical skills could well be a product of his truncated education.

2. ***Are signs of cranial nerve dysfunction present?***

His cranial nerve functions are intact.

3. ***Are there any changes in motor functions, such as reflexes, muscle tone, movement, or coordination?***

Limb strength was normal; however, he was slightly hypotonic, and his limbs appeared slack when not in motion. The deep tendon reflexes were slightly depressed, but the tendon taps were pendulent. He clearly was presenting with a movement disorder; the constant, jerky motion in the limbs is typical of a chorea. The insidious onset, his denial of the motion, and his attempts to hide involuntary movement with a more purposeful motion can occur in Huntington's disease. The cessation of involuntary movement with sleep, seen in this patient, is also typical of Huntington's disease.

4. ***Are any changes in sensory functions detectable?***

Note that movement disorders confined to the basal ganglia usually do not present with sensory loss. Sensory loss can present in unilateral basal ganglia movement disorders if the lesion has involved the internal capsule or thalamus.

5. ***At what level in the central neuraxis is this lesion most likely located?***

The gradual onset of an involuntary movement disorder consisting of continuous jerky movements superimposed on a background of writhing motions and

altered personality in the presence of no sensory loss is strongly suggestive of chorea such as that seen in Huntington's disease. Unfortunately, his family history does not allow confirmation of this diagnosis, since the father and grandparents either died young without expressing the disease or were not seen by a physician. The paternal grandfather's death is suspicious but lacks confirmation that it was related to a movement disorder.

6. ***Is the pathology focal, multifocal, or diffuse in its distribution within the nervous system?***

The presentation is bilaterally symmetric and involves the upper and lower limbs, suggesting a diffuse process.

7. ***What is the clinical–temporal profile of this pathology: acute or chronic; progressive or stable?***

This is of insidious onset. It is chronic, since it has lasted for months, and is progressive, since it seems to be getting worse.

8. ***Based on your answers to the previous two questions, decide whether the symptoms in this patient are most likely caused by a vascular accident, a tumor, or a degenerative or inflammatory process.***

The diffuse distribution, gradual onset, chronic duration, and progressive nature of the disease suggests a degenerative process

9. ***If you feel this is the result of a vascular accident, what vessels were most likely involved?***

The pathologic process is not of vascular origin.

10. ***What are the possible links between the patient's mental status and his motor disorder?***

The basal ganglia have long been known for their role in the modulation of motor activity, and degenerative diseases of these nuclei result in motor disorders of hypo- or hyperfunction. More recently, parallel circuits through the basal ganglia have been described that target the parietal, prefrontal, and cingulate cortex rather than the motor cortex. These circuits are believed to underlie a role for the basal ganglia in the modulation of cognitive thought processes and emotional behavior. These circuits utilize parallel structures and neurochemistry. Consequently, degenerative diseases of the basal ganglia would be expected to demonstrate inappropriate scaling of behavioral and cognitive functions similar to the inappropriate scaling that characterizes the disorders of the motor circuits.

11. ***Describe the pathophysiology of this disease in terms of the possible neural circuitry involved.***

A possible scenario for the pathophysiology of Huntington's disease is as follows:

The caudate and putamen demonstrate progressive loss of neurons in Huntington's disease. It has been shown that the acetylcholine neurons and the GABA/enkephalinergic neurons are affected the most in this loss. This would have the effect of reducing the outflow of the *indirect pathway* through the basal ganglia (see Fig. 10-5). The inhibitory influence of the striatum on the external segment of the globus pallidus would decrease, consequently increasing the external pallidal segment's inhibition of the subthalamic nucleus. Inhibition of the subthalamic input would thus allow greater inhibition of the internal segment by the *direct pathway*, creating an imbalance between the two systems.

With the indirect pathway turned down, the internal segment of the globus pallidus would no longer be excited by the subthalamic nucleus and, subsequently, could not express its inhibition on the ventral nuclei of thalamus. The release of inhibition of ventrolateral thalamus allows greater stimulation of the motor cortex. The end results are the release of hyperkinetic motor patterns such as those seen in Huntington's disease.

► Case Study 10-2

1. ***Does the patient exhibit a language or memory deficit or an alteration in consciousness or cognition?***

Other than the reduced volume in his speech he is not demonstrating any cognitive, memory, or language dysfunctions. However, he does demonstrate micrographia, which can present in Parkinson's disease.

2. ***Are signs of cranial nerve dysfunction present?***

His cranial nerve functions are intact.

3. ***Are there any changes in motor functions, such as reflexes, muscle tone, movement, or coordination?***

His strength and reflexes were within the normal range for a man of his age. He had a pronounced movement disorder consisting of bradykinesia, resting tremor, retropulsion, and postural embarrassment. This constellation of neurologic signs and symptoms is pathognomonic for Parkinson's disease.

4. ***Are any changes in sensory functions detectable?***

His sensory systems are intact (see question 4 in Study Case 10-1 for further comment).

5. ***At what level in the central neuraxis is this lesion most likely located?***

Movement disorders in the face of preserved strength and reflexes suggest the locus of damage involved the cerebellum, basal ganglia, or their connections, especially those in and around the thalamus. In this case, the disorder is one of intensity scaling rather than the timing of contractions, thus pointing to the basal ganglia. The diminished scale of movement (bradykinesia) with resting tremor, retropulsion, and postural embarrassment suggests Parkinson's disease, resulting from a loss of neurons in the substantia nigra of the midbrain.

6. ***Is the pathology focal, multifocal, or diffuse in its distribution within the nervous system?***

As Parkinson's disease progresses, the loss of neurons in the substantia nigra is usually bilateral, although it can initially present unilaterally. In addition, abnormal neuronal loss is seen in other nuclei of the brain: locus coeruleus, dorsal motor nucleus of the vagus, and basal forebrain areas. (Reviewed in Matzuk and Saper[16] and in Nakano and Hirano.[17]) Thus, this is a widespread, bilaterally symmetric or diffuse process.

7. ***What is the clinical–temporal profile of this pathology: acute or chronic; progressive or stable?***

This is a chronic, progressive disease.

8. ***Based on your answers to the previous two questions, decide whether the symptoms in this patient are most likely caused by a vascular accident, a tumor, or a degenerative or inflammatory process.***

The chronic, progressive, and diffuse properties characterize a degenerative process.

9. ***If you feel this is the result of a vascular accident, what vessels were most likely involved?***

The pathologic process is of nonvascular origin.

10. ***Describe the pathophysiology of this disease in terms of the possible neural circuitry involved.***

Parkinson's disease involves the degeneration of dopamine-producing neurons in the substantia nigra and the loss of dopamine-containing fibers in the corpus striatum. Normally, dopamine is excitatory to the direct pathway and inhibitory to the indirect pathway (see Fig. 10-5). With the loss of dopaminergic input, the balance between the indirect and direct pathway tips in favor of the indirect. Increased activity in the indirect pathway will excite the internal segment of the globus pallidus, thus increasing the inhibition on the ventrolateral nuclei of thalamus. The reduced output from ventrolateral thalamus to neocortex is one possible mechanism for producing the bradykinesia of Parkinson's disease.

► Case Study 10-3

1. ***Does the patient exhibit a language or memory deficit or an alteration in consciousness or cognition?***

   The patient's language skills, consciousness, and cognitive skills are intact.

2. ***Are signs of cranial nerve dysfunction present?***

   Although the examination is complicated by her movement disorder, there do not seem to be any detectable deficits involving the cranial nerve functions.

3. ***Are there any changes in motor functions, such as reflexes, muscle tone, movement, or coordination?***

   There could well be some residual hemiparesis from the initial stroke; however, it is not possible, given her violent movements, to examine the right limbs adequately. She is obviously presenting with a movement disorder. This is a disorder of intensity scaling rather than of timing, suggesting involvement of the basal ganglia. The violent flinging motion superimposed on a continuous writhing movement is called hemiballism.

4. ***Are any changes in sensory functions detectable?***

   Her sensory systems were intact.

5. ***At what level in the central neuraxis is this lesion most likely located?***

   Ballistic motion in a limb can be obtained in lesions involving the subthalamic nucleus on the contralateral side. The hemiparesis initially present most likely arises from infringement of the lesion on the adjacent internal capsule. The involvement of upper and lower extremities on the right in this process and the lack of language dysfunction are in agreement with the assumption that the lesion is not of cortical origin.

6. ***Is the pathology focal, multifocal, or diffuse in its distribution within the nervous system?***

   This is a unilateral event affecting a restricted area of the diencephalon; it is therefore a focal lesion.

7. ***What is the clinical–temporal profile of this pathology: acute or chronic; progressive or stable?***

   The initial stroke was of rapid onset and involved the subthalamic nucleus and adjacent internal capsule. As the edema and swelling recede, some of the surrounding tissue gradually begins to function again and the hemiparesis resolves. It is at this time that damage to the subthalamic nucleus, done in the initial stroke, is unmasked and can express itself. Thus, the pathology

is acute in onset and stable. The seemingly progressive expression of the movement disorder relates more to the repair process in the neural tissue than to a progressive, degenerative pathology.

8. ***Based on your answers to the previous two questions, decide whether the symptoms in this patient are most likely caused by a vascular accident, a tumor, or a degenerative or inflammatory process.***

   The rapid onset and stability indicate an infarctive vascular event in the vicinity of the subthalamic nucleus and adjacent internal capsule.

9. ***If you feel this is the result of a vascular accident, what vessels were most likely involved?***

   The subthalamic nucleus and adjacent internal capsule are supplied by the tuberothalamic branches of the posterior communicating artery (see Plates 21 and 22 and Chap. 7).

10. ***What is the most common etiology of this disease?***

    Posthemiplegic hemiballism is most often associated with a vascular lesions.[18]

11. ***Would you have expected to see language dysfunction with this right-handed person?***

    A lesion in the dominant side of the cerebral cortex that produces hemiparesis often associates with anterior aphasia. This lesion, although on the dominant side and presenting with hemiparesis, is in the internal capsule adjacent to the ventral portion of the thalamus. At this depth in the cerebrum there is less likelihood of language involvement.

12. ***Describe the pathophysiology of this disease in terms of the possible neural circuitry involved.***

    Hemiballism can arise from damage to the subthalamic nucleus. Normally, this nucleus is part of the indirect pathway of the basal ganglia and has an excitatory influence on the internal segment of the globus pallidus (see Fig. 10-5). The loss of this input would allow the inhibitory influence of the direct pathway to dominate the internal segment of the globus pallidus; consequently, the inhibitory input from palladium to ventrolateral thalamus is lifted. Based on this model, the thalamus would then be allowed to provide greater excitatory input to the cerebral cortex and the patient subsequently would express a hyperkinetic movement disorder.

► Case Study 10-4

1. ***Does the patient exhibit a language or memory deficit or an alteration in consciousness or cognition?***

   He is polylingual, with excellent memory and good cognition.

2. ***Are signs of cranial nerve dysfunction present?***

There is a slight loss of vibratory sense from the left side of the face; all other cranial nerve functions seem to be intact. This is most likely a residual from the previous stroke.

3. ***Are there any changes in motor functions, such as reflexes, muscle tone, movement, or coordination?***

He has a residual hemiparesis for the stroke consisting of elevated deep tendon reflexes and weakness in the upper and lower extremities on the left. A movement disorder is also apparent. The slow, writhing postural changes in the left upper extremity characterize athetotic movements. The tremor expressed in the upper right extremity is physiologic and will be discussed in question 11.

4. ***Are any changes in sensory functions detectable?***

Other than the mild loss of vibratory sense in the left face, all sensory systems appeared to be intact.

5. ***At what level in the central neuraxis is this lesion most likely located?***

The involvement of both limbs on the left in the initial stroke presentation coupled with the preserved cognitive, memory, and language skills argues that the lesion is below the level of the cerebral cortex in the internal capsule. The development of posthemiplegic athetosis suggests that the globus pallidus or the pallidothalamic tracts have been damaged. Thus, the lesion seems to be in the white matter of the internal capsule near the globus pallidus and its efferent pathways.

6. ***Is the pathology focal, multifocal, or diffuse in its distribution within the nervous system?***

The presentation is lateralized and relates to several structures in a circumscribed region, suggesting that it is focal.

7. ***What is the clinical–temporal profile of this pathology: acute or chronic; progressive or stable?***

The initial vascular accident was of acute onset. As the edema and swelling recede and some of the surrounding tissue gradually begins to function again, the hemiparesis resolves. It is at this time that damage to the globus pallidus or its efferent tracts, done in the initial stroke, is unmasked and can express itself. Thus, the pathology is acute in onset and stable. The seemingly progressive expression of the movement disorder relates more to the repair process in the tissue than to the initial pathology.

8. ***Based on your answers to the previous two questions, decide whether the symptoms in this patient are most likely caused by a vascular accident, a tumor, or a degenerative or inflammatory process.***

The rapid onset and stability indicate an infarctive vascular event in the vicinity of the globus pallidus, its efferent tracts, and adjacent internal capsule.

9. ***If you feel this is the result of a vascular accident, what vessels were most likely involved?***

The lateral striate arteries, branches of the middle cerebral artery, supply the posterior limb of the internal capsule as well as the globus pallidus and its efferent tracts (see Plates 22 to 25; Fig. 10-7).

10. ***What is the significance of the 10-Hz tremor experienced by this patient?***

The tremor seen in this patient is of the physiologic type, called essential tremor. It occurs when the extremity is stressed and disappears upon rest. It can be differentiated from the tremor of Parkinson's disease, since it is generally faster and does not occur at rest. It is distinguished from cerebellar tremor of intent, since it occurs in the outstretched (stressed) limb, whereas cerebellar tremor would occur during limb motion but cease when the limb reached its trajectory end point. The origin of essential tremor is not known; however, it does not seem to be related to the patient's poststroke syndrome.

Comment

Posthemiplegic athetosis is another unmasking syndrome, like that of posthemiplegic hemiballism seen in Case 10-3. It occurs following a lesion that has damaged the internal capsule and the globus pallidus or its efferent tracts. Initially, the patient expresses paralysis in the contralateral extremity. The movement disorder only comes to light as the paralysis begins to resolve.

► References

1. Plum F, Posner JB. The diagnosis of stupor and coma. Philadelphia: FA Davis, 1982.
2. Daube JR, Reagan TJ, Sandock BA, Westmoreland BF. Medical neurosciences. Boston: Little, Brown, 1986.
3. Roth G. The origin of fasciculations. Ann Neurol 1982;12:542–547.
4. Biller J, Brazis PW. The localization of lesions affecting the spinal cord. In: Brazis J, Masdeu JC, Biller J, eds. Localization in clinical neurology. Boston: Little, Brown, 1990:69–92.
5. Fisher CM, Karnes WE, Adams RD. Lateral, medullary infarction: the pattern of vascular occlusion. J Neuropathol Exp Neurol 1961;20:323.
6. Biller J, Brazis PW. The localization of lesions affecting the cerebellum. In: Brazis PW, Masdeu JC, Biller J. Localization in clinical neurology, 2nd ed. Boston: Little, Brown, 1990:287–298.
7. Duncan GW, Parker SW, Fisher CM. Acute cerebellar infarction in the PICA territory. Arch Neurol 1975;32:364–368.
8. Masdeu JC, Brazis PW. The anatomic localization of lesions in the thalamus. In: Brazis PW, Masdeu JC, Biller J, eds. Localization in clinical neurology, 2nd ed. Boston: Little, Brown, 1990:319–343.
9. Brazis PW. The localization of lesions affecting cranial nerve VII (the facial nerve). In: Brazis PW, Masdeu JC, Biller J, eds. Locali-

zation in clinical neurology, 2nd ed. Boston: Little, Brown, 1990:203–218.

10. Graff-Radford et al. Nonhemorrhage infarction of the thalamus: behavioral, anatomic, and physiologic correlates. Neurology 1984;34:14–23.

11. Masdeu JC, Brazis PW. The anatomic localization of lesions in the thalamus. In: Brazis PW, Masdeu JC, Biller J, eds. Localization in clinical neurology. Boston: Little, Brown, 1990:319–344.

12. Castaigne P, Lhermitte F, Buge A, Escourolle R, Hauw JJ, Lyon-Caen O. Paramedian thalamic and midbrain infarcts: clinical and neuropathological study. Ann Neurol 1981;10:127–148.

13. Shorvon SD. Classification of epilepsy. In: Asbury A, McKhann GM, McDonald WI, eds. Diseases of the nervous system. Philadelphia: WB Saunders, 1986:970–981.

14. Strub RL, Black FW. The mental status examination in neurology. Philadelphia: FA Davis, 1985.

15. Delgado-Escueta AV. Seizures. In: Kelly WN, ed. Textbook of internal medicine. Philadelphia: JB Lippincott, 1992:2220–2226.

16. Matzuk MM, Saper CB. Preservation of hypothalamic dopaminergic neurons in Parkinson's disease. Ann Neurol 1985;18:552–555.

17. Nakano I, Hirano A. Parkinson's disease: Neuron loss in the nucleus basalis without concomitant Alzheimer's disease. Ann Neurol 1984;15:415–418.

18. Fahn S. Huntington disease and other forms of chorea. In: Rowland LP, ed. Merritt's textbook of neurology. Philadelphia: Lea & Febiger, 1989:647–652.

SPINAL CORD &
BRAIN STEM
ATLAS

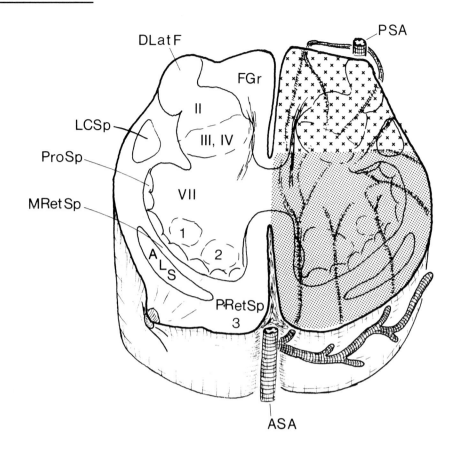

1 LMNu
2 MMNu
3 LVestSp

Plate 1

ALS Anterolateral System	IV Lamina IV	MRetSp Medullary Reticulospinal Tract
ASA Anterior Spinal Artery	LCSp Lateral Corticospinal Tract	PRetSp Pontine Reticulospinal Tract
DLatF Dorsolateral Funiculus	LMNu Lateral Motor Nucleus	ProSp Propriospinal Tract
FGr Fasciculus Gracilis	LVestSp Lateral Vestibulospinal Tract	PSA Posterior Spinal Artery
II Lamina II	MMNu Medial Motor Nucleus	VII Lamina VII
III Lamina III		

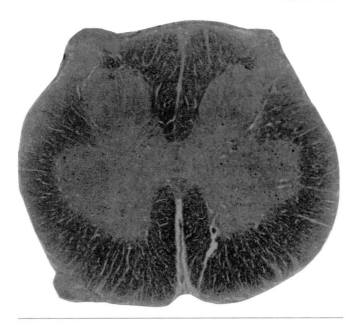

Plate 1

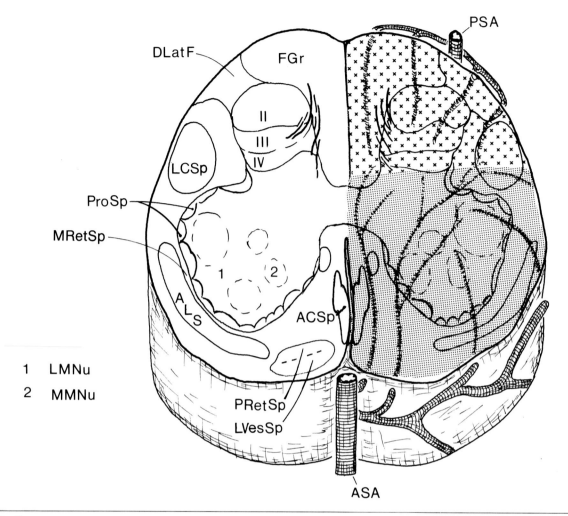

1 LMNu
2 MMNu

Plate 2

ACSp Anterior Corticospinal Tract
ALS Anterolateral System
ASA Anterior Spinal Artery
DLatF Dorsolateral Funiculus
FGr Fasciculus Gracilis
II Lamina II

III Lamina III
IV Lamina IV
LCSp Lateral Corticospinal Tract
LMNu Lateral Motor Nucleus
LVestSp Lateral Vestibulospinal Tract
MLF Median Longitudinal Fasciculus

MMNu Medial Motor Nucleus
MRetSp Medullary Reticulospinal Tract
PRetSp Pontine Reticulospinal Tract
ProSp Propriospinal Tract
PSA Posterior Spinal Artery

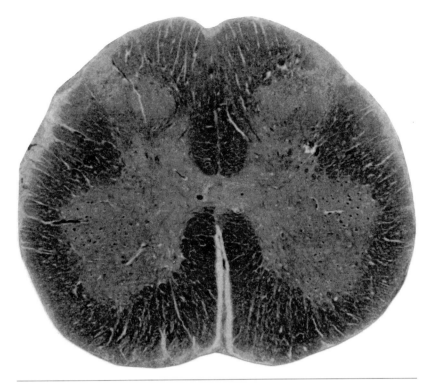

Plate 2

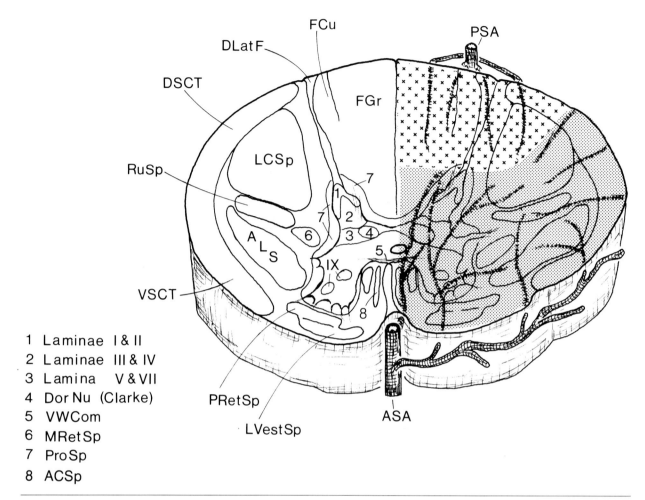

1 Laminae I & II
2 Laminae III & IV
3 Lamina V & VII
4 Dor Nu (Clarke)
5 VWCom
6 MRetSp
7 ProSp
8 ACSp

Plate 3

ACSp Anterior Corticospinal Tract
ALS Anterolateral System
ASA Anterior Spinal Artery
DLatF Dorsolateral Funiculus
DorNu Dorsal Nucleus of Clarke
DSCT Dorsal Spinocerebellar Tract

FCu Fasciculus Cuneatus
FGr Fasciculus Gracilis
IX Lamina IX
LCSp Lateral Corticospinal Tract
LVestSp Lateral Vestibulospinal Tract
MRetSp Medullary Reticulospinal Tract

PRetSp Pontine Reticulospinal Tract
ProSp Propriospinal Tract
PSA Posterior Spinal Artery
RuSp Rubrospinal Tract
VSCT Ventral Spinocerebellar Tract
VWCom Ventral White Commissure

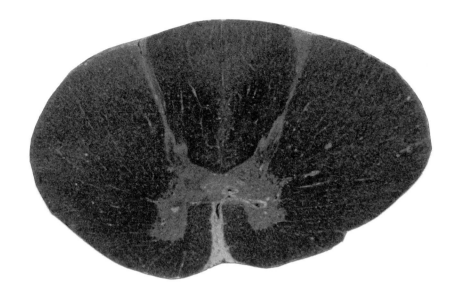

Plate 3

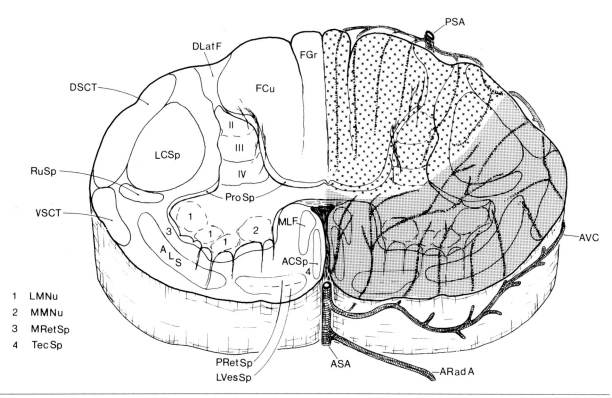

Plate 4

ACSp Anterior Corticospinal Tract	**FGr** Fasciculus Gracilis	**MMNu** Medial Motor Nucleus
ALS Anterolateral System	**II** Lamina II	**MRetSp** Medullary Reticulospinal Tract
ARadA Anterior Radicular Artery	**III** Lamina III	**PRetSp** Pontine Reticulospinal Tract
ASA Anterior Spinal Artery	**IV** Lamina IV	**ProSp** Propriospinal Tract
AVC Arterial Vasocorona	**LCSp** Lateral Corticospinal Tract	**PSA** Posterior Spinal Artery
DLatF Dorsolateral Funiculus	**LMNu** Lateral Motor Nucleus	**RuSp** Rubrospinal Tract
DSCT Dorsal Spinocerebellar Tract	**LVestSp** Lateral Vestibulospinal Tract	**TecSp** Tectospinal Tract
FCu Fasciculus Cuneatus	**MLF** Medial Longitudinal Fasciculus	**VSCT** Ventral Spinocerebellar Tract

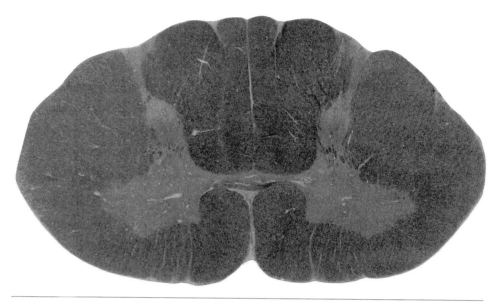

Plate 4

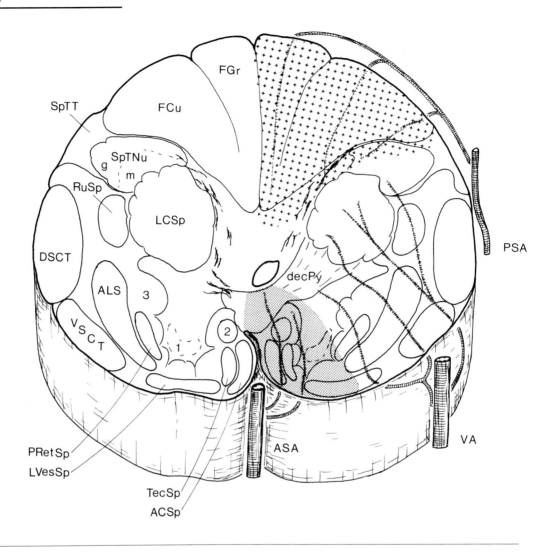

1   Acc Nu
2   MLF
3   MRetSp

Plate 5

AccNu Accessory Nucleus
ACSp Anterior Corticospinal Tract
ALS Anterolateral System
ASA Anterior Spinal Artery
decPy Decussation of the Pyramidal Tract
DSCT Dorsal Spinocerebellar Tract
FCu Fasciculus Cuneatus
FGr Fasciculus Gracilis

LCSp Lateral Corticospinal Tract
LVestSp Lateral Vestibulospinal Tract
MLF Medial Longitudinal Fasciculus
MRetSp Medullary Reticulospinal Tract
PRetSp Pontine Reticulospinal Tract
PSA Posterior Spinal Artery
RuSp Rubrospinal Tract
SpTNu Spinal Trigeminal Nucleus

SpTNu, g Spinal Trigeminal Nucleus, pars gelatinosia
SpTNu, m Spinal Trigeminal Nucleus, pars magnocellularis
SpTT Spinal Trigeminal Tract
TecSp Tectospinal Tract
VA Vertebral Artery
VSCT Ventral Spinocerebellar Tract

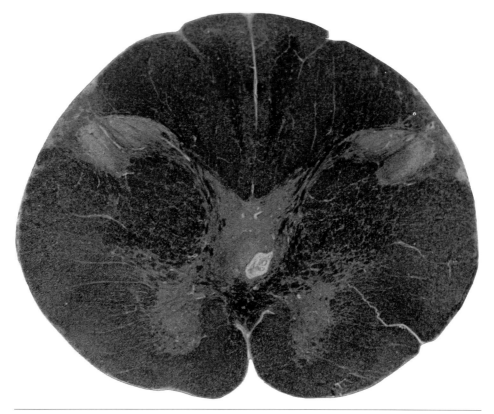

Plate 5

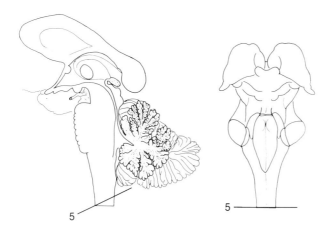

5 _____

5 _____

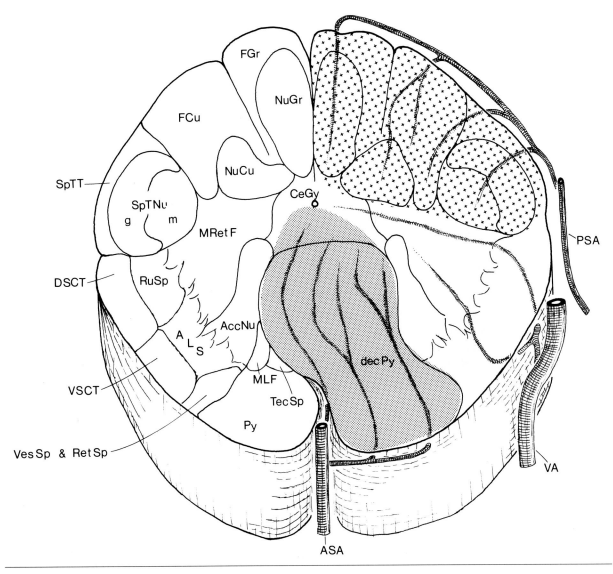

Plate 6

AccNu Accessory Nucleus	**NuCu** Nucleus Cuneatus	**SpTNu, m** Spinal Trigeminal Nucleus, pars
ALS Anterolateral System	**NuGr** Nucleus Gracilis	magnocellularis
ASA Anterior Spinal Artery	**PSA** Posterior Spinal Artery	**SpTT** Spinal Trigeminal Tract
CeGy Central Gray	**Py** Pyramidal Tract	**TecSp** Tectospinal Tract
decPy Decussation of the Pyramidal Tract	**RetSp** Reticulospinal Tract	**VA** Vertebral Artery
DSCT Dorsal Spinocerebellar Tract	**RuSp** Rubrospinal Tract	**VesSp** Vestibulospinal Tract
FCu Fasciculus Cuneatus	**SpTNu** Spinal Trigeminal Nucleus	**VSCT** Ventral Spinocerebellar Tract
FGr Fasciculus Gracilis	**SpTNu, g** Spinal Trigeminal Nucleus, pars	
MLF Medial Longitudinal Fasciculus	gelatinosia	
MRetF Medullary Reticular Formation		

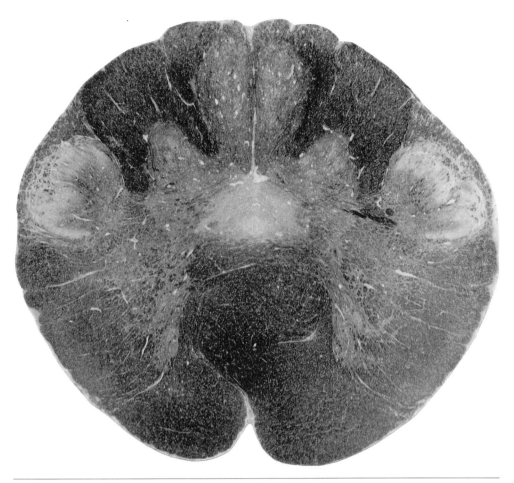

Plate 6

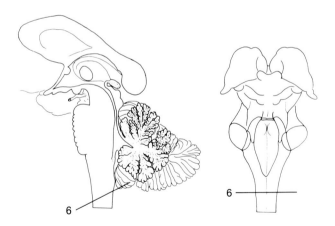

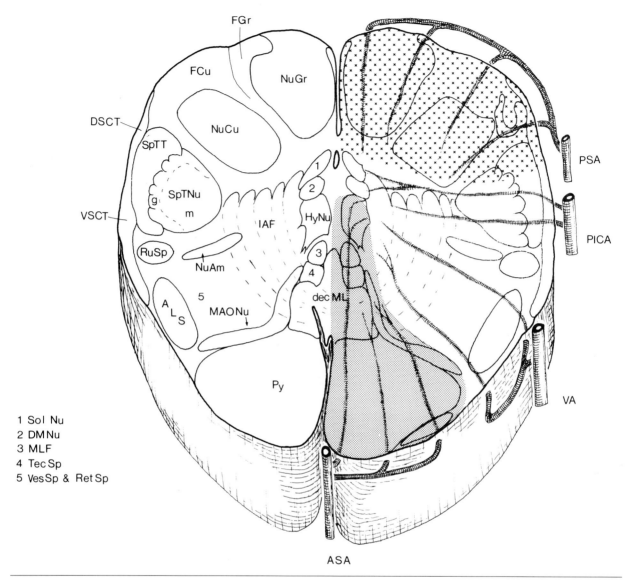

Plate 7

ALS Anterolateral System
ASA Anterior Spinal Artery
decML Decussation of the Medial Lemniscus
DMNu Dorsal Motor Nucleus
DSCT Dorsal Spinocerebellar Tract
FCu Fasciculus Cuneatus
FGr Fasciculus Gracilis
HyNu Hypoglossal Nucleus
IAF Internal Arcuate Fibers
MAONu Medial Accessory Olivary Nucleus
MLF Medial Longitudinal Fasciculus

NuAm Nucleus Ambiguus
NuCu Nucleus Cuneatus
NuGr Nucleus Gracilis
PICA Posterior Inferior Cerebellar Artery
PSA Posterior Spinal Artery
Py Pyramidal Tract
RetSp Reticulospinal Tract
RuSp Rubrospinal Tract
SolNu Solitary Nucleus
SpTNu Spinal Trigeminal Nucleus

SpTNu, g Spinal Trigeminal Nucleus, pars gelatinosia
SpTNu, m Spinal Trigeminal Nucleus, pars magnocellularis
SpTT Spinal Trigeminal Tract
TecSp Tectospinal Tract
VA Vertebral Artery
VesSp Vestibulospinal Tract
VSCT Ventral Spinocerebellar Tract

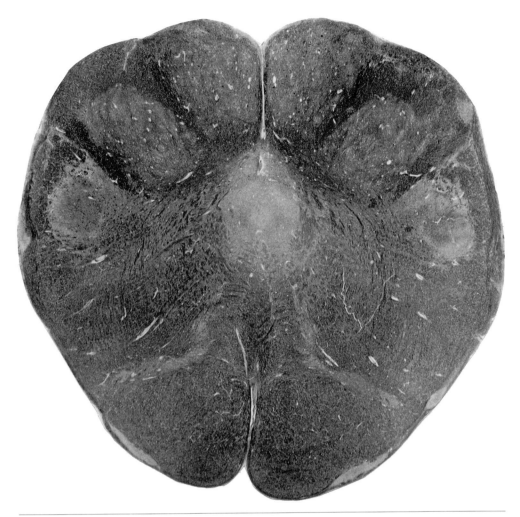

Plate 7

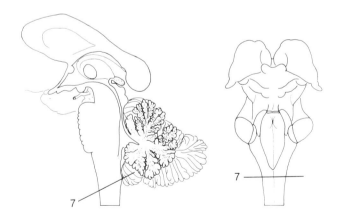

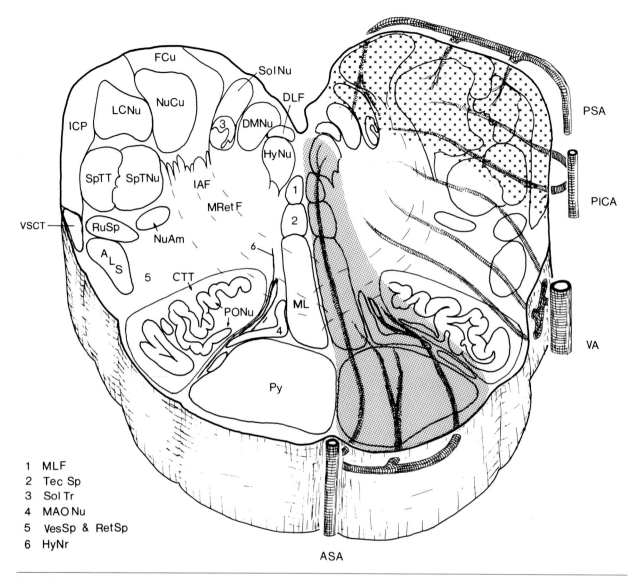

1 MLF
2 Tec Sp
3 Sol Tr
4 MAO Nu
5 VesSp & RetSp
6 HyNr

Plate 8

ALS Anterolateral System
ASA Anterior Spinal Artery
CTT Central Tegmental Tract
DLF Dorsal Longitudinal Fasciculus
DMNu Dorsal Motor Nucleus
FCu Fasciculus Cuneatus
HyNu Hypoglossal Nucleus
HyNr Radiations of Hypoglossal Nerve
IAF Internal Arcuate Fibers
ICP Inferior Cerebellar Peduncle
LCNu Lateral Cuneate Nucleus

MAONu Medial Accessory Olivary Nucleus
ML Medial Lemniscus
MLF Medial Longitudinal Fasciculus
MRetF Medullary Reticular Formation
NuAm Nucleus Ambiguus
NuCu Nucleus Cuneatus
PICA Posterior Inferior Cerebellar Artery
PONu Principal Inferior Olivary Nucleus
PSA Posterior Spinal Artery
Py Pyramidal Tract
RetSp Reticulospinal Tract

RuSp Rubrospinal Tract
SolNu Solitary Nucleus
SolTr Solitary Tract
SpTNu Spinal Trigeminal Nucleus
SpTT Spinal Trigeminal Tract
TecSp Tectospinal Tract
VA Vertebral Artery
VesSp Vestibulospinal Tract
VSCT Ventral Spinocerebellar Tract

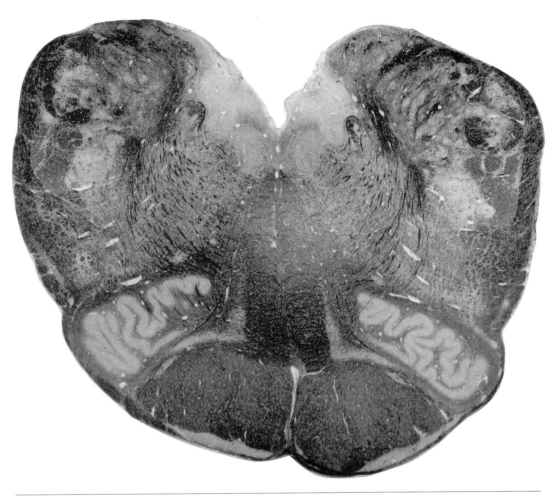

Plate 8

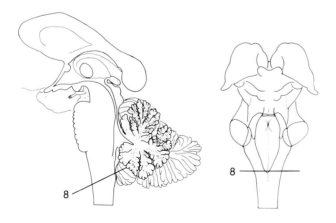

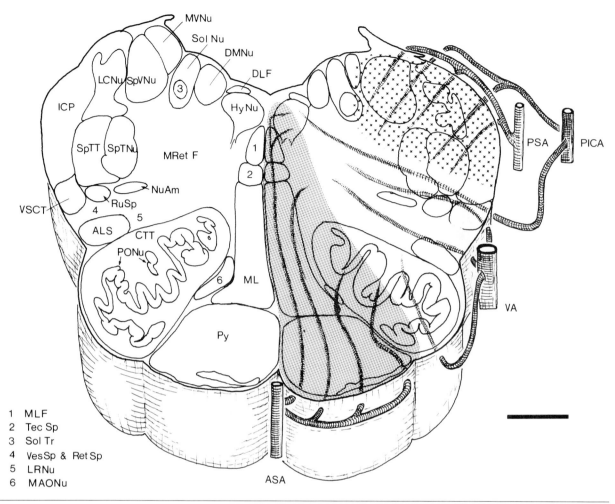

1 MLF
2 Tec Sp
3 Sol Tr
4 VesSp & Ret Sp
5 LRNu
6 MAONu

Plate 9

ALS Anterolateral System	**ML** Medial Lemniscus	**RuSp** Rubrospinal Tract
ASA Anterior Spinal Artery	**MLF** Medial Longitudinal Fasciculus	**SolNu** Solitary Nucleus
CTT Central Tegmental Tract	**MRetF** Medullary Reticular Formation	**SolTr** Solitary Tract
DLF Dorsal Longitudinal Fasciculus	**MVNu** Medial Vestibular Nucleus	**SpTNu** Spinal Trigeminal Nucleus
DMNu Dorsal Motor Nucleus	**NuAm** Nucleus Ambiguus	**SpTT** Spinal Trigeminal Tract
HyNu Hypoglossal Nucleus	**PICA** Posterior Inferior Cerebellar Artery	**SpVNu** Spinal Vestibular Nucleus
ICP Inferior Cerebellar Peduncle	**PONu** Principal Inferior Olivary Nucleus	**TecSp** Tectospinal Tract
LCNu Lateral Cuneate Nucleus	**PSA** Posterior Spinal Artery	**VA** Vertebral Artery
LRNu Lateral Reticular Nucleus	**Py** Pyramidal Tract	**VesSp** Vestibulospinal Tract
MAONu Medial Accessory Olivary Nucleus	**RetSp** Reticulospinal Tract	**VSCT** Ventral Spinocerebellar Tract

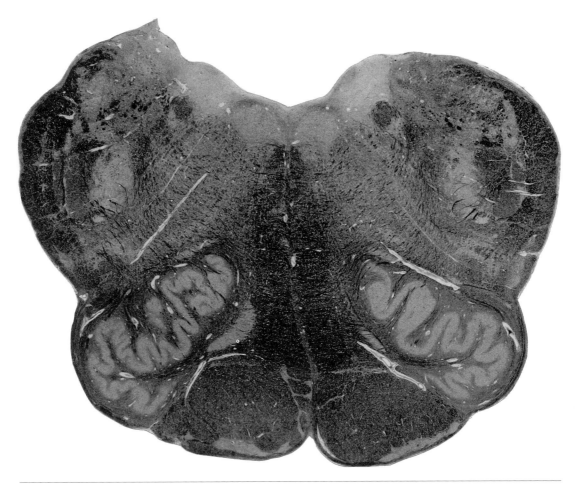

Plate 9

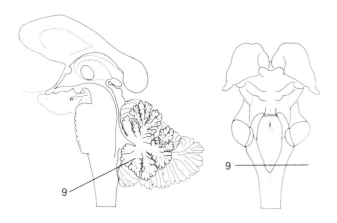

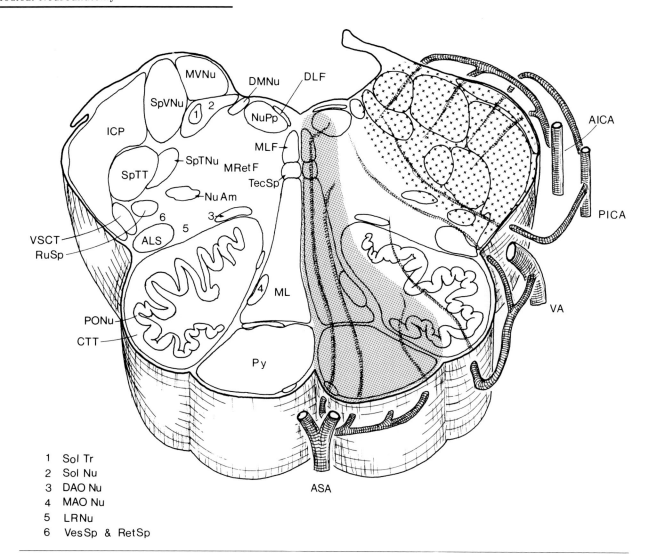

1 Sol Tr
2 Sol Nu
3 DAO Nu
4 MAO Nu
5 LRNu
6 Ves Sp & Ret Sp

Plate 10

AICA Anterior Inferior Cerebellar Artery
ALS Anterolateral System
ASA Anterior Spinal Artery
CTT Central Tegmental Tract
DAONu Dorsal Accessory Olivary Nucleus
DLF Dorsal Longitudinal Fasciculus
DMNu Dorsal Motor Nucleus
ICP Inferior Cerebellar Peduncle
LRNu Lateral Reticular Nucleus
MAONu Medial Accessory Olivary Nucleus

ML Medial Lemniscus
MLF Medial Longitudinal Fasciculus
MRetF Medullary Reticular Formation
MVNu Medial Vestibular Nucleus
NuAm Nucleus Ambiguus
NuPp Nucleus Prepositus
PICA Posterior Inferior Cerebellar Artery
PONu Principal Inferior Olivary Nucleus
Py Pyramidal Tract
RetSp Reticulospinal Tract

RuSp Rubrospinal Tract
SolNu Solitary Nucleus
SolTr Solitary Tract
SpTNu Spinal Trigeminal Nucleus
SpTT Spinal Trigeminal Tract
SpVNu Spinal Vestibular Nucleus
TecSp Tectospinal Tract
VA Vertebral Artery
VesSp Vestibulospinal Tract
VSCT Ventral Spinocerebellar Tract

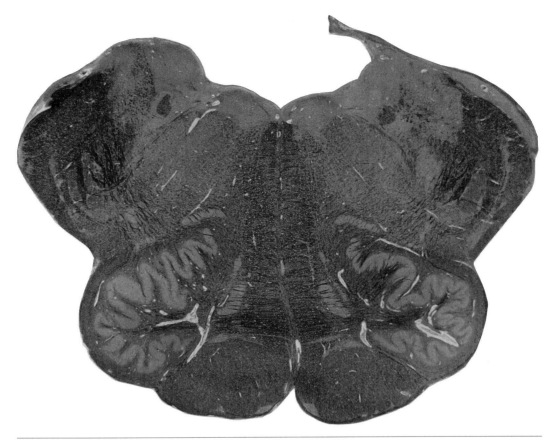

Plate 10

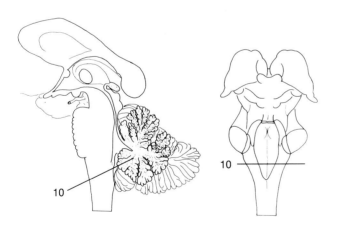

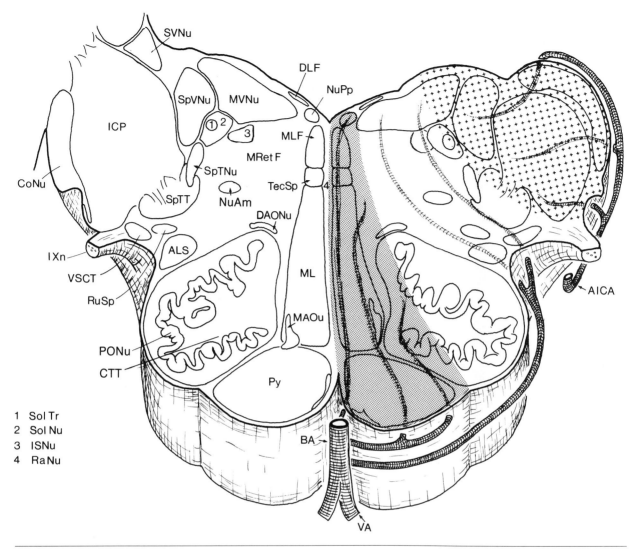

1 Sol Tr
2 Sol Nu
3 ISNu
4 RaNu

Plate 11

AICA Anterior Inferior Cerebellar Artery	**MAONu** Medial Accessory Olivary Nucleus	**RuSp** Rubrospinal Tract
ALS Anterolateral System	**ML** Medial Lemniscus	**SolNu** Solitary Nucleus
BA Basilar Artery	**MLF** Medial Longitudinal Fasciculus	**SolTr** Solitary Tract
CoNu Cochlear Nucleus	**MRetF** Medullary Reticular Formation	**SpTNu** Spinal Trigeminal Nucleus
CTT Central Tegmental Tract	**MVNu** Medial Vestibular Nucleus	**SpTT** Spinal Trigeminal Tract
DAONu Dorsal Accessory Olivary Nucleus	**NuAm** Nucleus Ambiguus	**SpVNu** Spinal Vestibular Nucleus
DLF Dorsal Longitudinal Fasciculus	**NuPp** Nucleus Prepositus	**SVNu** Superior Vestibular Nucleus
ICP Inferior Cerebellar Peduncle	**PONu** Principal Inferior Olivary Nucleus	**TecSp** Tectospinal Tract
ISNu Inferior Salvatory Nucleus	**Py** Pyramidal Tract	**VA** Vertebral Artery
IXn Glossopharyngeal Nerve	**RaNu** Raphe Nucleus	**VSCT** Ventral Spinocerebellar Tract

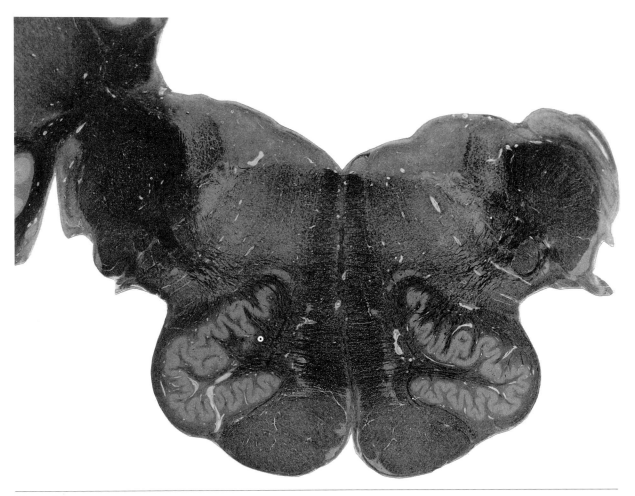

Plate 11

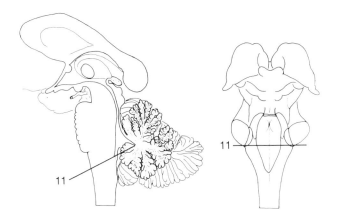

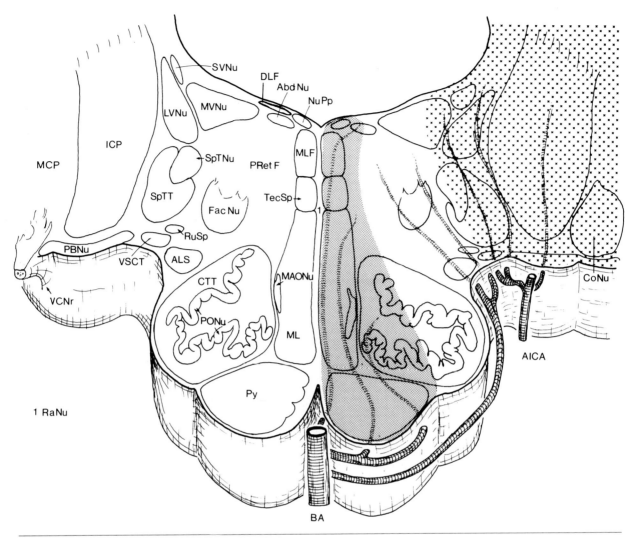

Plate 12

AbdNu Abducens Nucleus
AICA Anterior Inferior Cerebellar Artery
ALS Anterolateral System
BA Basilar Artery
CoNu Cochlear Nucleus
CTT Central Tegmental Tract
DLF Dorsal Longitudinal Fasciculus
FacNu Facial Nucleus
ICP Inferior Cerebellar Peduncle
LVNu Lateral Vestibulospinal Nucleus

MAONu Medial Accessory Olivary Nucleus
MCP Middle Cerebellar Peduncle
ML Medial Lemniscus
MLF Medial Longitudinal Fasciculus
MVNu Medial Vestibular Nucleus
NuPp Nucleus Prepositus
PBNu Pontobulbar Nucleus
PONu Principal Inferior Olivary Nucleus
PRetF Pontine Reticular Formation

Py Pyramidal Tract
RaNu Raphe Nucleus
RuSp Rubrospinal Tract
SpTNu Spinal Trigeminal Nucleus
SpTT Spinal Trigeminal Tract
SVNu Superior Vestibular Nucleus
TecSp Tectospinal Tract
VCNr Vestibuiocochlear Nerve
VSCT Ventral Spinocerebellar Tract

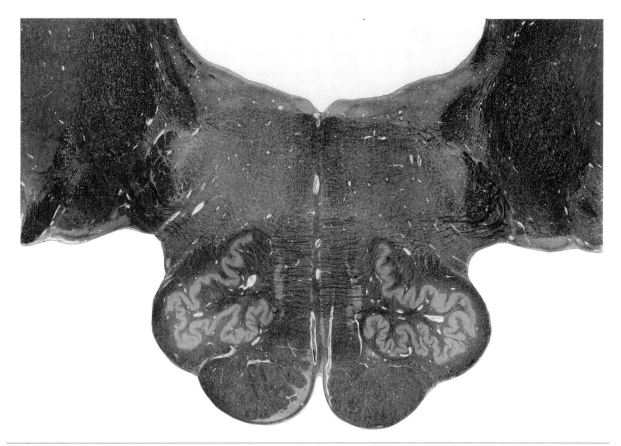

Plate 12

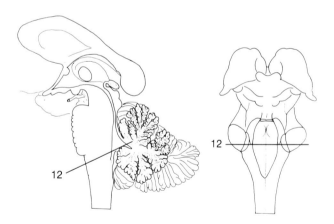

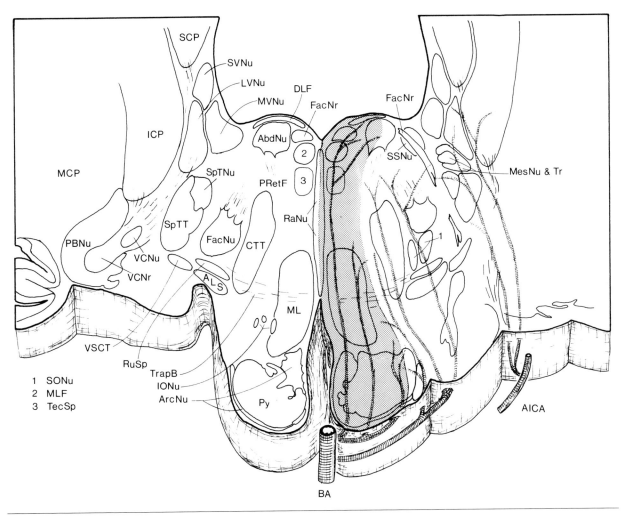

SCP

SVNu

LVNu

DLF

MVNu

FacNr

FacNr

ICP

AbdNu

2

SSNu

MesNu & Tr

MCP

SpTNu

PRetF

3

RaNu

SpTT

1

PBNu

FacNu

CTT

VCNu

VCNr

ALS

ML

VSCT

RuSp

TrapB

IONu

Py

ArcNu

AICA

1 SONu
2 MLF
3 TecSp

BA

Plate 13

AbdNu Abducens Nucleus
AICA Anterior Inferior Cerebellar Artery
ALS Anterolateral System
ArcNu Arcuate Nucleus
BA Basilar Artery
CTT Central Tegmental Tract
DLF Dorsal Longitudinal Fasciculus
FacNr Radiations of the Facial Nerve
FacNu Facial Nucleus
ICP Inferior Cerebellar Peduncle
IONu Inferior Olivary Nucleus
LVNu Lateral Vestibulospinal Nucleus

MCP Middle Cerebellar Peduncle
MesNu&Tr Mesencephalic Trigeminal Nucleus
 & Tract
ML Medial Lemniscus
MLF Medial Longitudinal Fasciculus
MVNu Medial Vestibular Nucleus
PBNu Pontobulbar Nucleus
PRetF Pontine Reticular Formation
Py Pyramidal Tract
RaNu Raphe Nucleus
RuSp Rubrospinal Tract
SCP Superior Cerebellar Peduncle

SONu Superior Olivary Nucleus
SpTNu Spinal Trigeminal Nucleus
SpTT Spinal Trigeminal Tract
SSNu Superior Salvitory Nucleus
SVNu Superior Vestibular Nucleus
TecSp Tectospinal Tract
TrapB Trapezoid Body
VCNr Vestibulocochlear Nerve
VCNu Ventral Cochlear Nucleus
VSCT Ventral Spinocerebellar Tract

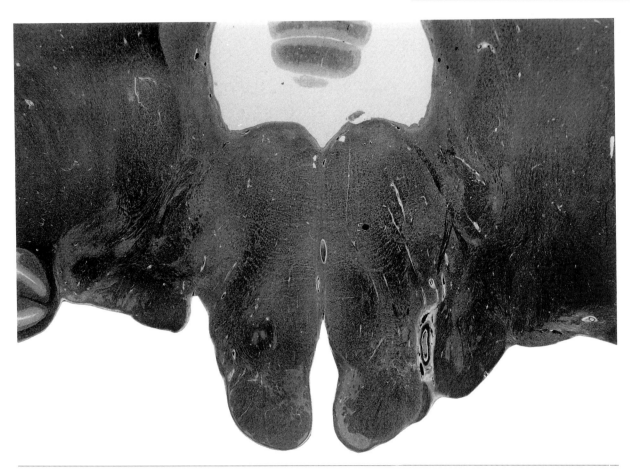

Plate 13

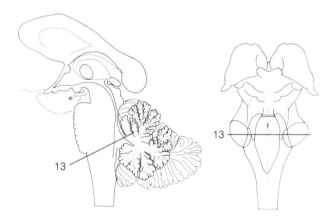

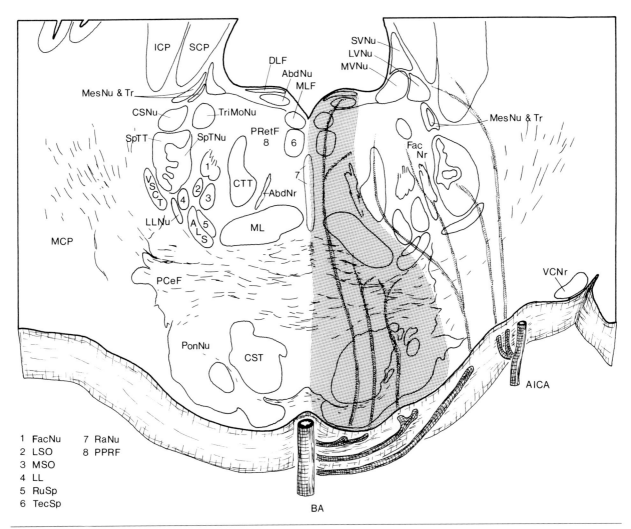

Plate 14

AbdNr Radiations of the Adbucens Nerve
AbdNu Abducens Nucleus
AICA Anterior Inferior Cerebellar Artery
ALS Anterolateral System
BA Basilar Artery
CSNu Chief Trigeminal Sensory Nucleus
CST Corticospinal Tract
CTT Central Tegmental Tract
DLF Dorsal Longitudinal Fasciculus
FacNr Radiations of the Facial Nerve
FacNu Facial Nucleus
ICP Inferior Cerebellar Peduncle
LL Lateral Lemniscus

LLNu Nuclei of the Lateral Lemniscus
LSO Lateral Superior Olivary Nucleus
LVNu Lateral Vestibulospinal Nucleus
MCP Middle Cerebellar Peduncle
MesNu&Tr Mesencephalic Trigeminal Nucleus
& Tract
ML Medial Lemniscus
MLF Medial Longitudinal Fasciculus
MSO Medial Superior Olivary Nucleus
MVNu Medial Vestibular Nucleus
PCeF Pontocerebellar Fibers
PonNu Pontine Nuclei
PPRF Paramedian Pontine Reticular Formation

PRetF Pontine Reticular Formation
RaNu Raphe Nucleus
RuSp Rubrospinal Tract
SCP Superior Cerebellar Peduncle
SpTNu Spinal Trigeminal Nucleus
SpTT Spinal Trigeminal Tract
SVNu Superior Vestibular Nucleus
TecSp Tectospinal Tract
TriMoNu Trigeminal Motor Nucleus
VCNr Vestibulocochlear Nerve
VSCT Ventral Spinocerebellar Tract

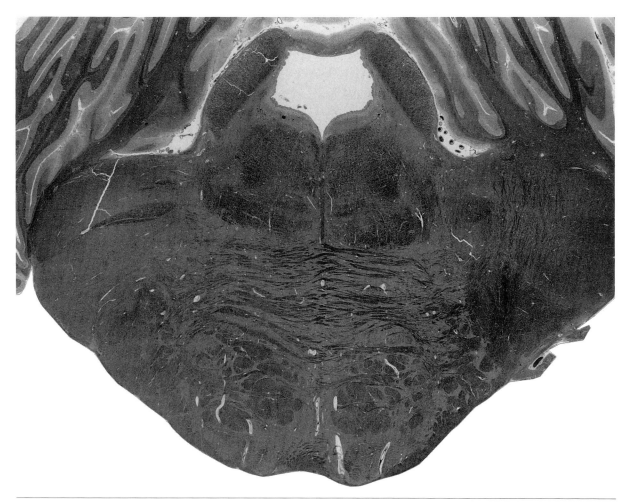

Plate 15

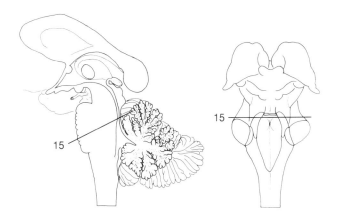

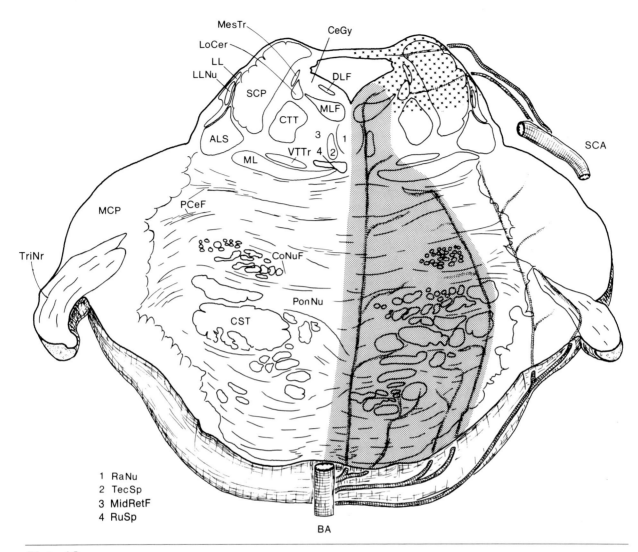

MesTr
LoCer
LL
LLNu
CeGy
DLF
SCP
MLF
CTT
ALS
3 1
VTTr 4 2
ML
SCA
MCP
PCeF
TriNr
CoNuF
PonNu
CST
1 RaNu
2 TecSp
3 MidRetF
4 RuSp
BA

Plate 16

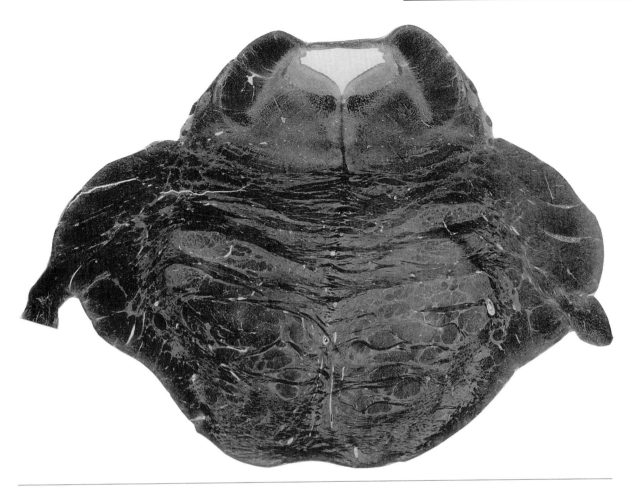

Plate 16

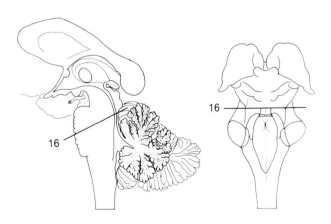

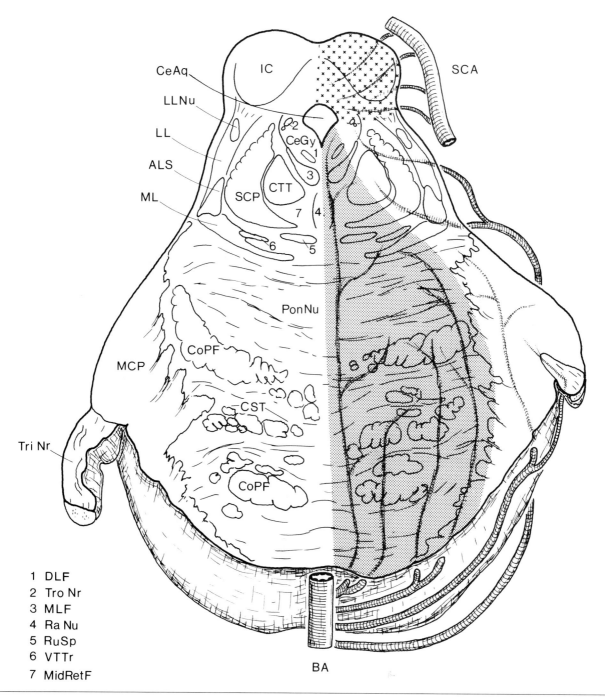

CeAq
LLNu
LL
ALS
ML

IC
CeGy
CTT
SCP

SCA

PonNu

CoPF

MCP

CST

Tri Nr

CoPF

BA

1 DLF
2 Tro Nr
3 MLF
4 Ra Nu
5 RuSp
6 VTTr
7 MidRetF

Plate 17

ALS Anterolateral System
BA Basilar Artery
CeAq Cerebral Aqueduct
CeGy Central Gray
CoPF Corticopontine Fibers
CST Corticospinal Tract
CTT Central Tegmental Tract
DLF Dorsal Longitudinal Fasciculus

IC Inferior Colliculus
LL Lateral Lemniscus
LLNu Nuclei of the Lateral Lemniscus
MCP Middle Cerebellar Peduncle
MidRetF Midbrain Reticular Formation
ML Medial Lemniscus
MLF Medial Longitudinal Fasciculus
PonNu Pontine Nuclei

RaNu Raphe Nucleus
RuSp Rubrospinal Tract
SCA Superior Cerebellar Artery
SCP Superior Cerebellar Peduncle
TriNr Trigeminal Nerve
TroNr Radiations of the Trochlear Nerve
VTTr Ventral Trigeminothalamic Tract

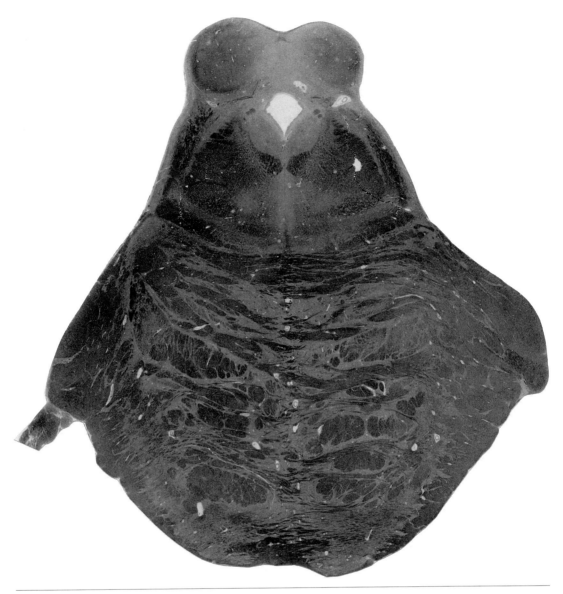

Plate 17

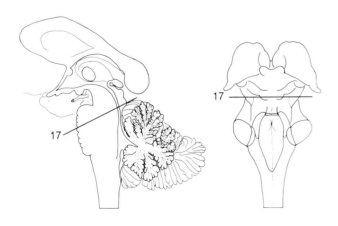

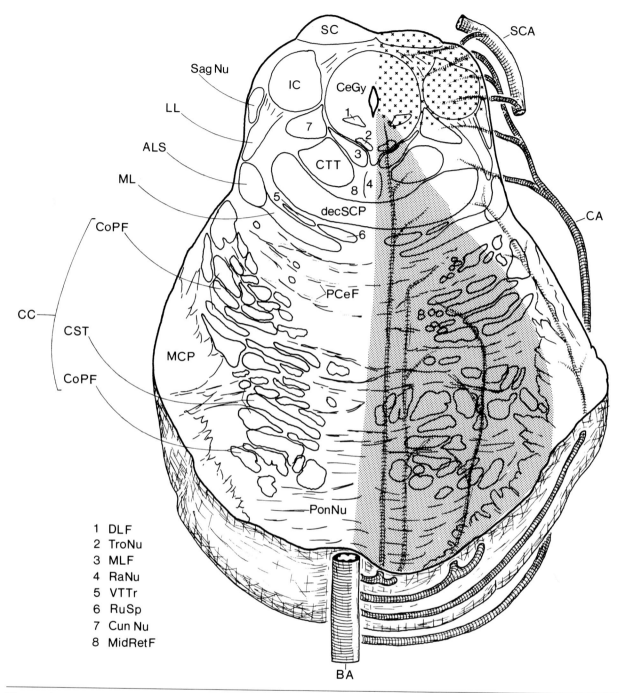

1 DLF
2 TroNu
3 MLF
4 RaNu
5 VTTr
6 RuSp
7 Cun Nu
8 MidRetF

Plate 18

ALS Anterolateral System
BA Basilar Artery
CA Collicular Artery
CC Crus Cerebri
CeGy Central Gray
CoPF Corticopontine Fibers
CST Corticospinal Tract
CTT Central Tegmental Tract
CunNu Cuneiform Nucleus

decSCP Decussation of the Superior Cerebellar Peduncle
DLF Dorsal Longitudinal Fasciculus
IC Inferior Colliculus
LL Lateral Lemniscus
MCP Middle Cerebellar Peduncle
MidRetF Midbrain Reticular Formation
ML Medial Lemniscus
MLF Medial Longitudinal Fasciculus

PCeF Pontocerebellar Fibers
PonNu Pontine Nuclei
RaNu Raphe Nucleus
RuSp Rubrospinal Tract
SagNu Nucleus Sagulum
SC Superior Colliculus
SCA Superior Cerebellar Artery
TroNu Trochlear Nucleus
VTTr Ventral Trigeminothalamic Tract

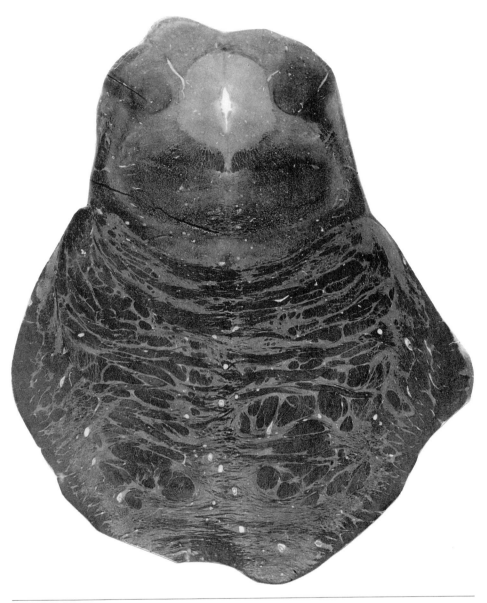

Plate 18

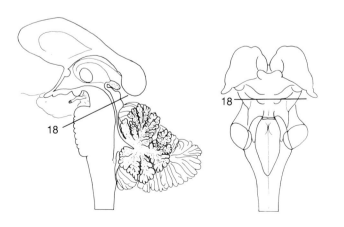

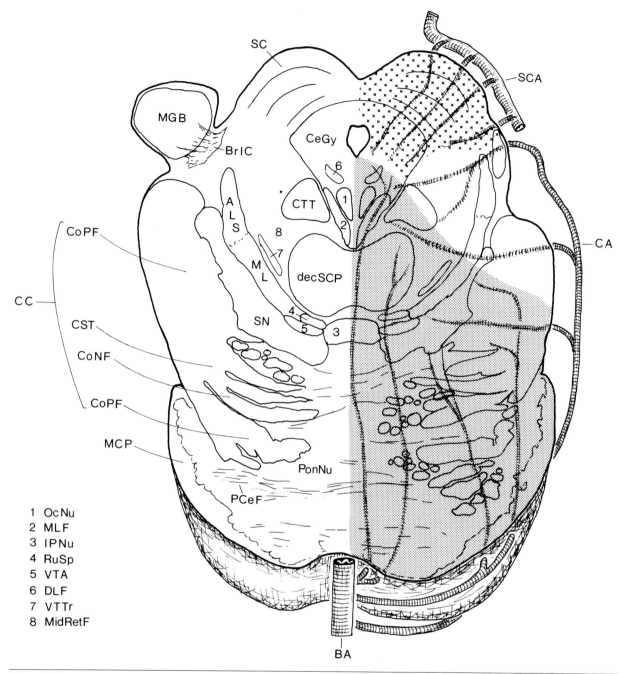

1 OcNu
2 MLF
3 IPNu
4 RuSp
5 VTA
6 DLF
7 VTTr
8 MidRetF

Plate 19

ALS Anterolateral System
BA Basilar Artery
BrIC Brachium of the Inferior Colliculus
CA Collicular Artery
CC Crus Cerebri
CeGy Central Gray
CoNF Corticonuclear Fibers
CoPF Corticopontine Fibers
CST Corticospinal Tract
CTT Central Tegmental Tract

decSCP Decussation of the Superior Cerebellar Peduncle
DLF Dorsal Longitudinal Fasciculus
IPNu Interpeduncular Nucleus
MCP Middle Cerebellar Peduncle
MGB Medial Geniculate Body
MidRetF Midbrain Reticular Formation
ML Medial Lemniscus
MLF Medial Longitudinal Fasciculus
OcNu Oculomotor Nucleus

PCeF Pontocerebellar Fibers
PonNu Pontine Nuclei
RuSp Rubrospinal Tract
SC Superior Colliculus
SCA Superior Cerebellar Artery
SN Substantia Nigra
VTA Ventral Tegmental Area
VTTr Ventral Trigeminothalamic Tract

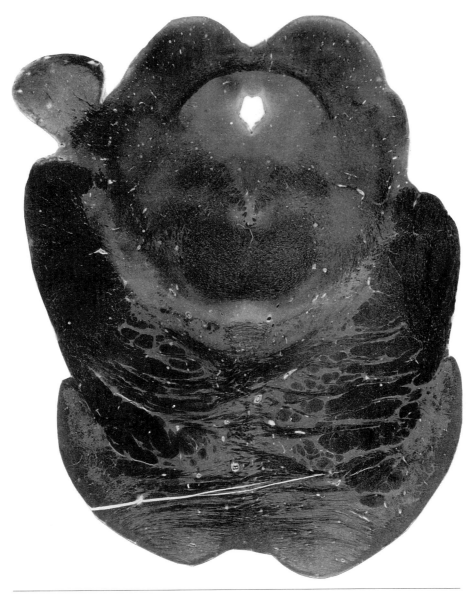

Plate 19

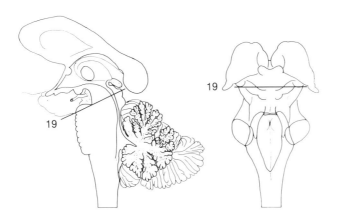

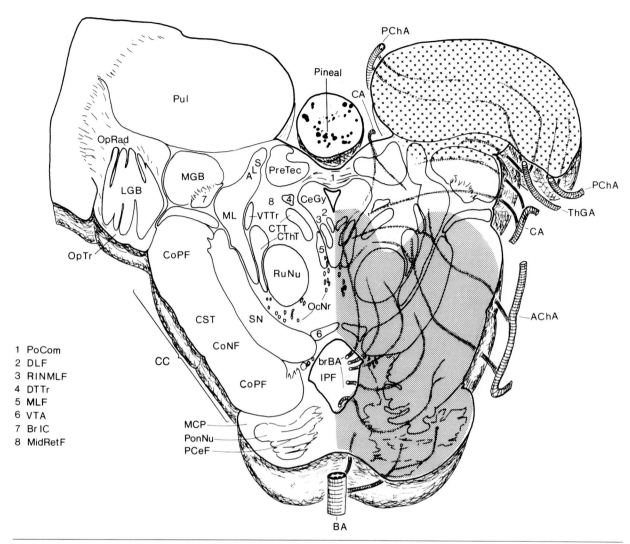

1 PoCom
2 DLF
3 RINMLF
4 DTTr
5 MLF
6 VTA
7 Br IC
8 MidRetF

Plate 20

AChA Anterior Choroidal Artery
ALS Anterolateral System
BA Basilar Artery
brBA Paramedian Branches of Basilar Artery
BrIC Brachium of the Inferior Colliculus
CA Collicular Artery
CC Crus Cerebri
CeGy Central Gray
CoNF Corticonuclear Fibers
CoPF Corticopontine Fibers
CST Corticospinal Tract
CThT Cerebellothalamic Tract
CTT Central Tegmental Tract

DLF Dorsal Longitudinal Fasciculus
DTTr Dorsal Trigeminothalamic Tract
IPF Interpeduncular Fossa
LGB Lateral Geniculate Body
MCP Middle Cerebellar Peduncle
MGB Medial Geniculate Body
MidRetF Midbrain Reticular Formation
ML Medial Lemniscus
MLF Medial Longitudinal Fasciculus
OcNr Radiations of the Oculomotor Nerve
OpRad Optic Radiations
PCeF Pontocerebellar Fibers
PChA Posterior Choroidal Artery

PoCom Posterior Commissure
PonNu Pontine Nuclei
PreTec Pretectal Nuclei
Pul Pulvinar Nucleus
RINMLF Rostral Interstitial Nucleus of the
    Medial Longitudinal Fasciculus
RuNu Red Nucleus
SN Substantia Nigra
ThGA Thalamogeniculate Artery
VTA Ventral Tegmental Area
VTTr Ventral Trigeminothalamic Tract

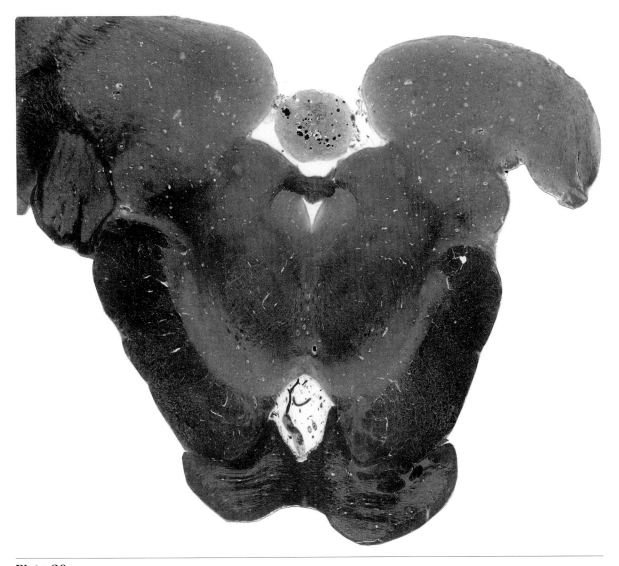

Plate 20

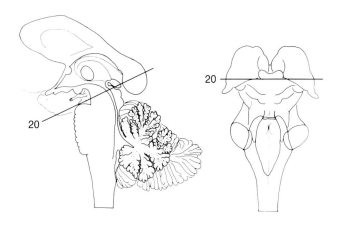

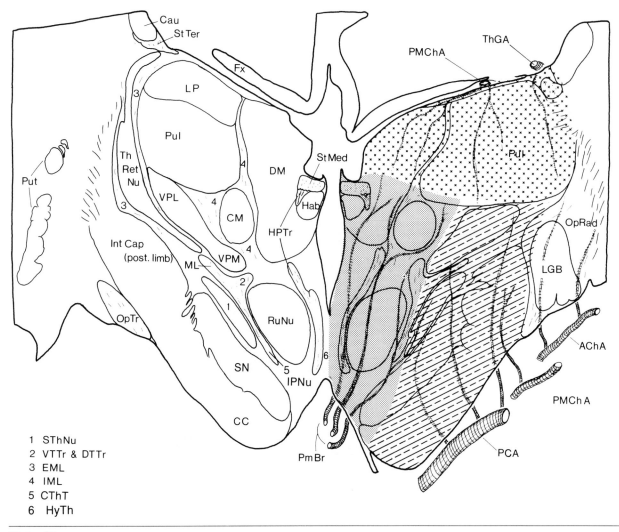

1 SThNu
2 VTTr & DTTr
3 EML
4 IML
5 CThT
6 HyTh

Plate 21

AChA Anterior Choroidal Artery
Cau Caudate
CC Crus Cerebri
CM Centromedian Nucleus
CThT Cerebellothalamic Tract
DM Dorsomedial Nucleus
DTTr Dorsal Trigeminothalamic Tract
EML External Medullary Lamina
Fx Fornix
Hab Habenular Nucleus
HPTr Habenulopeduncular Tract

HyTh Hypothalamus
IML Internal Medullary Lamina
IntCap Internal Capsule
IPNu Interpeduncular Nucleus
LGB Lateral Geniculate Body
LP Lateral Posterior Nucleus
ML Medial Lemniscus
OpRad Optic Radiations
OpTr Optic Tract
PCA Posterior Cerebral Artery
PmBr Paramedian Branches
PMChA Posteromedial Choroidal Artery

Pul Pulvinar Nucleus
Put Putamen
RuNu Red Nucleus
SN Substantia Nigra
SThNu Subthalamic Nucleus
StMed Stria Medullaris
StTer Stria Terminalis
ThGA Thalamogeniculate Artery
ThRetNu Thalamic Reticular Nucleus
VPL Ventroposterior Lateral Nucleus
VPM Ventroposterior Medial Nucleus
VTTr Ventral Trigeminothalamic Tract

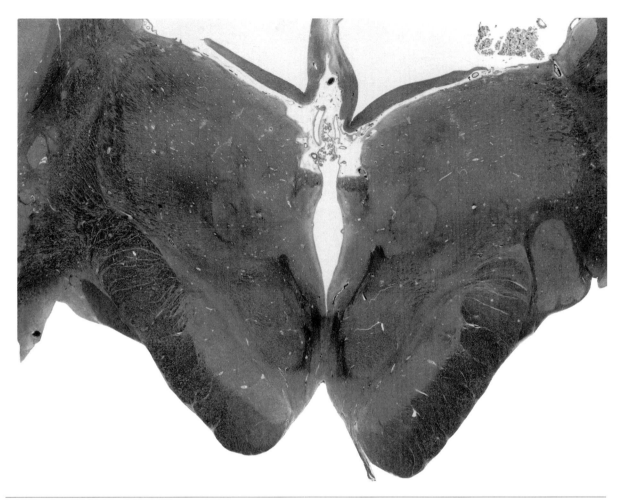

Plate 21

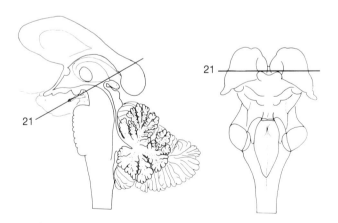

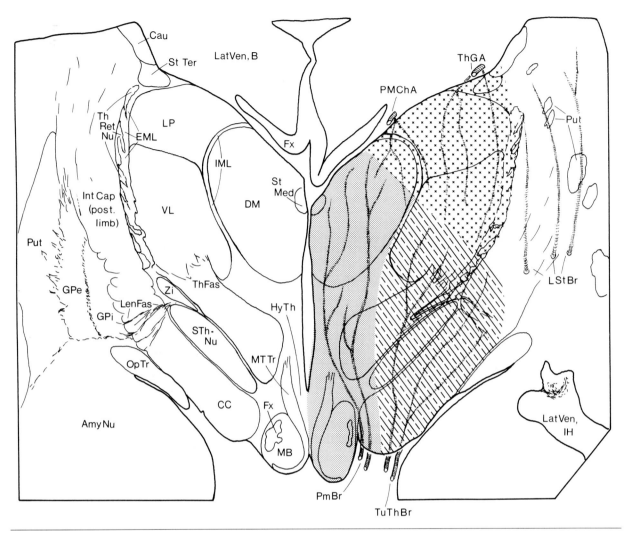

Plate 22

AmyNu Amygdaloid Nucleus
Cau Caudate
CC Crus Cerebri
DM Dorsomedial Nucleus
EML External Medullary Lamina
Fx Fornix
GPe Globus Pallidus, External Segment
GPi Globus Pallidus, Internal Segment
HyTh Hypothalamus
IML Internal Medullary Lamina
IntCap Internal Capsule

LatVen,B Lateral Ventricle, Body
LatVen,IH Lateral Ventricle, Inferior Horn
LenFas Lenticular Fasciculus
LP Lateral Posterior Nucleus
LStBr Lenticulostriate Branches
MB Mammillary Bodies
MTTr Mammillothalamic Tract
OpTr Optic Tract
PmBr Paramedian Branches
PMChA Posteromedial Choroidal Artery
Put Putamen

SThNu Subthalamic Nucleus
StMed Stria Medullaris
StTer Stria Terminalis
ThFas Thalamic Fasciculus
ThGA Thalamogeniculate Artery
ThRetNu Thalamic Reticular Nucleus
TuThBr Tuberothalamic Branches
VL Ventrolateral Nucleus
Zi Zona Incerta

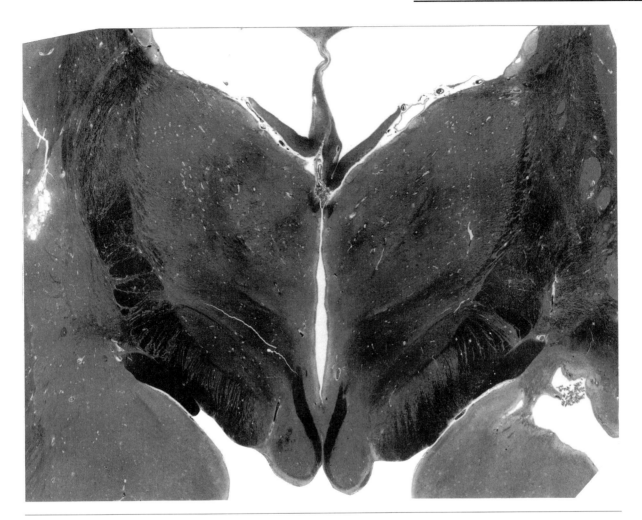

Plate 22

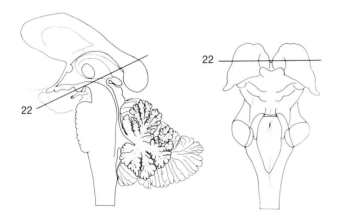

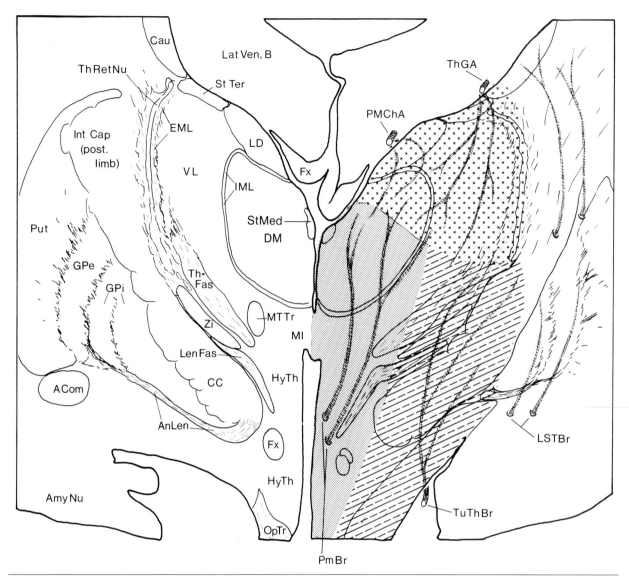

Plate 23

ACom Anterior Commissure	**IML** Internal Medullary Lamina	**Put** Putamen
AmyNu Amygdaloid Nucleus	**IntCap** Internal Capsule	**StMed** Stria Medullaris
AnLen Ansa Lenticularis	**LatVen,B** Lateral Ventricle, Body	**StTer** Stria Terminalis
Cau Caudate	**LD** Laterodorsal Nucleus	**ThFas** Thalamic Fasciculus
CC Crus Cerebri	**LenFas** Lenticular Fasciculus	**ThGA** Thalamogeniculate Artery
DM Dorsomedial Nucleus	**LStBr** Lenticulostriate Branches	**ThRetNu** Thalamic Reticular Nucleus
EML External Medullary Lamina	**MI** Mass Intermedia	**TuThBr** Tuberothalamic Branches
Fx Fornix	**MTTr** Mammillothalamic Tract	**VL** Ventrolateral Nucleus
GPe Globus Pallidus, External Segment	**OpTr** Optic Tract	**Zi** Zona Incerta
GPi Globus Pallidus, Internal Segment	**PmBr** Paramedian Branches	
HyTh Hypothalamus	**PMChA** Posteromedial Choroidal Artery	

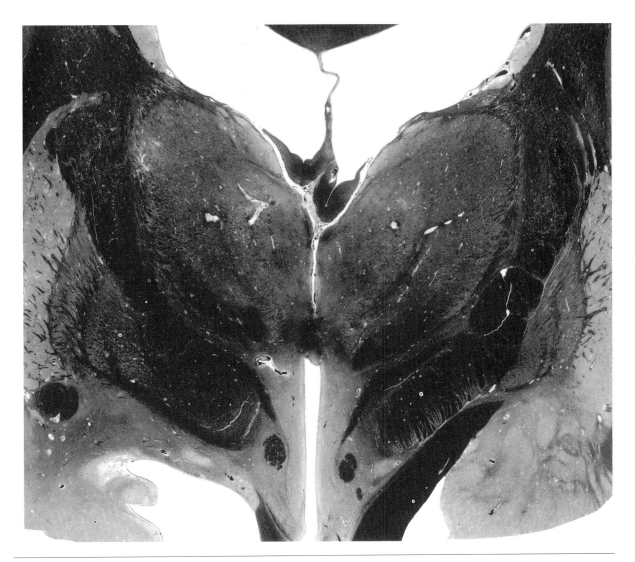

Plate 23

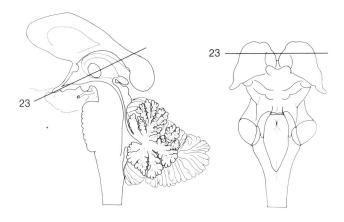

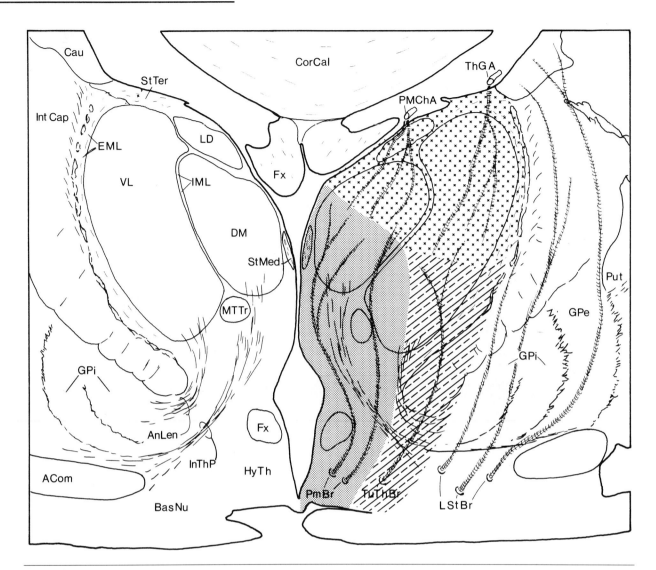

Plate 24

ACom Anterior Commissure	**GPi** Globus Pallidus, Internal Segment	**PMChA** Posteromedial Choroidal Artery
AnLen Ansa Lenticularis	**HyTh** Hypothalamus	**Put** Putamen
BasNu Basal Nucleus	**IML** Internal Medullary Lamina	**StMed** Stria Medullaris
Cau Caudate	**IntCap** Internal Capsule	**StTer** Stria Terminalis
CorCal Corpus Callosum	**InThP** Inferior Thalamic Peduncle	**ThGA** Thalamogeniculate Artery
DM Dorsomedial Nucleus	**LD** Laterodorsal Nucleus	**TuThBr** Tuberothalamic Branches
EML External Medullary Lamina	**LStBr** Lenticulostriate Branches	**VL** Ventrolateral Nucleus
Fx Fornix	**MTTr** Mammillothalamic Tract	
GPe Globus Pallidus, External Segment	**PmBr** Paramedian Branches	

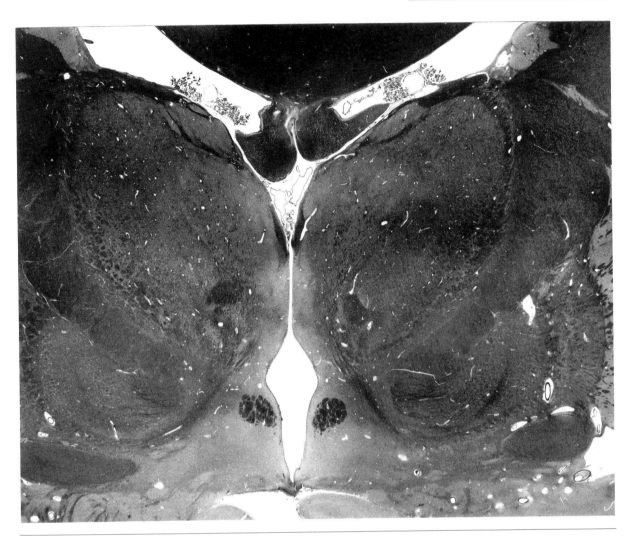

Plate 24

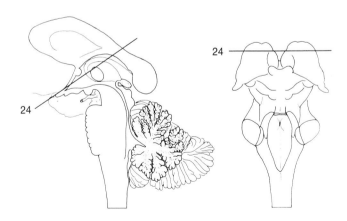

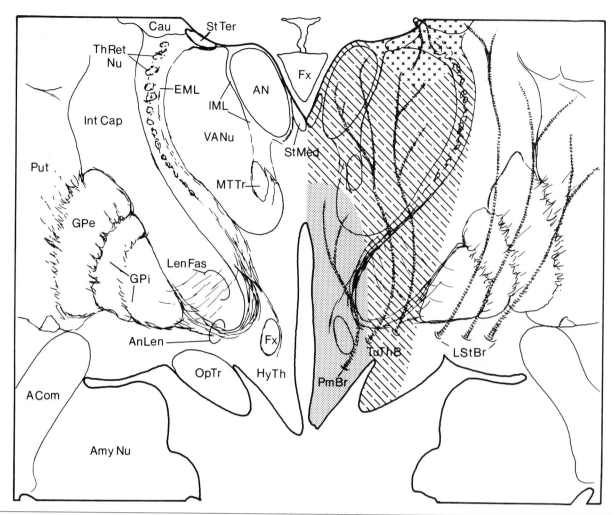

Plate 25

ACom Anterior Commissure
AmyNu Amygdaloid Nucleus
AN Anterior Nucleus
AnLen Ansa Lenticularis
Cau Caudate
EML External Medullary Lamina
Fx Fornix
GPe Globus Pallidus, External Segment

GPi Globus Pallidus, Internal Segment
HyTh Hypothalamus
IML Internal Medullary Lamina
IntCap Internal Capsule
LenFas Lenticular Fasciculus
LStBr Lenticulostriate Branches
MTTr Mammillothalamic Tract
OpTr Optic Tract

PmBr Paramedian Branches
Put Putamen
StMed Stria Medullaris
StTer Stria Terminalis
ThRetNu Thalamic Reticular Nucleus
TuThBr Tuberothalamic Branches
VANu Ventroanterior Nucleus

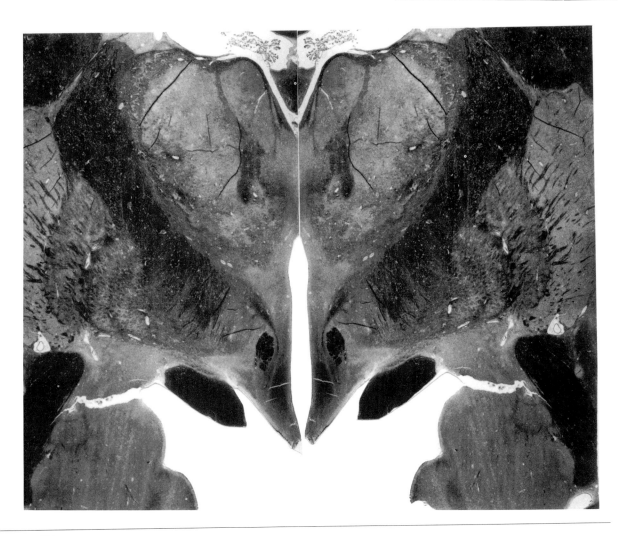

Plate 25

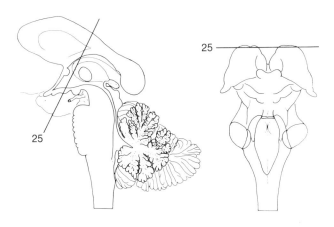

INDEX

Page numbers followed by *f* indicate illustrations; *t* following a page number indicates tabular material.

Vasocorona, arterial, 47, 260*f*–261*f*
VCNr. *See* Vestibulocochlear nerve
    root
VCNu. *See* Vestibular cochlear nucleus
Ventral cochlear nucleus, 82*f*
Ventral corticospinal tract, 40,
    256*f*–263*f*
Ventral funiculus, 32, 40–41
    clinical deficit, 40
    deep, 40–41, 254*f*–273*f*, 276*f*–285*f*
    superficial, 40, 254*f*–281*f*, 288*f*–291*f*
Ventral horn, of spinal cord, 7, 24, 28
    clinical deficit, 28
Ventral lateral nucleus of thalamus, an-
    terior division of, 212*f*
Ventral median fissure, 6*f*
Ventral pallidum, 208
Ventral posterior nucleus of thalamus,
    53*f*
Ventral root(s), of spinal cord, 6*f*, 7
Ventral spinocerebellar tract (VSCT),
    36, 56, 89, 258*f*–283*f*
Ventral striatum, 208, 215*f*
Ventral tegmental area (VTA), 124, 192,
    290*f*–293*f*
    clinical deficit, 124
Ventral trigeminothalamic fibers, 84*f*
Ventral trigeminothalamic tract (VTTr),
    84*f*, 88–89, 282*f*–295*f*
    clinical deficit, 89
Ventral white commissure (VWCom),
    57*f*, 258*f*–259*f*
Ventricle
    fourth, 8–9, 11
    third, 12, 136*f*
Ventroanterior thalamic nucleus (VA),
    143*f*, 147*f*, 153, 210*f*, 215*f*,
    300*f*–301*f*

Ventrolateral thalamic nucleus (VL),
    143*f*, 147*f*, 150, 210*f*, 215*f*,
    296*f*–301*f*
    clinical deficit, 150
Ventromedial motor column, 28
Ventroposterior nuclei (VPL and VPM),
    146, 294*f*–295*f*
    clinical deficit, 146
Ventroposterolateral nucleus (VPL),
    143*f*, 146, 147*f*, 294*f*–295*f*
Ventroposteromedial nucleus (VPM),
    143*f*, 294*f*–295*f*
Verbal auditory agnosia, auditory cor-
    tex lesions and, 173
Vermis, of cerebellum, 11, 104, 104*f*
Vertebral artery(-ies) (VA), 14, 14*f*,
    113*f*, 178, 179*f*, 262*f*–275*f*
Vertebral compartment, 5, 6–7
VesSp. *See* Vestibulospinal tract
Vestibular nucleus
    lateral, 67, 276*f*–281*f*
        clinical deficit, 67
    medial, 65, 270*f*–281*f*
    spinal, 65, 270*f*–271*f*
        clinical deficit, 65
    superior, 66, 274*f*–284*f*
Vestibular tract, lateral, 254*f*–263*f*
Vestibulocerebellum, 104, 105*f*, 106,
    110*f*
Vestibulocochlear nerve, 8, 9*f*,
    10*f*, 11
Vestibulocochlear nerve root (VCNr),
    67, 276*f*–281*f*
    clinical deficit, 67
Vestibulocochlear nucleus (VCNu), 79,
    276*f*–277*f*, 278*f*–279*f*
    clinical deficit, 79

Vestibulospinal tract (VesSp), 56–58,
    264*f*–273*f*
    clinical deficit, 56–58
    lateral, 40, 254*f*–281*f*
        clinical deficit, 40
    medial, 40–41
Visual cortex, 181*f*
VL. *See* Ventrolateral thalamic nucleus
VPL. *See* Ventroposterolateral nucleus
VPM. *See* Ventroposteromedial nucleus
VSCT. *See* Ventral spinocerebellar
    tract
VTA. *See* Ventral tegmental area
VTTr. *See* Ventral trigeminothalamic
    tract
VWCom. *See* Ventral white commissure

W

Weber's syndrome, 130, 131, 131*t*
Wernicke's speech area, 169*f*, 172,
    182*f*
    clinical deficit, 172
White commissure of spinal cord
    anterior, 38
    ventral, 57*f*, 258*f*–259*f*
Willis, circle of, 14, 14*f*, 135, 179*f*,
    180

X

Xanthochromia, subarachnoid hemor-
    rhage and, 17

Z

Zona incerta (Zi), 150, 296*f*–299*f*